56 · press-ganging not practiced in Dutch Republic.

67ff medicine chest contents

Ship's Surgeons of the Dutch East India Company

74– disagreeable voyage

80ff– malaria in Batavia re

128 The collapse of the golden century in the 18th

179. illiterate young uneducated barbers as ship surgeons is a myth

Ship's Surgeons of the Dutch East India Company

Commerce and the Progress of Medicine in the Eighteenth Century

Iris Bruijn

Leiden University Press

The publication of this book is made possible by a grant from Stichting Historia Medicinae, Stichting dr Hendrik Muller's Vaderlandsch Fonds, and the Directie der Oostersche Handel en Reederijen

Cover design: Maedium, Utrecht
Lay-out: ProGrafici, Goes

ISBN 978 90 8728 051 2
e-ISBN 978 90 4850 657 6
NUR 685

To my mother

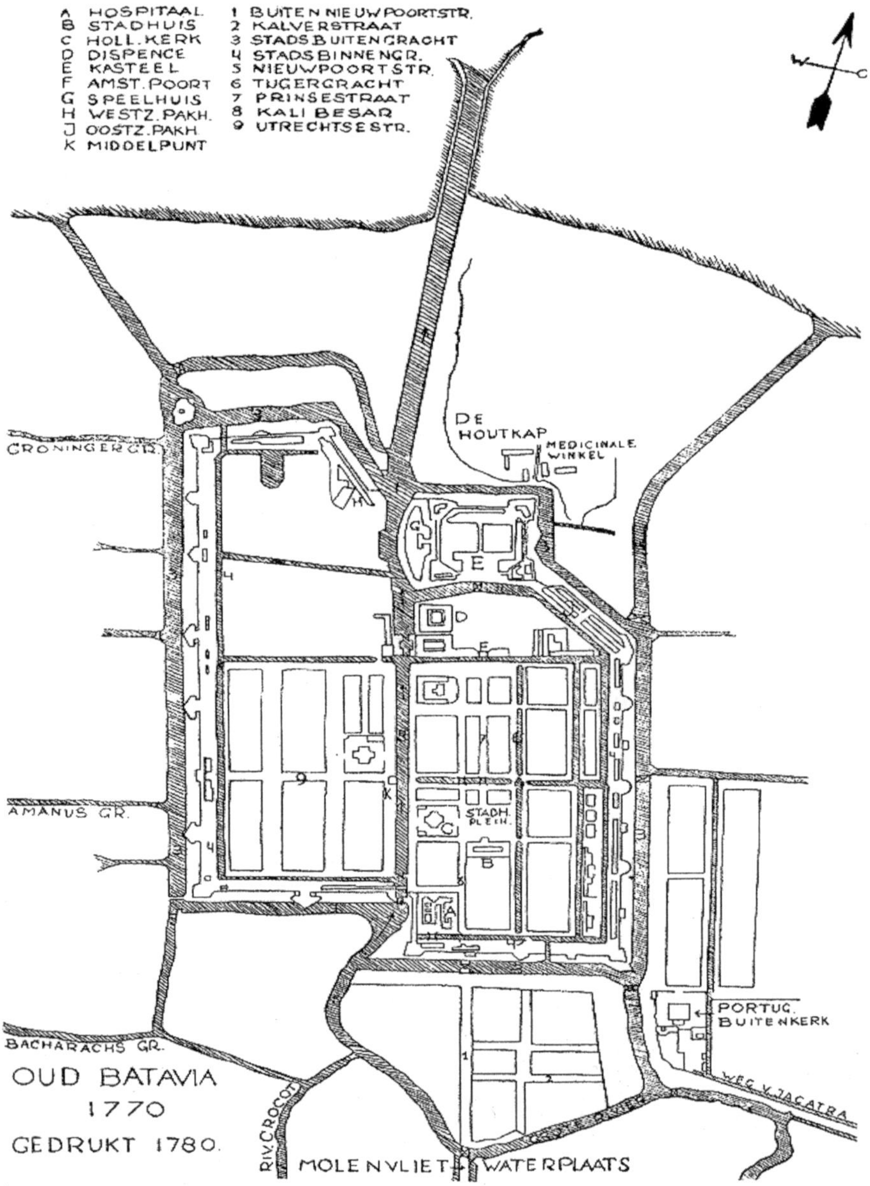

OUD BATAVIA
1770
GEDRUKT 1780.

Table of contents

List of tables, graphs and maps 9
Acknowledgements 13

Introduction: Coping with a black legend 15
1. The surgeon's tale: The development of surgery 23
2. The world of the East India Company surgeon 49
3. The medical service of the Dutch East India Company 85
4. The geographic origin of the Company's surgeons 125
5. The career of the Company surgeons 169
6. 'Great expectations'! 209
Conclusion: The surgeon's legacy 245

Appendix 1. Methods, statistical account, graphs and tables pertaining to chapters 4-6 259
Appendix 2. Maps 283
Appendix 3. Notaries used by the Company's surgeons in Batavia 1600-1800 305
Appendix 4. Ship's surgeons who died on board and whose collection of books is listed 307
Appendix 5. Ship's surgeons who died on board and were in the possession of instruments 309

Archives and bibliography 315
Notes 339
Indices 375

List of tables, graphs and maps

Chapter 2

Table T2.1 : Estimation of people employed in the Dutch seafaring industries 57
Table T2.2 : Possession of razors 66
Table T2.3 : Company personnel outward-bound to Asia and their mortality rates 75
Table T2.4 : Mortality rates Asia-Cape of Good Hope 76

Chapter 3

Table T3.1 : Wages of the Amsterdam Chamber medical staff in Dutch guilders 89
Table T3.2 : Number of Company surgeons in Batavia around 1700 101
Table T3.3 : Company personnel in Asia during the eighteenth century 111
Table T3.4 : Mortality in Batavia 1714-1744 114

Chapter 4

Table T4.1 : Estimate of sailors on Dutch vessels 134
Table T4.2 : Geographic origins of Company sailors and craftsmen in percentages 136
Table T4.3 : Non-Dutch Company surgeons within the sample 140
Table T4.4 : Geographical origins of the Company's surgeons in the eighteenth century 141
Table T4.5 : Ratio between ships and surgeons supplied to the ships per chamber 141
Table T4.6 : Geographical origins of the Company's sea surgeons around 1699/1700 and 1789/1790 142
Table T4.7 : Recruitment of Dutch surgeons per area 143
Table T4.8 : Surgical recruitment in North Holland 148
Table T4.9 : Surgical recruitment in South Holland 149
Table T4.10 : Geographical origins of recruited surgeons of the Zeeland Chamber 150
Table T4.11 : Surgeons from Zeeland 151
Table T4.12 : Geographical origins of recruited surgeons of the Amsterdam Chamber 153
Table T4.13 : Geographical origins of recruited surgeons of the Hoorn and Enkhuizen Chambers 154
Table T4.14 : Geographical origins of recruited surgeons of the Delft and Rotterdam Chambers 155
Table T4.15 : German surgical participation 157
Table T4.16 : Regional German surgical participation 158

Table T4.17 :	Sampled ship's surgeons from Lower Saxony	161
Table T4.18 :	Surgical participation from Belgium, Scandinavia, Switzerland, and France	162
Table T4.19 :	Geographical recruitment of surgeons in the eighteenth century	164
Table T4.20 :	Dutch and non-Dutch surgeons per Chamber	164
Graph G4.1 :	Total number of persons on board the Dutch East Indiamen (1602-1795)	135
Graph G4.2 :	Surgical recruitment per area	152

Chapter 5

Table T5.1 :	Level of education at first contract during the eighteenth century	176
Table T5.2 :	Span of time between apprenticeship and first VOC contract	179
Table T5.3 :	Average age per period of sampled surgeons (Group A)	180
Table T5.4 :	Average age first ship's surgeon top of career (Group A)	180
Table T5.5 :	Number of sampled surgeons and their departures per Chamber	181
Table T5.6 :	Eighteenth-century VOC captains (skippers) and first ship's surgeons	181
Table T5.7 :	The earnings of Adriaan van Brakel	184
Table T5.8 :	Annual incomes of master surgeons in Amsterdam	186
Table T5.9 :	Sampled surgeons repatriated within five years never to take service again	191
Table T5.10 :	Surgeons who died within five years after first departure	192
Table T5.11 :	Promotion to First Surgeon (Group E)	193
Table T5.12 :	Promotion to Surgeon's Mate (Group E)	194
Table T5.13 :	Not promoted surgeons (Group E)	194
Table T5.14 :	Surgeon's Mates promotions (Group E)	195
Table T5.15 :	Surgeon's Mates not promoted (Group E)	195
Table T5.16 :	The mortality of ship's surgeons during their VOC-tenure	199
Table T5.17 :	Average age at demise of sampled surgeons	200
Table T5.18 :	Surgeons' mortality on further voyages (Group I)	201
Table T5.19 :	Average life span (Group I)	202
Table T5.20 :	Survival rates after first departure (Group S)	202
Table T5.21 :	Ship's surgeons' mortality over time	204
Graph G5.1 :	Survival rates after first departure (Group S)	203

Chapter 6

Table T6.1 :	Ranks of surgeons drawing up a legal deed	221
Table T6.2 :	Married surgeons	223
Table T6.3 :	Wives of surgeons	224
Table T6.4 :	Sums of lawful shares	228
Table T6.5 :	Prices of surgical books in the Dutch Republic	233

Table T6.6 :	Kruijs voyages for the Company	238
Table T6.7 :	The debts (investments ?) incurred by Frederik Kruijs	239
Table T6.8 :	The career of B.J. Engelbert	241
Graph G6.1 :	Number of surgeons whose legal deed was deposited at the Batavian Weeskamer	222

Appendix 1

Table TA1 :	Financial books and number of sampled surgeons	262
Table TA2 :	Verified birthplaces	264
Table TA3 :	Number of surgeons and birthplaces	265
Table TA4 :	Geographic origins of VOC surgeons	267
Table TA5 :	Researched sources	268

Appendix 2

Map A2.1 :	Surgical recruitment from the northern area	283
Map A2.2 :	Surgical recruitment from the eastern and central area	284
Map A2.3 :	Surgical recruitment from the southern area	285
Map A2.4 :	Surgical recruitment from North Holland	286
Map A2.5 :	Surgical recruitment from South Holland	287
Map A2.6 :	Surgical recruitment from Zeeland	288
Map A2.7 :	Surgical recruitment in the Dutch Republic 1700-1795	289
Map A2.8 :	German surgical recruitment 1700-1795	291
Map A2.9 :	Surgical recruitment from Lower Saxony	293
Map A2.10 :	Surgical recruitment from Saxony	294
Map A2.11 :	Surgical recruitment from Saxony-Anhalt	295
Map A2.12 :	Surgical recruitment from Westphalia	296
Map A2.13 :	Surgical recruitment from Brandenburg	297
Map A2.14 :	Surgical recruitment from Mecklenburg-Vorpommern	298
Map A2.15 :	Surgical recruitment from Schleswig-Holstein	299
Map A2.16 :	Surgical recruitment from Hessen	300
Map A2.17 :	Surgical recruitment from Thuringia	301
Map A2.18 :	Surgical recruitment from Rheinland-Pfaltz	302
Map A2.19 :	Surgical recruitment from Bavaria	303
Map A2.20 :	Surgical recruitment from Baden-Württemberg	304

Acknowledgements

I first made my acquaintance with the ship's surgeons of the Dutch East India Company when I was searching for a subject to conclude my study of history at the Leiden University. I then submitted a pilot study on ship's surgeons as my master's thesis. Afterwards, it was my father who kept my interest in these surgeons alive. He accompanied me on many, many visits to the National Archives in The Hague and organised my trip to the National Archives of Indonesia. Alas, he died too soon to see the dissertation completed and it must now serve as an encomium to his never-failing support. Gratitude is too small a word to express what I owe him and which he would not have wanted to be owed: he needed not to be mentioned.

The study presented in the following pages is the result of the input of many people to whom I would like to express my deep thanks. For instance, those who answered to my queries on birth dates, which I listed in genealogical e-mail groups; most of them are mentioned in appendix 1. And although I have never met Herman de Wit, his website on genealogical source material of the Netherlands is second to none. Furthermore, the personnel at the National Archives in The Hague have been invaluable: Saturday after Saturday they ensured that hundreds of the Company financial records were brought to me.

Peter Poortvliet and Dick van Zuidam have each spared me at least months of work by generously supplying me with their data pertaining to surgeons from the provinces of Zeeland, Gelderland, and Overijssel. H. de Vos introduced me to the interesting aspect of job interviews at the Company's chamber of Enkhuizen. Pim Sterk was invaluable with his able and convincing demonstrations of the practical side of barbering.

Ab Leestemaker was a pretty unique person in showing his ready understanding when I talked to him about my daily experiences with (the construction of) databases and computerprograms. Dr. Nico Nagelkerke possessed an angelic patience in initiating me into the mysteries of statistics. Time and again, I intruded into his temple of ciphers, like one who had to solve the Enigma code without any clues, and came out feeling only more bewildered, my head stuffed with 'Chi-square tests', 'Kaplan-Meier things' (but perhaps they are people) and words which sounded like 'Confidence interval'. Mine seemed to take a long holiday.

I am very grateful to the institute of Nederlands Wetenschappelijk Onderzoek (NWO) which granted me a six-month scholarship.

The erudite Amsterdam notary R. van Helden explained to me many aspects of inheritance law and practice of the seventeenth and eighteenth centuries. Rosemary Robson saw to it that I did not entirely ruin the English language. Dr. Carla Musterd rigorously pointed out all inconsistencies. G.J. de Moor helped me on many geographical aspects and produced all the maps. Alice van Waveren, Juliette Jonker, Margot van IJlzinga Veenstra, and Theo Kliebisch sustained me with wine and lunches over the years, and Christina Ericson with chicken (boiled, baked, grilled, stuffed and unstuffed). I am truly blessed with them as friends.

Last but never least, I dedicate this book to my mother, Rosemary Bruijn-Koolschijn.

Introduction: Coping with a black legend

Minorca, April 1800. War has been raging between England and France since 1793. Much of it fought at sea, and if it is to be concluded triumphantly for England, many men and vessels will be needed for the Royal Navy. Naval Captain Jack Aubrey, R.N., freshly appointed master and commander of His Majesty's Sloop *Sophie*, stationed in the Mediterranean, and faced with the dire need to complement the ranks on board, asks the physician Stephen Maturin to join his crew as ship's surgeon. But Maturin hesitates to accept the offer and mutters something like 'not being qualified enough' as a naval surgeon, knowing nothing of naval hygiene or about the particular maladies of seamen. Captain Aubrey, however, is not put off and replies, 'Think of what we are usually sent – surgeon's mates, wretched half-grown stunted apprentices that have knocked about an apothecary's shop just long enough for the Navy Office to give them a warrant. They know nothing of surgery, let alone physic; they learn on the poor seamen as they go along, and they hope for an experienced loblolly boy or a beast-leech or a cunning-man or maybe a butcher among the hands – the press brings in all sorts ...'.[1] Thus, through the words of Captain Aubrey, Patrick O'Brian expresses the public's opinion of ship's surgeons in his novels, summarising an *idée réçue* which had been passed down through many centuries. The ship's surgeon is generally depicted as a mere village barber, a good-for-nothing and an illiterate by his contemporaries as well as by modern authors. This is the universally shared opinion in the history of the European seafaring countries.

The ship's surgeons of the Dutch Republic do not escape this stereotypical image. The seventeenth-century captain Willem IJsbrantsz Bontekoe (1587-1657), who sailed to Asia in the service of the Dutch East India Company and whose journal of his voyage has become an integral part of the Dutch cultural heritage, tells us that the ship's surgeons 'after they had wandered the high seas and, like executioners, had tormented and ill-treated the miserable crews, such bunglers consider their education to be complete and dare to establish themselves as qualified masters in the home-country'.[2] Indeed, in sharp contrast to the academically schooled physician, the (ship's) surgeon was largely trained empirically. In the eighteenth century, when Paulus de Wind (1714-1771), physician in Middelburg in the province of Zeeland and Dutch translator of William Harvey, acted in the capacity of examiner of the ship's surgeons to the Dutch East India Company, he complained that the ship's surgeons suffered from 'extreme incompetence and had a very limited intelligence; moreover, they were young boys, some thirteen years old, without any knowledge of anatomy, surgery and medicines'.[3] The physician and botanist Jacob Voegen van Engelen (1756-*circa* 1796) described his contemporary Dutch ship's surgeons as follows: 'In our country, where surgery is practised on a contemptible level, and only upheld by a few worthy and experienced surgeons in the distinguished cities, our ship's surgeons start their schooling with the shaving of beards to be followed by the smearing of plasters and the letting of blood; the patron [the master surgeon] gives his pupil a short tract on surgery; a good memory and the spilling of some mutilated Latin jargon serves to round off his education. A sorry examination then follows, some money is paid, and there is our *Aesculaepius* who has been provided with a certificate which gives him the licence to treat all our sailors throughout the entire world until they are cured or die.'[4]

The eighteenth-century traveller Jacob Haafner was amazed that the Dutch East India Company (hence, VOC or the Company) employed so many ignorant surgeons. Accordingly, he was not surprised by the high mortality rates on board the Company vessels. He had seen – he wrote – many a soldier or sailor fall victim to the stupidity and negligence of these surgeons and their mates.[5] Haafner described the typical career of a ship's surgeon as follows. 'The ship's surgeon is a village barber aged twenty or so, who makes a lightning career on his way to Asia. He starts the outward-bound voyage as third surgeon. But because of the [un]timely demise of the first surgeon and the surgeon's mate, he is appointed first surgeon by the ship's council, thereby bypassing the obligatory examination. Upon his arrival in Asia, in no time at all he will be appointed physician of the Company hospital and, a few months later, he will find himself promoted to chief physician of the entire infirmary. Now his fortune is made, although hardly on the basis of his surgical skills.'[6] In Haafner's eyes, because of the ignorant surgeons these Company hospitals were no better than murderers' dens. The hospitals had as bad a name as the surgeons who worked there.

In Europe too, the reputation of the hospitals was rather ghastly. In general, European hospitals offered refuge to the poor, the orphaned, the widowed, the elderly, and even the occasional pauper-traveller. There, the major context of the provision of health care was, in the words of a modern medical historian, a 'refuse-heap relief', which has to be seen within the context of the ideology of the Reformation; it was more concerned with the providing of a social safety net than providing medical or surgical care.[7] As such, these 'hospitals' created a Black Legend, that is the argument that hospitals were 'mere gateways to death' and cesspools of infection, and that the hospital surgeons were merely the gatekeepers. The hospitals of the Dutch East India Company in Asia, however, were not founded on any charitable Christian emotion. Nevertheless, each of the above-quoted authors tarred the Company surgeons and the Company hospitals with the same brush as that used to blacken the name of their counterparts in Europe; they too were part and parcel of the 'Black Legend'. The one hospital that was considered synonymous with this stereotype was the Batavian City Hospital (*Binnenhospitaal*).

More recent authors have joined the ranks of the critics. The twentieth-century historian of pharmacy, P.H. Brans, informed his readers that the ship's surgeons' skills were as a rule 'very limited'.[8] And even the prestigious handbook of maritime history of the Netherlands (*Maritieme Geschiedenis der Nederlanden*), confirms this view.[9] Modern fiction writers, such as Patrick O'Brian, faithfully echo this historical opinion. Of course, he cast no such aspersion on his fictional hero Stephen Maturin as he was a physician. European physicians usually had a much higher standing than Europe's surgeons.

Because so many German ship's surgeons entered the Dutch East India Company's service, it is perhaps interesting to investigate how their image was presented. Not much has been written about them and, sadly, what there is does not differ much from what has been said about their Dutch colleagues; perhaps the picture is even blacker. According to one historian, the (German) physician was still carefully distinguished from the surgeon, who, until the end of the eighteenth century, with few exceptions, was a man of little education and ranked no higher than a skilled artisan, trained as he was like a craftsman by apprenticeship in a guild.[10] He adds that '[German] surgery was particularly backward, the empiric skills of the surgeons being seldom backed by any theoretical knowledge'.[11] And, according to another historian, the German surgeons were 'dishonourable in certain regions of the empire', while in other regions they were socially 'vulnerable and of low standing'.[12]

This then is the portrait we have of the men whose duty it was to accompany so many Europeans to Asia on the vessels of the Dutch East India Company during the seventeenth and eighteenth centuries, charged with keeping the seafarers' health up to par. It is not a very generous picture. But, more importantly, is it a true one? That question will be the material point in the coming pages.

The ship's surgeons of the Dutch East India Company were responsible for the health of circa one million men who sailed to Asia. This huge number did not consist of sailors alone. Many of the men were soldiers, needed to defend the Dutch trading empire, stretching from the Cape of Good Hope to Japan. And other professionals were necessary too, as territories were to be conquered and defended, trade agreements to be made, cities to be built, hospitals to be constructed, epidemics to be combatted, and personnel to be cured. All as efficiently, speedily, and cheaply as possible to serve the needs of the Company.

Right from its inception, the Company provided a health-care service by employing ship's surgeons on its vessels and at its settlements in Asia and the Cape of Good Hope. Their task was a daunting one. The crowded vessels created ideal breeding grounds for epidemics; disorders resulting from malnutrition flared up as a result of the lack of vitamins in the diet on board; unhygienic conditions caused diseases such as dysentery to spread like wildfire. The various climates experienced by the seafarers gave rise to colds, pneumonia, and sunburn. Added to these natural hazards were the duties of the sailors, which often caused contusions, ulcers, broken arms and legs, and inflammations. The European surgeon was trained to treat the skin and the bones, as opposed to the physician who thought about the cause and cure of fevers. Physicians, however, were rarely found in the Dutch settlements of its trading empire, so it was the surgeons employed in the Company hospitals who faced typhus, dysentery, malaria, beriberi and the like.

Why choose to devote a detailed study to the ship's surgeons of this epoch since they were, according to their contemporaries and later historians, such an ignorant and vulgar lot? Small talented, greatly opportunistic, and largely inferior to the great minds and powerful figures of the heroic scientific age such as Nicolas Copernicus, Tycho Brahe, William Harvey and Isaac Newton, are not these surgeons worth only a short and insignificant footnote in what is often portrayed as the exciting annals of the birth of modernity? To my knowledge, no specific study has yet been conducted in order to establish whether these negative opinions were actually based on verified facts or might merely turn out to be preconceived inferences based on hearsay, or, even worse, fiction.[13] This is rather surprising because it stands to reason to assume that this category of Company employees, entrusted with duties that required seasoned skills and an educated sense of responsibility, would stand a fair chance of being excluded from such ideas and not be indiscriminately lumped together with the motley crowd of unsavoury individuals who may have formed a considerable part of the crews of the Company vessels. Although this may seem to be a logical assumption, the commonly shared idea among historians is that they, the surgeons, were also poor and ill educated. Why else would they enlist for arduous voyages, full of hardship, unknown dangers, gruesome diseases and frequently of fatal destiny?

The public, then and today, remains rather ignorant when it comes to the ship's surgeons. What usually springs to the mind is 'scurvy', which is often associated with the ship's surgeon. Even though scurvy has vanished from the modern world, its memory remains a vivid reminder of the seventeenth and eighteenth centuries. The memory of scurvy completely eclipses the fact that these 'quacks' stood on the front line of the war against tropical diseases, bureaucratic inefficiency and miserly funding. It was these surgeons who accompanied the crews employed in pursuing the expansion of world trade, encountering and battling malignant unspecified fevers as well as having to tackle the ravages of scurvy. In the period between the scientific revolution of the sixteenth and seventeenth centuries and the medical breakthroughs of the nineteenth century, it was the surgeons on board and in faraway places who were left with the challenges of circumstances and exotic diseases with which they would not have had to deal with at home in Europe.

The diseases they dealt with have been amply described in studies made many decades ago, such as D. Schoute's *Occidental Therapeutics in the Netherlands East Indies during three centuries of Netherlands settlement (1600-1900)* (1937), or by L.S.A.M. von Römer in his compilation of *Historical sketches: An introduction to the Fourth Congress of the Far Eastern Association of Tropical Medicine* (1921), or in J.M.H van Dorssen's *De lepra in Nederlandsch Oost-Indië tijdens de zeventiende en achttiende eeuw* (1897) ('Leprosy in the Dutch East Indies during the seventeenth and eighteenth centuries'). These studies, solid as they were, nowadays seem rather old-fashioned and written in the tradition of the history of medicine recorded by physicians. Even the most recent study of the Dutch ship's surgeons, A.E. Leuftink's *Harde Heelmeesters. Zeelieden en hun dokters in de 18de eeuw* (1991, 'Tough Healers. Sailors and their doctors in the eighteenth century'), continued along this same trend. Today, the emphasis of the history of medicine has shifted from disease and the physician towards health and the patient as a result of which medical history has changed beyond recognition over the past couple of decades. Actually, present medical history no longer belongs to the discipline of medicine, but to that of social history.

As a disciple of this modern school of social medical history, Mary Lindemann argues that it was in the military hospitals that hospital medicine first emerged. Certain factors were significant in this development such as the founding of specialised hospitals, the requirement that a qualified staff be employed; and the subsequent elevation of the status of the medical corps. The military hospitals provided many patients for empirical research; in these hospitals, surgeons and physicians alike were able to make bedside observations undisturbed; and plenty of corpses were used for medical autopsies. According to Lindemann, England and the Dutch Republic lagged far behind in the establishment of such efficiently organised hospitals.[14]

The study presented here is concerned with the history of the (predominantly) Dutch ship's surgeons employed by the Dutch East India Company in the eighteenth century. At that time, the schism between medicine (*geneeskunde*) as exercised by physicians, and surgery (*heelkunde*) as exercised by surgeons, still existed in Northwestern Europe. Surgeons were neither academically educated nor solely empirically schooled. They did not belong to the top of the medical echelon – the physicians – nor to the bottom, made up of 'quacks' or empiricists, and 'wise' men or women. Limited work at best has been done on the social background of (sea) surgeons. Certainly none has been carried out to delve into their careers, their demographic origins, their education, their motives, and their private lives; at least not systematically. Contrary to Mary Lindemann's theory, an argument will emerge from these pages that postulates that the Dutch

East India Company hospitals were the first to undergo a transformation and to professionalise into general modern *Krankenhäuser*, guided in their metamorphosis by the ships' surgeons under the aegis of the Company. These hospitals employed surgeons who treated malaria, beriberi, typhoid fever, as well as turning their attention to broken bones and open ulcers. Medical frontiers were broken down; unknown diseases described; details of indigenous treatments published; and tropical plants catalogued and sent to Europe. All done by these 'ignorant village barbers', who went to Asia in the wake of commerce. As a result, surgery became medicine, and medicine was practised by surgeons; the twin branches of the medical tree, medicine and surgery, gradually coalesced. Could it be that there was more to these surgeons than meets the eye?

In short, it is high time we examine the image and the myth – and indeed a myth it will prove to be – of the 'poor ignorant village barber' who served as a surgeon on the Company vessels and at the Company trading posts during the eighteenth century. To that end, we have to go straight to the sources, to the ship's surgeons themselves. In all likelihood, there must have been some twelve thousand surgeons altogether in the employ of the Dutch East India Company during the two centuries of the Company's existence. Archival material about them for the seventeenth century is rather sparse. Therefore, the emphasis in this study is on the eighteenth-century surgeons, precisely during the period in which the 'Black Legend' acquired its momentum. A sample of nearly 3,000 ship's surgeons will form the core of the present study. The sample is extracted from the Company's financial books, or muster rolls (*scheepssoldijboeken*), which every vessel possessed to keep track of a crew member's career in order to pay him according to his rank and length of tenure. To place this group of surgeons in their time, the opening chapters (chapters 1 and 2) of this book provide a background to medicine and surgery up to and including the early modern period, although the question of whether the surgeons in the pre-antiseptic and the pre-anaesthesia-era played an effective and decisive role in the treatment of their patients will not be studied in depth. In chapter 2, the environment of the ship's surgeon on the long-distance voyages will be examined and set against the sea surgery of the other European maritime powers of the time.

The third chapter focuses mainly on the organisation of the Company's health care in its overseas trading settlements. It is essentially based on the ordinances issued by the Company's headquarters in Batavia and on resolutions made by the general management of the Company in the Republic. Although the usefulness of such materials in exploring the health-care organisation of the Company may well be questioned, as these documents are, prima facie, indicative only of the policies and programmes of the Company's authorities, these ordinances and resolutions offer much more information than that. They are, in fact, extraordinarily finely tuned to the problems of the day with respect to shipboard- and hospital diseases, hospital beds, mortality on board and in the hospitals of Asia, and to surgical personnel. The ordinances and resolutions are reactions to these problems, which allow us to envisage what exactly these threats were and how the authorities thought they should be dealt with. The manner in which they reacted to these threats tells a tale all of its own. As we will see, the Company authorities in the Republic, and even more particularly in Batavia, were acutely aware when and if any crisis was about to descend upon them, and they were intelligent enough to ask for advice from those who worked daily with such problems, namely the surgeons themselves.

The sample of 3,000 ship's surgeons figures prominently in chapters 4-6. Chapter 4 examines the motives and the geographical origins of the surgeons. Why did they seek service in the Dutch East India Company? What did they hope to gain from this employment? Was the Company surgeon the lowest detritus from Europe's surgical society and/or was the Company an outlet for his talents because he was the proverbial jack-of-all-trades and the master of none, which made a professional future in Europe impossible for him to contemplate? Was it because of mere traditional reasons, such as family traditions, that they became surgeons? Or did they simply take part in the main labour streams of north-western Europe? In other words, did the Company's surgeons belong to the streams generated, inter alia, by areas of economic backwardness, on the one hand, and areas with opportunities and (envisaged) wealth, on the other? Chapter 5 examines the surgeon's education, his career, and mortality during his Company tenure. Not much material exists about the surgeons' (working) lives in general. In nineteenth- and twentieth-century historiography, specific diseases from which the Company's personnel suffered, as well as some deserving Company's surgeons, have been highlighted and brought to the attention of a greater audience.[15] The anonymous body of Company's ship's surgeons, however, has not been so fortunate, even though it was that body that shaped the medical organisation in Batavia and elsewhere, and which raised, in all likelihood, medical care and medical science to a more advanced level. Questions pertaining to their schooling, their possible career options in the context of the Company and the time-span allowed to these men in which they could make a career, and to their qualifications for the task they were called upon to perform, are investigated in this chapter. The surgeons' social origins, as well as their ages when they started their Company service, and their level of education will be examined in order to provide some answers to these questions. Besides this, their number of voyages in relation to promotions and mortality will be looked into. Chapter 6 deals with their networks and their acquired wealth or straightened circumstances during their tenure, for which source material derived from the National Archive in Jakarta, Indonesia has been used. A detailed explanation of the methodology as well as of the background to any graph presented is given in appendix 1.

This book gravitates towards the eighteenth century although some excursions into the seventeenth century will be made. The reasons for this are simple and clear. For one thing, the source-materials on which the sample is based cover mainly the eighteenth century. For another thing, the sordid image of the Company's ship's surgeons really materialised in the eighteenth century. Then the Company faced – alongside its financial crisis – severe health crises on the ships and at the settlements, for which, as we will see, the surgeons had to bear the brunt of the blame. This book will deal neither with diseases in particular, nor with any individual physician or surgeon of the Company. Its theme is primarily to paint a true picture of a group so often abused, a group which was crucial to the professionalisation of hospitals in Asia.

1. The surgeon's tale: The development of surgery

'To speke of phisik and of surgerye'

Amongst the company of Geoffrey Chaucer's pilgrims there was a fascinating man of outstanding qualities. To get acquainted, it is best to quote Chaucer in full:

> With us ther was a Doctour of Physik,
> In al this world ne was ther noon hym lik-
> To speke of phisik and of surgerye;
> For he was grounded in astronomye.
> He kepte his pacient a ful greet deel
> In houres, by his magyk natureel;
> wel koude he fortunen the ascendent
> of his ymages for his pacient;
> He knew the cause of everick maladye-
> Were it hoot or cold, or moyste or drye-
> And where they engendred, and of what humour,
> He was a verray parfit practisour.
> The cause yknowe, and of his harm the roote,
> Anon he yaf the sike man his boote.
> Ful redy hadde his apothecaries;
> To sende him drogges, and his lectuaries;
> For ech of him made oother for to wynne-
> Hir frendschipe nas nat new to bigynne.
> Wel knew he the olde Esculapius,
> And Deyscordes, and eek Rufus,
> Old Ypocrase, Haly and Galyen,
> Serapion, Razis and Avycen,
> Averrois, Damascien, and Constantyn;
> Bernard, and Gatesden, and Gilbertyn...[1]

Chaucer (*circa* 1340-1400) provides us here with a picture of the typical medieval European physician as seen by a layman. His physician has been educated by reading the classical giants such as Dioscorides (*Deyscordes*), Hippocrates (*Ypocras*), and Galen (*Galien*), as well as Avicenna (*Avycen*). The theory of humours is known to him, '*were it hoot or cold, or moiste or drye*', and his reference to astrology shows the Arabic influence: '*well coulde he fortunen the ascendent ...*'.

His physician speaks of medicine and surgery '*for he was grounded in astronomy*', believing he knows the cause of every illness. Chaucer's subtle irony can hardly escape us here. William Shakespeare, almost two centuries later, suffered even less scruples. When Falstaff demands his page the physician's opinion of Falstaff's water, the page answers: 'He said, Sir, the water itself was a good healthy water; but for the party who owed it, he might have more diseases than he knew of',[2] leaving no doubt about Shakespeare's opinion of the physician's (uroscopal) theories (and his patient).

The university-trained physician of early modern times was generally seen as an insufferable prig and pedant, his practice formalized and circumscribed by custom and tradition. Even some centuries later, this picture had not changed much if we may believe another literary witness, the French playwright Molière (1622-1673). Quite brusque, he made no bones about the medical profession in his *Le Malade Imaginaire*. The candidate for the doctor's degree answers every question during his examination: '*Clisterium donare; postea seignare; ensuitta purgare*' to which the examinators responded: '*Bene, bene, bene, bene respondere; Dignus, dignus est intrare; In nostro docto corpere*'.[3]

This – hardly kind – opinion, shared by so many of the European intellectual elite, may well have been prompted by the fact that a physicians' education and methods were based on the twin pillars of interpretation and prognosis, of observation and speculation, tested against the humoral theory of Hippocrates and Galen, and against the logic of Aristotle. The physician, learned in philosophy and skilled in humoral medicine, knew how the body was constituted and how it varied according to age, climate, and sex. He knew how a particular patient reacted to the factors that caused illness. His reasoned treatment was mainly concerned with diet, and he could prescribe theory-based interventions and medicines.[4] As such, his advice was not always impressive in the eyes of the patient, who, perhaps, would have been more content with an immediate, if drastic, intervention.

Nonetheless, this physician, learned as he may have been, was not the only kind of medical practitioner in Western Europe. The practice of 'external' medicine (*heelkunde*) was exercised by others, among them the (barber-)surgeons, midwives, 'specialists', and apothecaries. In the pages which follow, we will concern ourselves with the first-mentioned category, that of the surgeons. As these surgeons worked within a – probably collectively held – Galenic concept of mind, it is necessary to sketch the general medical landscape in Europe in this chapter. However, the surgeon's tale will remain central in the following exposé: What kind of treatment did he apply; how did he learn his profession; and in which medical and social context did he work?

The development of medicine

Geoffrey Chaucer started writing his *Tales* around 1387. At that time, Europe had just witnessed the age of the creation of hospitals (1200-1350). The medieval term 'hospital' embraced four main types of institutions: leper houses; almshouses; hospices for poor wayfarers and pilgrims; and institutions that cared for the indigent sick. In general, they provided no medical care as such. The treatments most likely to have been available to the ill were bed rest, warmth, relative cleanliness, and an adequate diet. The medieval conception of death as the collected destiny of man did not motivate an impassioned fight against disease. Death was the law of nature.[5]

Only members of marginal groups went to a hospital such as low-ranked military personnel; single apprentices and journeymen; the poor within the purview of a charity organization; the aged and the infirm without family; and lower-class groups who could not avoid the hospital. They had no other choice when they became seriously ill. It was certainly not meant for the upper and middle classes of society.[6]

The provision of shelter was the traditional function of the hospitals although it is a common assumption among historians that the advent of the Black Death and leprosy led to an increased 'medicalisation' of the hospital.[7] However, even in the seventeenth and eighteenth centuries, diseases were still seen as the will of God, and thus inevitable. They represented individual or collective (in the case of epidemics) punishments for sins committed, certainly in Protestant societies.[8] It would only be the late eighteenth or even the early nineteenth century which would see the reform of the hospitals in Europe. Only then, as a result of various forces, did the European hospital transform itself from a multi-purpose institution into a place designated to heal the sick.[9]

Also in Chaucer's time, the first universities were created in Italy, Spain, France, and England, and there medicine occupied a prominent place from the very beginning. In all probability, although the process has never satisfactorily been explained, it was Chaucer's Europe that saw the beginning of the schism between medicine and surgery, only to be bridged again in the nineteenth century. Before the eleventh century, Europe possessed only a rudimentary knowledge of the scientific ideas of the Greeks and Romans. Europe became strongly affected by the impact of the Arab translations, incorporating Aristotelian philosophical learning, the introduction of Arab medicine, and the subsequent re-acquaintance with Greek medicine, which influence was coined by Charles Haskins as the *Renaissance of the Twelfth Century*. By the end of the fourteenth century, medicine in Europe had become a blend of Greek, Roman, and Arab knowledge, founded and developed by venerated medical authorities such as Hippocrates (460-377 BC), Galen (131-200), and Avicenna (980-1037). The theoretical part of medicine (and that of science in general) became more important to its practitioners than the practical part.

The Hippocratic theory attributed all diseases to a disordered balance of the body fluids. According to the Hippocratic corpus, the four elements of nature (fire, air, water and earth) and the four qualities of hot, cold, moist, and dry corresponded to the varying mixture of the fluids, or humours: blood; phlegm; yellow and black bile. Hippocrates did not attribute disease to the vindictiveness or malevolence of the gods. Instead, he emphasised the clinical method in which the careful observation of the patient played a primary role.[10] The interpretation and prognosis of the disease was based on this observation. Accordingly, a certain diet and/or medicines were prescribed, and sometimes operations were advised, usually executed by specialists.

Galen of Pergamon had elaborated Hippocrates' system of humoral pathology into an exact science in which anatomy, physiology as well as pathology, therapy and prophylaxis were clearly defined. The four humours of man played a significant role in the interpretation of health and disease: it was thought that the proportional mixture of these fluids in relation to factors such as age and season determined health. If the fluids were balanced, a man was healthy, but the balance was different for every person. Disease was the result of a seriously disturbed balance of humours.

It was after the death of Galen that his theories became predominant, and a systematisation or 'Galenism' reached its apogee with Avicenna.[11] The Arabs gave Greek medicine new impulses and developed it further by the translation of those Greek texts, which already existed in a Persian edition. The seventh-century Arab expansion created a new culture which extended from Persia to the Pyrenees in which Arabic became the language of science mainly as a result of this translation movement. The Persian Avicenna represents the zenith of Islamic medical literature. His *Canon Medicinae* provides a complete system of medicine according to the principles of Galen (and Hippocrates).[12] To a considerable extent, Galenism was able to play a dominant role during the late Middle Ages and Renaissance through the mediation of Avicenna. For the European and Muslim world, the theories of Galen and Avicenna assumed a canonical status.[13]

Scholasticism may have been a major cause for the schism between medicine and surgery. In medieval Europe, scholasticism reigned supreme. This emphasised a universe of law and order as well as offering the possibility of understanding that order through logical thinking. Galenism appealed to this universe of law and order as this rationalism of sorts accepted certain authorities as final and emphasised the role of logical thinking at the expense of observation and experience.[14] Theory and an appeal to the classic authorities as the basis of the study of science reached its climax in the scholastic period of the thirteenth and fourteenth centuries.[15] Surgery as a practical art lost much of its status at least partly as a result of this scholasticism, and Galenism was able to maintain its position as the major medical theory for hundreds of years. Therefore, the Western medical tradition was largely based on Hippocrates and Galen.

Physicians, apart from diagnosing the disturbance of the humoral balance, tried to remedy it by the revulsion or derivation of humours. Therapies consisted of giving advice about special diets, of bloodletting, sweating cures, purging, medicines, or, sometimes as a last resort, of an operation. Bloodletting was done using a lancet or sharp knife to open a vein, allowing 'dirty' blood and 'evil fluids' to escape, or by means of cupping or the use of leeches. It was regarded as a preventive measure as well. Cupping served the same purpose: by placing heated glasses on the skin, and, after a pause of a couple of minutes and the removal of the glass, a small incision was made, and the 'dirty' blood spurted out. Purging through laxatives and clystering (using an enema or syringe) was thought to achieve the same result. The evil fluids were removed and consequently the disturbed balance should and would eventually restore itself.

Although progress was and would be made in anatomy, in the refinement of medical instruments, in medicines, and although new schools of thought would criticise Galenism, for many of the medical practitioners, the treatment of diseases largely adhered to Galenic principles well into the nineteenth century as a large part of the European medical body firmly believed in Galen and in Galenism. Physicians, (barber-)surgeons, and the empirics tried to keep the body fluids in balance. The methods prescribed by physicians and exercised by surgeons for a long time remained *seignare, purgare et clysterium donare*: bloodletting, purging, and clystering. On the other hand, considerable improvements were made in the technique of major operations such as amputations and herniotomy, in the diagnosis and treatment of fractures, diseases of the joints and urinary apparatus, of the eye, ear, and the teeth. And above all, the second half of the eighteenth century witnessed an increased determination of surgeons to save organs and their functions and to limit mutilating or cruel operations.[16] European medical and surgical practitioners would not break with Galenism, there was no need to as in time they would simply outgrow Galenism.

The emergence of medical schools and its relation to surgery

The European universities proved to be essential to the development and progress of medicine. The first were founded in Italy at the beginning of the twelfth century. Anatomy was studied at the medical school of Salerno once again and dissection was practised on animals. For the first time since the fall of the Roman Empire, classical Greek medicine was taught as a science at a university, enriched by the texts transmitted by the Arabs. Salerno's influence spread to other Italian cities like Bologna, where for the first time in about a thousand years a human body was dissected in 1302. It was also in Bologna in 1315 that a modest start was made with the teaching of anatomy using human subjects.[17] Within a hundred years, the methods of the Salernitan school spread to the universities of Paris and Montpellier.

While in Italy and Spain lectures in surgery were given at the universities, this subject was rarely included in the university curricula of northern Europe. There, surgical practice was largely organised on a guild basis.[18] Paris in particular would develop into the leading centre to study surgery (at the Hôtel Dieu) but this occurred outside the structures of the university. Surgery did not succeed in obtaining a structural place in the curriculum of the universities in northwestern Europe, where it was only occasionally tutored in special courses. Although the breach between the two branches of medicine was never absolutely conclusive, the (university-schooled) physicians claimed that their education, knowledge, and licence were all-encompassing and complete. Therefore, they claimed control over the other medical practitioners, and as a result the surgeons too eventually found themselves subordinated to the doctors.[19]

Changing charity

According to the Parisian medical faculty, the Black Death (1347-1351) had been caused by the special conjunction of the planets Saturn, Jupiter and Mars on 24 March 1345, which had heated the air, with pestilence as a result. So it advised Philippe VI in 1348.[20] The plague may have killed off as much as one-third of Europe's population. It had a tremendous impact on medieval European society. For one thing, based on contemporary notions of miasma and contagion, plague management relied on cleansing efforts to purge all corrupted humours. The goal of early public health measures in the face of an epidemic was to protect the healthy. Municipal authorities constructed pest houses (lazaretto's); they appointed (in Italian city-states) special, temporary health committees to deal with epidemics; and they introduced land and marine quarantines. Meanwhile, as the European population recovered, many young adults could no longer make a living in their own villages and so they flocked to the cities. These new 'immigrant' poor, it was felt, often turned to theft, prostitution, and begging and came to be viewed as potential criminals.[21] As a result, a growing emphasis on law and order in daily life (already expressed in scholasticism) tended to displace the traditional Christian welfare schemes.[22]

This ideology of law and order also fit in with the doctrine of the Reformation. By attacking the begging and the mendicant orders, the Protestant Reformation added emphasis to the already widespread concerns about the growing ranks of idle vagrants. The ideology of the Reformation was more concerned with the providing of a social safety net then with medical and/or social care.[23] Now, instead of donations to charitable institutions as an instrument of salvation (which was the rationale of Catholic charity), charity was channelled through existing social structures.[24] The providing of a municipal safety net was the result of a slow mental transformation, which may well have been rooted in the age of the Black Death. In the northern European countries, this transformation blossomed in the ideology of the Reformation. Moreover, as donations dwindled, the gradual decrease in income forced the securitization of the traditional hospital system, which helped transform charity from a religious obligation into a social duty. For Protestants, charity became a Christian obligation within the civic Christian community. In exchange, the poor belonging to the (Dutch) Reformed communities were expected to refrain from begging in return for the relief provided by their community.[25]

The rise of the surgeons

While physicians, who diagnosed according to Galen's doctrine, tutored at the universities, the barber-surgeons practiced external medicine such as bloodletting, the treatment of wounds, ulcers, skin diseases, hernias, and contusions.[26] These barber-surgeons organised themselves into guilds, which were medieval European associations of merchants and craftsmen, created for mutual aid and protection and for the promotion of their professional interests. They set and maintained standards for the quality of goods and the integrity of their practices. A guild was often associated with a patron saint, and a local guild would maintain a chapel in the parish church to be used by its members.

The guilds were hierarchical institutions organised on the basis of the apprenticeship system. The members of a guild were divided into a hierarchy of masters, journeymen, and apprentices. The master was an established craftsman of recognised abilities who took on journeymen and apprentices. The latter were boys in late childhood or early adolescence who boarded with the master's family and were trained by him in the rudiments of his trade or craft. The apprentices were provided with food, clothing, shelter, and an education by the master; in return, they worked for him without payment. After completing a fixed term of service (four to nine years), an apprentice could become a journeyman, i.e., a craftsman who continued to work for the same or another master and was then paid. A journeyman, who produced his masterpiece as proof of his technical competence (the 'master's examination') might rise in the guild to that of master status, whereupon he could set up his own workshop and hire and train apprentices.[27] Because both were arts of the knife, surgery and barbering (the first having grown out of the second) were yoked together within the guild system. The surgeon's status remained humbler than that of the physician. His was a manual craft rather than an intellectual science with its emphasis on logical reasoning, involving the hand and not the head. His job was treating external complaints, setting bones and performing simple operations. For this, surgical anatomical knowledge was restricted to the bones and the veins; more was not needed.

In England, the barbers of London were first organised as a religious guild but were granted a charter for their own proper guild by Edward IV in 1462. This guild was amalgamated with the Fellowship of Surgeons in 1540 (Act of Union) under a charter granted by Henry VIII. From then on, the London surgeons were legally restricted to the practice of surgery, whilst in the countryside, surgeons could practise more generally, together with apothecaries, empirics, and physicians.[28] In fact, according to English common law, anyone could practise medicine as long as the patient consented.[29] In 1563, Elizabeth I's Statute of Artificers and Apprentices laid down that the apprentices must be under twenty-one years of age on entry, must serve for seven years, and must have attained the age of twenty-four before they could be licensed.[30] Thus, after 1563, the age upon entry of an average apprentice was seventeen, prior to which he attended his local grammar school, or one of the few remaining schools associated with the churches in London. Most of the apprentice's instruction was practical, for he assisted his master in bleeding, administering clysters, applying ointments or splints, suturing wounds, removing foreign bodies, and, on rare and exciting occasions, he might help to hold a limb or a patient down during an amputation. His theoretical knowledge depended largely on himself, for it came principally from books. Upon completion of his seven years of study, the London apprentice was brought to the hall by his master, who had to testify to his faithful service, to be examined on anatomy and surgery.[31]

For surgeons and surgery things started to change in the course of the fourteenth century. It was in France that surgeons were for the first time formally appreciated by royal favour. A royal decree of 1383 declared that 'the king's first barber and valet' was to be the head of the barbers and surgeons of the entire kingdom. Thus, the rise of surgical standing in northern Europe started in France. Paris developed into the leading centre for the study of surgery; surgery was entirely in French hands until far into the eighteenth century. Surgery could be properly studied at the Hôtel Dieu, although still outside the purlieus of the university of Paris.[32] It was there that ligature (the clamping off of the major vessels and arteries before amputation) and sewing (of skin flaps) had already become routine medical practice by the end of the sixteenth century as opposed to cauterisation (using a hot iron or boiling oil). Among those French surgeons who bridged the transition from classical to modern surgery, several stood out. First, there was Guy de Chauliac (1300-1368), whose *Chirurgia Magna* (1363) was often reprinted, for example, four times in the Netherlands alone between 1509 and 1646, and which remained a classic work on surgery until well into the seventeenth century. Although still written in the tradition of the classics – in fact, Galen's ideas were Chauliac's parameters – and although not based on any anatomical dissections by the author himself, *Chirurgia Magna* was based on observation and experience.[33]

Meanwhile, Ambroise Paré (1510-1590), the *primus inter pares* of the empirically minded surgeons, came to Paris in 1529 as a barber's apprentice, at the age of nineteen. He received his early surgical training as a dresser at the Hôtel Dieu.

During the Italian campaign of 1536 to 1545, he served as a military surgeon and gained most of his vast surgical experience on the battlefield. It was there that he began to question the rules of established classical treatment. During one particularly heavy and lengthy battle, Paré ran out of boiling oil used for the treatment of gunshot wounds. He had to improvise and thus concocted a cocktail of egg yolk, attar of roses, and turpentine in which he drenched the bandages to spread over the wounds. The next morning, he found his patients, who already felt relieved at not having been exposed to the torture of cauterisation, in much better condition than he had expected.[34] Broadly speaking, radical surgery was rare. It was mostly performed by military surgeons like Paré and ship's surgeons.[35] Paré recorded his experiences in a large number of books. The Dutch translation of Paré's collected works, which comprised 28 volumes, was published in 1592.

As a result of various factors such as technical improvements in surgery and the development of private courses in the seventeenth century, surgery rose in professional standing, a chance occurring, again, first in France through royal favour.[36] These private courses, which usually took three months and during which anatomy, lithotomy, the couching of the cataract, and herniotomy were taught, represented a higher surgical education. Given that the gap between surgeons and physicians was wide, there were also many French physicians who were interested in surgery, especially in the seventeenth and eighteenth centuries such as Francois Poupart (1616-1708), a physician, and Alexis Littre (1658-1726), an anatomist and surgeon. From the early eighteenth century, surgery began to be taught in Paris in lectures and demonstrations, at the Académie Royale de Chirurgie, founded in 1731. Accordingly, the status of surgeons achieved equality with that of physicians. A further step was taken in 1768, when the conventional surgical training by apprenticeship was definitely abolished in Paris.[37]

A similar development occurred in Denmark and Spain. Danish surgeons received an excellent training in eighteenth century Copenhagen. The city had boasted a school for surgeons, the *Theatrum Anatomico-Chirurgicum*, since 1736, which elevated the position of the surgeons. In 1774, the surgeons of this school, after an additional course at the medical faculty, were allowed to practise as physicians. Even this extra course was no longer necessary after the foundation of a surgical Academie in 1785.[38] The Surgical School attached to the Cadiz Hospital in Spain, established in 1748 and founded by the army and the naval surgeon Pedrol Virgili, offered anatomical instruction to prospective ship's surgeons. This school, falling under the patronage of the Spanish crown, was endowed with its own building, anatomical theatre, library and botanical garden, and by 1757, the crown gave this college the right to confer the degree of Latin Surgeon, which could formerly only have been granted by the Spanish universities. [39]

Progress in medicine and surgery

Apart from Guy de Chauliac and Ambroise Paré, there were several others who contributed to the advance of medicine and surgery. Andreas Vesalius (1514-1564), born in Brussels, laid the foundations for modern anatomy in his book *De humani corporis fabrica libri septem* (1543). Five years' experience as a public demonstrator at Padua, where he taught students to dissect and inspect the parts in situ, culminated in this Fabrica. With first-hand knowledge of the dissected human body, the *Fabrica* corrected Galen's osteology and muscular anatomy and recreated the gross anatomy of the human body. Galenic errors, as in Adam's missing rib, were swept aside: the rib was there after all.[40] Vesalius's work represents the culmination of the humanistic revival of ancient learning, the introduction of human dissection into medical curricula, and the growth of a European anatomical literature. After Vesalius, anatomy became a scientific discipline, with far-reaching implications not only for physiology but for all biology, and certainly for surgery and the surgeon's practice.

The German-Swiss physician and alchemist Paracelsus (Aureolus Theophrastus Bombastus van Hohenheim, 1493-1541) joined, at the age of fourteen, the many vagrant youths who swarmed across Europe during the Renaissance, seeking famous teachers at one university after another. During the next five years Paracelsus is said to have attended the universities of Basel, Tübingen, Vienna, Wittenberg, Leipzig, Heidelberg, and Cologne, but was disappointed in them all. He later wrote that he wondered how 'the high colleges managed to produce so many high asses'. He is one of the few writers who advanced medicine by quarrelling with it. In 1527, as a lecturer in medicine at the University of Basel, he burned the books of Avicenna and those of Galen in front of the university, scandalising city authorities. He stressed the healing power of nature and raged against those methods of treating wounds, such as padding with moss or dried dung that prevented natural drainage. The wound must drain, he insisted, because, if the infection could be prevented, nature would heal the wound. He venomously attacked many of the other medical malpractices of his time and jeered at worthless pills, salves, infusions, balsams, electuaries, fumigants, and drenches. As far as he was concerned, knowledge was experience and his concept of disease was the disharmony of normal functions. He discarded the four humours, attacked the idea of witchcraft, opposed uromancy and star craft, taught the unity of medicine and surgery and introduced the use of chemical drugs in the place of herbal remedies.[41] He is sometimes called the 'father of chemistry', as he introduced laudanum, mercury, lead arsenic, copper sulphate, tinctures and alcoholic extracts into the pharmacopeia. In *Der grossen Wundartzeney* (1536), he appears to have written the best contemporary clinical description of syphilis, maintaining that it could be successfully treated by carefully measured doses of mercury compounds taken internally.

Next to the field of humoral pathology, an iatrochemical school arose, of which Paracelsus was the founding father. Later, the Leiden professor Franciscus De le Boë Sylvius (1614-1672) developed this school further.[42] The iatrochemists explained the greater part of physiology and pathology in terms of acids and alkalines and based their therapies on them. The iatrophysicists subsequently began using mechanics in the study of the human body based on René Descartes' (1578-1657) view that the human body was a machine and that it functions mechanically. They were not only interested in the form of a human body but also in its function (physiology) in terms of the laws of physics and mechanics. William Harvey (1578-1657) was an exponent of this school. In 1628, he published his classic *De Motu Cordis* in which he definitively demonstrated the circulation of the blood, a landmark in medical progress. The Leiden professor Herman Boerhaave (1668-1738) was also an iatrophysicist.

Once the dismantling of Galenism had begun, there was no stopping it. Prohibitions on the dissection of human bodies were lifted, albeit slowly. The zeal for observation and independent conclusions began to outweigh the slavish devotion to the study of the giants of antiquity. A new scientific spirit revolted against the old system and new medical goliaths stood up. Vesalius questioned Galen, and Paracelsus opposed the whole scholastic tradition in medicine by claiming that disease was caused by an entity invading the human body.[43] In seventeenth-century Europe, medical thinking no longer displayed the intellectual and methodological coherence which had been characteristic of scholasticism since late Antiquity. Now, alongside Galenism, other schools of thought began to emerge like that of the iatrochemists. This intellectual crisis led some to believe that medicine was not part of reasoned knowledge, but an empirical art, such as surgery, depending solely on experience and observation.[44]

The eighteenth century would prove to be the age of the surgeon in Europe. Technical improvements in surgery were small but steady, including the treatment of bladder stones, in military surgery, and in eye operations. Mercury became a basic ingredient in the *materia chirurgica* as syphilis was usually treated by the surgeon. Qualified surgeons increasingly earned their university doctorates. Physicians became interested in surgery, and it began to be taught at the universities. The social and professional standing of the surgeon slowly rose.

Developments in the Netherlands

The Union of Utrecht in 1579 laid the foundations of the new state of the United Provinces of the Netherlands (later: the Dutch Republic). It included those provinces and towns that were committed to carrying on the resistance to Spanish rule. The primary power of the Government of the United Provinces lay in its provinces (Holland, Zeeland, Utrecht, Gelderland, Overijssel, Friesland, and

Groningen), ruled by assemblies of Provincial States who represented the towns and landed nobility. Provincial delegates formed the central government in the body of the States General, in which the province of Holland, because of the wealth of its cities, became the most influential. Each province was allowed to have one university and Franeker (1585), Groningen (1614), Utrecht (1637), and Harderwijk (1645) were founded accordingly, Leiden University had already been established in 1575. Although, as elsewhere in Europe, the practice of surgery was detached from medicine, surgery was taught at the Dutch universities and could be chosen as a subject for specialisation.

Joannes Groenevelt, for instance, was a medical student of Leiden who graduated with a degree in a surgical subject. He was born in Deventer in 1648, where he attended the local grammar school (gymnasium) and the Illustrious School. He matriculated in the medical faculty of the Leiden University in 1667. The first year medical students could be taught a variety of subjects such as rhetoric, philosophy, classical languages, history and mathematics. After this so-called propaedeuse year, the actual study of medicine began.[45] In the first decades after the founding of the Leiden University, the most renowned in the Dutch Republic, teaching was still based on the classics, Hippocrates and Galen. This changed with the arrival of Professor Le Boë Sylvius. After 1636, clinical lessons began being offered in Leiden's hospital, the St. Caecilia Gasthuis, along with anatomical dissections. The addition of clinical and chemical training to the standard lecturing and debating curriculum in Leiden, made the medical faculty of Leiden University unusual and outstanding. Furthermore, it boasted an excellent botanical garden which introduced Groenevelt to the plants used in medicines. During his lifetime, Leiden led the field in anatomy with professors such as Le Boë Sylvius, Boerhaave and Bernhard Siegfried Albinus (1697-1770), who became a professor of anatomy and surgery in 1718.[46] Albinus had succeeded the physician Johannes Rau, formerly a surgeon, as professor of medicine, anatomy, and surgery in Leiden. Although the Dutch Republic had its surgical guilds, clearly quite a few of the physicians (some of whom had been surgeons) devoted themselves to anatomy and surgery (which was also the case in France). In the eighteenth century, the propaedeuse lectures embraced chemistry, physics, the sciences, botany, pharmacology, anatomy, physiology, and zoology.

Groenevelt was taught by Le Boë Sylvius, as well as by Joannes van Horne (anatomy and surgery), Florentius Schuijl (who taught theoretical medicine and botany), and Charles Drélincourt (anatomy, a former royal physician to Louis XIV). His studies were focused on gaining medical experience at the St. Caecilia Gasthuis under Le Boë Sylvius, in the anatomy theatre, in the botanical garden, and in the chemical laboratory, and he coupled this with Hippocratic method and Cartesian natural philosophy. He finished his studies with a thesis on bladder stones in 1670. He then moved to Amsterdam, to find an appointment. Naturally, he was interested in bladder stones. The problem was that physicians as a rule did not practise surgery, which meant he had to enter into a kind of association with a surgeon. He met Henricus Velthuis, a specialist in the cutting of bladder stones. In his capacity as physician and member of the Amsterdam *Collegium Medicum*, Groenevelt recommended his patients to Velthuis if they needed surgery, and Velthuis would return the courtesy by having Groenevelt confirm his diagnosis in order to fulfil the municipal requirement before such an operation.[47]

Another exceptional physician with an eye for surgery and surgeons appears to have been Johannes de Gorter (1689-1762), born in Enkhuizen, who became the rector magnificus of Harderwijk University in 1748. De Gorter combined his enormous theoretical knowledge with his practical experience as a surgeon and physician in Enkhuizen. He also wrote some books in the vernacular especially for army and ship's surgeons.[48] He moved to Harderwijk in 1725, where he was offered a professorship at the university. He accepted the position of city physician of Harderwijk, where he examined the Harderwijk-trained future surgeons and midwives. In 1746, De Gorter asked the trustees of Harderwijk University that surgeon's mates be taught anatomy and surgery in the vernacular (as opposed to Latin), as De Gorter believed that surgical science had declined in the Dutch Republic. He thought that if surgery were taught in Dutch (as it was done in French in Paris and in German in Berlin) it would be absorbed better.

Medical regulations

While the guilds regulated the quality and number of the surgeons in the Dutch cities, in the villages this task was supposed to be performed by local authorities, although some of them never took the trouble to do so. In the village of Graft, for instance, there were no regulations governing surgeons at all, as a result of which every practitioner could settle there as such and hang out his shingle. In 1680, five surgeons were practising in Graft.[49] At the time, the relationship between the supplier of medical services and the patient was still a simple and direct one. A large variety of practitioners offered their medical services to the patient, each one of them competing with the others for the favours of the patients.[50] During the sixteenth century, we see the first signs of interference in this relationship: the medical and surgical bodies in the towns tried to gain more control over the business of the irregulars and of that of the various herbalists, druggists, chemists, and apothecaries. They did this via the *Collegium Medicum*. The *Collegium anatomico-chirurgicum Medioburgence* of Middelburg (Zeeland), founded in 1658, consisting of three physicians and two surgeons, organised public anatomical demonstrations to educate surgeons.[51] In Amsterdam, the *Collegium Medicum*, consisting mainly of physicians and apothecaries, was especially concerned with the supervision of the dispensing of medicines. It must be kept in mind that the physician was not only the supervisor of the surgeon, but also of the apothecary. Like the surgeon, the apothecary kept a shop and pursued a trade, while his education, via an apprenticeship, was largely practical. The physician prescribed and supervised while the apothecary dispensed prescriptions.

The Amsterdam *Pharmacopeia Amstelredamensis* of 1636 decided which herbs and other *materia medica* should be available on the premises of the apothecary.[52] This was regularly checked by the *Collegium Medicum*, which decided that druggists and surgeons were not allowed to sell composita or even prepare the prescriptions listed in the pharmacopeia. It was under its auspices that the Pharmacopeia was kept up to date, it organized regular anatomical lessons for the surgeons of the Amsterdam guild, and it inspected the apothecaries.[53] Among its many functions, the Collegium regulated the entrance of new physicians to the town, it regulated the future apothecaries and midwives, it advised municipal officials whenever the town was struck by an epidemic, and it gave permission for travelling empirics to practise in town.[54]

Here, too, no uniformity existed in the Republic. In other cities, the mountebanks, the travelling empirics, and the performers of operations such as cataract couchers (*staarstekers*), masters of the stone and inguinal ruptures or hernia (*steen- en breuksnijders*), cupping mistresses (*koppenzetsters*), tooth masters (*tandmeesters*), bonesetters (usually done by executioners), cancer masters (*kankermeesters*), tumour masters (*fijtmeesters*, derived from ficus), head masters (*hoofdmeesters*), masters of scofula (*meesters van scrofulen en glandulen*), none of them organised, had to ask the guilds or mayors, or collegia medica for permission to practise as well as whatever institutions existed locally. Usually, one member of the surgeon's guild (if present in the particular city) attended operations carried out by these empirics.[55] After 1700, these operations were increasingly performed by the surgeons, and the operating empirics either managed to integrate more and more into the surgeon's guilds or slowly faded away.[56] Hendrik Velthuis, for instance, was not only a fully licensed surgeon in Amsterdam, he was also a 'specialist' as a stonecutter, for which, however, permission from a physician of the *Collegium Medicum* (Joannes Groenevelt) was required.

These *collegia medica* existed in other European countries as well, with more or less the same function: to exercise control on behalf of the local government. In Cleves (Kleve) for example, a 1685 edict ordered authorised surgeons and barbers to practice only if they had successfully passed an examination. They were not allowed to treat internal diseases or provide medicines. The edict of 1725 authorised that only surgeon-apprentices with an experience of at least seven years were to take the master proof.[57] In London, the formal entry qualification for admission into the London Company, or into its equivalent in other corporate towns, lay in serving an indentured apprenticeship, normally for a period of seven years.[58] Many more examples could be quoted from the various countries, but this system was more or less the same throughout Western Europe, with small differences due to national, regional, and local traditions.

Surgeon's guilds in the Republic

Barbers presumably practised on a large scale in the Netherlands during the Middle Ages. They were needed for shaving, bloodletting, and minor surgery. The first distinctions between the barbers and the surgeons are found in the fourteenth century. Count Jan of Bloys, Lord of Gouda (1308-1356), had a barber in his employ to bleed him after copious dinners. For the treatment of his hunting accidents, however, a surgeon was called in, while the barber played the role of assistant.[59] Around the middle of the fifteenth century, indications show that they began joining an existing guild. A century later, surgeons often were forming their own barber/surgeons guilds.[60] In Gorinchem, a surgeon's guild had already been founded in 1465; in Middelburg by 1500; in Deventer in 1513; in Veere in 1520; in Amsterdam in 1552; in Groningen, the surgeon's guild was founded in 1597; in Vlissingen in 1606; and in Gouda only in 1660. Surgeon's guilds tended to be found only in the larger towns.[61]

As noted, the essence of guild organization was regulation. By controlling the entrance regulations for a craft, guilds limited the labour supply. By defining wages, hours, tools, and techniques, they regulated both working conditions and the production process. The barber/surgeon-to-be had to follow the path of the apprenticeship system: from pupil or apprentice (*leerknecht*), starting in Amsterdam, for example, at around the age of fifteen but in Groningen as young as ten, via journeyman (*knecht*) eventually to master (*meester*). The quality of the education depended on the master in whose house the pupil lodged. The pupil's work usually consisted of the shaving of beards, the powdering of hair, the cleaning of the master's shop and instruments, as well as observing and assisting when the master was practising his surgical skills like treating skin conditions, boils, wounds, and injuries.[62] At the end of this learning period, the master provided the pupil with a *leerbrief* (apprenticehip's paper), a certificate stating that the apprentice had satisfactorily performed the first half of his training and had finished his articles. The *leerbrief* also served as a certificate of good behaviour. Shown to the local guild, it was a prerequisite for becoming a journeyman and for preparing the masterpiece, or rather, in the case of surgeons, the master's examination (*huisproef*). The learning period of a pupil usually ranged from two to three years.

The curriculum in Amsterdam, for instance, provided that the apprentice assisted his master daily, and an obligatory attendance at a *practicum* which consisted of practical lessons in the Gasthuis, where the apprentice learned to dress wounds, crucial to any surgeon's education. The municipal authorities occasionally provided cadavers to be dissected at the *Theatrum Anatomicum*. The pupils were expected to attend the dissections. Moreover, there were lessons in the Hortus Medicus, the 'medical gardens', for which the pupil paid a fee at the beginning of his apprenticeship (*hortus-penning*). Demonstrations in herbs were given in these gardens and the apprentice learned how to make ointments and drugs.[63]

In 1556, the Amsterdam surgeon's guild acquired the privilege of disposing of a body (once belonging to a criminal) for anatomical purposes from Philip II. Soon thereafter, anatomical lessons were being offered twice a week in the *Theatrum Anatomicum*, which was compulsory for all Amsterdam surgeons and immortalised by Rembrandt's 'Anatomical Lesson by Dr. Nicolaes Tulp'. A great number of anatomical theatres were established in the seventeenth century. The most famous one, in Leiden, had already opened in 1593. Between 1615 and 1649, all universities in the Republic followed Leiden's example. For the extramural tuition of surgeons and midwives, theatres were established by city authorities. They appointed physicians of medicine as special lectors in anatomy. Their lessons, given in the vernacular, were primarily meant for surgeons and their apprentices.[64] At the Amsterdam Binnengasthuis, a dissecting room was made available to physicians and surgeons. The *knechten* (journeymen) were obliged to follow lessons in the anatomical theatre, in the Amsterdam Gasthuis and in the botanical garden.

The anatomical lessons were theoretical as well as practical, and the Gasthuis proved to be a capital supplier of dead foreigners, their corpses unclaimed by family members. There was a tremendous interest in these practica, noisy sessions as they were, not only from the medico-surgical body of Amsterdam, but also from other inhabitants of the town. They were permitted to join these demonstrations against payment of a sum. The places were arranged according to a hierarchical scheme: the first row was reserved for municipal authorities, the inspectors of the *Collegium Medicum*, and older physicians. The second row was reserved for the other physicians, the officials of the surgeon's guild, and for the elderly master surgeons. Then a couple of rows for the other master surgeons and finally, the rows for the *knechten*, packed in like herrings in a barrel (but less quiet), with those behind them pushing, and everybody struggling and shouting to those around the table whose heads interfered with their line of vision.

A candidate for the master's examination had to register twice for the guild: once as a pupil (*leerknecht*) for at least two to three years, then as a journeyman (*knecht*) for at least two to three years, a total of a minimum of five years. The requirements for the master examination's had already been mandatory in the earliest surgeon's guilds. During the Middle Ages, the barbers joined other craftsmen, such as shoemakers, to form a guild. During this period, the requirements for barbers were limited to the candidate's ability to let blood properly and the fashioning of a lancet from raw iron and being able to sharpen it. These barbers can only be defined as barbers in the narrowest sense of the word.[65] As a result of the reorganisation of the guilds in Amsterdam in 1552, the other craftsmen were purged from this guild in which only the barbers and surgeons remained, and a formal distinction was drawn between the two. The requirements for a barber-master candidate, which included the shaping of some pieces of iron into lancets as well as the letting of blood with these self-made lancets, was broadened to include some theoretical background, which consisted of Avicenna's *Fleubotomia*. The master surgeon candidate was required to have a theoretical knowledge of bloodletting, unnatural growths, wounds, ulcers and fractures, the *Materia chirurgica*, and also had to demonstrate his knowledge in a practical examination during which he had to trephine a skull. These examination requirements seem to be based on the *Chirurgia Magna* of Guido de Chauliac (1315).[66] The 1552 Amsterdam ordinance specifically forbade those with only a barber's certificate to perform surgery in the wider sense.[67] The barbers were only allowed to pursue shaving and bloodletting.

The master's examination in Arnhem of 1620 consisted of the practical part which required the preparation of two lancets as well as the phlebotomy itself, and a theoretical part that embraced general anatomy, a knowledge of veins and arteries that could be used for the letting of blood, complicated wounds, fractures, and dislocations.[68] The examination in Middelburg in 1501, consisted of the shaping of three pieces of irons into lancets as well as the phlebotomy test. In the seventeenth century, this examination was expanded to include extirpation (amputation), trepanation of the skull, the treatment of a contusion, and a theoretical examination on anatomy, including the making of lancets and the phlebotomy test, which became only a preliminary step towards the master's examination.[69] The candidate was then required to know about unnatural growths, suppurating ulcers, sores, and their treatment. Ulcers were particularly common. The humoral theory taught that ulcers were the result of an accumulation of acrid humours in the blood, and the ulcers themselves acted as drains through which such humours could escape.[70] The master surgeon candidate had to know how to distinguish wounds and fractures, and how to treat them.[71] He had to be able to amputate, as amputation was the most common treatment for a severe limb injury. Finally, he had to be able to trephine a skull. By the eighteenth century, the surgeon-master's examination reached its full maturity and, in the larger cities, included practical bandaging at the hospital or Gasthuis, which formed part of his examination, as did the application of the trephining of a skull. Finally, the theoretical knowledge and the *materia chirurgica* were examined.[72]

The case of Isaac Olthof is one example of many that illustrates the elaborate process of examining master-surgeon candidates. He wanted to become a master surgeon in Haarlem in 1699, for which he had to pass the master's examination. He appeared no less than five times at the surgeon's guild within a two-week period. The first time, the members of the guild read the statutes of the surgeon's guild to him. The second time, a week later, Olthof showed his *burgerceel*, a certificate which proved his burghership of the town of Haarlem. Subsequently, he was examined on the surgeon's handbook and about 'the inner and outer accidents of the body of the human being as well as on the bandaging of these accidents'.[73] Four days later, he was examined on anatomy by the guild. He paid six guilders and six *stuivers* for the privilege of this examination. The next day, Olthof performed a bloodletting on a hand and a foot, and the fifth and last day he was promoted to master, for which privilege he paid another six Dutch guilders, and no less than 240 guilders in tax (a year's income for a master surgeon in Haarlem at the time).[74]

Surgery was never identical with major operative surgery. The practice of a master surgeon existed much more for the everyday cure of wounds, inflammations, ulcers, dislocations, and fractures. Moreover, the surgeon removed foreign bodies, catheterized, and treated scurvy, diseases of the eye and ear, skin diseases, and venereal diseases. Of course, surgical infections occurred frequently, although not as often as is commonly assumed, provided that the treatment took place outside the large hospitals. It may well be possible that his treatment of external disorders was therapeutically more effective than the physician's treatment of internal diseases.[75]

Surgeons retained their right to exercise barbering until the beginning of the nineteenth century; hairdressing and shaving contributed a substantial additional income to many a surgeon or were even his principal source of income.

Professional literature

We have already seen above that Avicenna's *Fleubotomia* was obligatory reading for the aspiring barber surgeon. This poses the question which scientific professional literature was significant to the education of the surgeon. It is not an easy question to answer, as education differed from region to region and country-to-country. In England, for example, during the early Tudor period, some authors – mostly of non-English descent – seem to have been favourites amongst England's surgeons.[76] The *Buch der Wundartzney* (Strasbourg, 1497), a book on wound surgery by Hieronymous Brunschwig (Heinrich Braunschweig), was published in English translation in 1525 and widely used. It contained the first detailed account of gunshot wounds in medical literature. In performing amputations, Brunschwig still applied the actual cautery or boiling oil to check haemorrhaging from the stump. And so did Giovanni di Vigo (1460-1520), physician to Pope Julius II, who taught in his *Practica* (1514) that gunshot wounds were poisonous and should be treated with a dressing of boiling oil. This (Arab) technique is not found in another popular book on military surgery in England written by Hans von Gersdorff: *Feldtbuch der Wundartzneij* (Strasbourg, 1517). In amputating, Gersdorff discarded cautery and enveloped the limb in a styptic of his own devising. Guy de Chauliac was also an English favourite; his *Chirurgia* appeared in an English translation in 1541. Besides this continental contribution, the English surgeons were taught from the works of two English authors, Dr Andrew Boorde's *Dyetary* and Thomas Vicary's anatomical treatise of 1548. Dr Andrew Boorde (149?-1549) was a physician and traveller who put his medical knowledge and experience within reach to the middle classes of England by publishing his *Compdyous Regyment* or a *Dyetary of Health*. This treatise on the cultivation of health is one of the earliest composed in English. Vicary became surgeon to King Henry VIII and was subsequently appointed to King Edward IV, Queen Mary, and Queen Elizabeth I. His first book, *A Profitable Treatise of the Anatomy of Man's Body*, was published in 1577, but was little more than a compilation of older writers. He was, in other words, still a pre-Vesalian anatomist.

In the Netherlands, Brunschwig, Di Vigo, and Von Gersdorff were certainly read, but it was Avicenna's *Fleubotomia* (an abstract of the chapter on venesection in the *Canon*), which provided the basic knowledge for any barber and surgeon. Guy de Chauliac was also popular in the Low Countries. Paracelsus had already been translated into Dutch in 1556. Modern French surgery made its entry into Holland towards the end of the sixteenth century when Paré's work, in which the modern anatomy of Vesalius was included, was translated in 1592.[77] There were practical books for the surgeons such as Carel Baten's *Handboec der chirurgyen*, first published in 1590, which was especially written in the vernacular for the benefit of surgeons.[78] Sixteenth-century surgical knowledge seems to have been based on the *Chirurgia Magna* of De Chauliac.

The surgical guilds acquired medical libraries for the benefit of patients and apprentices, and they kept their collections up to date. For instance, in 1654, the Rotterdam guild bought *De anatomi Spigeli* for twenty-six guilders; the *Anatomi Bartolin* for five guilders; all the works of Dr Beverwijck, and some by Felix Würtz. *De anatomi Spigeli* must be a work by Adriaan van den Spiegel (1578-1625), a Flemish anatomist and botanist, probably the *De humani corporis Fabrica libri X tabulis aere icisis exeronati* (1627), a lengthy and detailed anatomy text. Spiegel is considered to be the last of the great Paduan anatomists. The *Anatomi Bartolin* refers to the Dane Thomas Bartholinus (1616-1680) who was a very popular medical author in the Republic during the seventeenth century, principally because of his *Historiarum anatomicarum centuria*. Jan van Beverwijck (1594-1647) was a Dutch physician working in Dordrecht as *praelector anatomiae* and as city physician. His *Opera Omnia* included *De calculo renum et visicae (Steen-stuck*, 1638) and *Heelkonste* ('Surgery', 1645).[79] Felix Würtz's *Practica der Wundartzney* (1563) was also a favourite surgical book in the Republic. A Dutch translation of the work by Würtz, who was a German follower of Paracelcus, was published in 1621.

In 1655, the Rotterdam guild bought, *inter alia*, a book on the plague by the physician Nicolaas Zas (1610-1663), which had just been printed (*Pest-weeringh of verhandelinge van de besmettlijke vijerige sieckte ende des selven genesinge* (Rotterdam, 1655). It also acquired 'a book written by Ambroise Paré' (1510-1590),[80] and a *medicijnboek* (a book on medicines) by Oswalt Gabelhoven.[81] In 1656, the guild acquired the 'comments of Fabritius Hildanus' (1560-1634);[82] a book by Barbette (1619-1665)[83] was purchased in 1661, as well as *Het welwater*, again by Dr Zas;[84] and the *opera omni* of Master De Bils (1624-1669);[85] in 1662, *'t licht der apothekers; den Amsterdamschen farmacopeus;*[86] Carolum Battum,[87] Pieter Pigre,[88] *anatomie gelee;*[89] *de bloemen van Guido* ('the flowers of Guy de Chauliac'?). In the same year, the guild gave orders for the *Opera Paracelsi*[90] to be newly bound because they had fallen apart as a result of intensive consultation.[91]

It is obvious that the Rotterdam guild did its utmost to keep the professional knowledge of its surgeons up to date. This was rather easy, since the Dutch Republic was a centre of printing and publishing in Europe. The Middelburg surgeon's guild, which possessed five, mostly anatomical, books in 1608 (the *Opera Adriani Spigeli*, the *Herbarius Rembertus Dodoneus Cruijtboeck,*[92] *the Anatomia Lourentius*, the *Anatomia Vesalius*, and a book which showed the 'fabric of the human body'), was the proud owner of some 150 medical and surgical works in 1746.[93] Post-fifteenth century (medical and) surgical education featured the presence of medical and surgical texts as a result of the advent of printing and the subsequent decline in the cost of books. There were many surgical books available in the Republic, such as the treatises of Guy de Chauliac and the works by Ambroise Paré, but also a classic work such as Hippocrates' treatise on head injuries. Many Italian authors were read, including Giovanni di Vigo, Gabrielle Fallopio (1523-1562, one of the most prominent anatomists of his time), Fabricius ab Aquapendante (professor of anatomy in Padua), and Marcus Aurelius Severinus (1580-1656). Apart from German authors such as Wilhelmus Fabricus Hildanus, Johannes Sculteus (1595-1645, author of *Armamentorium chirurgicum*), and Felix Würtz (1518-1574), some Danish (Thomas Bartholinus), and, as we saw, a number of Dutch authors, such as the physicians Jan van Beverwijck, Paulus Barbette and Cornelis van Solingen (1641-1687) were read.[94] Salomon van Rustingh (1650-after 1700), a former army surgeon, recommended the books by Sculteus and Van Solingen to apprentice surgeons. Textbooks in the form of Questions and Answers were sometimes composed particularly for apprentices. Those written by Cornelis Herls, who published *Examen der Chirurgie* (Surgical Examination) in 1678 and *Chirurgijns Scheepskist* (Surgeon's Sea chest) in 1664, and Cornelis van de Voorde (*circa* 1630-1678) whose *Lichtende fakkel der cheirurgia* appeared in 1664 were extremely popular.[95]

Of the eighteenth-century Dutch surgical literature, the *Nieuwe Gezuiverde Heelkonst* (1746), by the Harderwijk professor, Johannes de Gorter was translated from the Latin into Dutch for surgeons. The author addressed, amongst other matters, the disputes between the physician and the surgeon. De Gorter answered this problem as follows: 'Although the physician has precedence in reporting, he does not have more credibility in judgment. The reporting should be done on the basis of capability and knowledge of anatomy and not because of precedence. Therefore, a capable surgeon should be believed more than an incapable physician'".[96] In the *Gezuiverde geneeskonst, of Kort onderwijs der meeste inwendige ziekten, ten nutte van de chirurgijns* (1744), which De Gorter composed particularly for the surgeons, in the preface of which he wrote that, although medicine and surgery were taught separately, the surgeons who served in the army or on board ship should practise both. De Gorter then listed the principal diseases, which should be cured by internal medicines for the benefit of those surgeons. His first book, *De gezuiverde heelkonst, ter onderwijzingen van den leerenden en konstoeffenenden heelmeester t'zamengestelt* (1735) was also written especially for surgeons.

Unfortunately, our knowledge of the possible private libraries of the surgeons remains scant. Private libraries might have been even more important to the professional education and skills of surgeons than those of the guilds. We will come back to this issue in the last chapter.

Hospitals and medical poor relief

The first hospitals in the Netherlands were founded in the twelfth and thirteenth centuries. They, as elsewhere, had come into being as charitable institutions. There appear to be many indications that the Netherlands have not been struck by the Black Death as severely as the other European countries except for hard-hit areas like the east of the Netherlands and the south of Belgium (i.e., the Austrian Netherlands). Plague epidemics occurred later in the Netherlands.[97] At the end of the Middle Ages, city physicians and city surgeons were appointed and charged with the medical and surgical care of the poor. They were early 'medical officers of health' and were appointed in all probability as a measure against the idle sick and poor. Zwolle was one of the few cities struck by the Black Death. The city of Zwolle had already employed a city physician by 1399.[98] Arnhem appointed a city physician in 1412, and in 1527 both a city physician and city surgeon were employed by the city.[99] In Rotterdam, a city surgeon practised as early as in 1426.[100] In Kampen, a city physician is mentioned in 1434.[101] We know that in Gouda, at the beginning of the fifteenth century, the authorities appointed a city surgeon for the care of poor burghers and the city's prisoners.[102] For the local gasthuis, Gouda appointed other surgeons, as it did for the plague hospital (Pesthuis) and the lepers hospital (*leproserie*). Amsterdam lagged somewhat behind as it was 1515 before a city surgeon was appointed. This surgeon was not only responsible for the care of the indigent sick and prisoners, but also for the patients in the Gasthuis. During the sixteenth century, the responsibility for the complete surgical care of all the Amsterdam poor was squarely placed on the shoulders of this man.[103] The municipality of Hoorn employed no less than three city physicians around 1600. Such a city physician (*medicus civilis*) or a city surgeon (*chirurgicus civilis*) were, in the Republic, contracted by the local municipality, received a regular salary, and had to observe a binding set of instructions delineating a series of duties.[104]

In 1589, the Binnengasthuis of Amsterdam appointed its own surgeon; and only its own physician as late as 1661. By the end of the eighteenth century, the hospital employed two physicians and two surgeons, whereas the town employed five physicians, five surgeons, three hernia masters (*breukmeesters*), two obstetricians (*vroedmeesters*), and eighteen midwives.[105] This expansion of the medical system was to a considerable extent attributable to the economic prosperity and population growth of the city. In the seventeenth century, Amsterdam's population increased from circa 60,000 in 1600 to circa 200,000 in 1700, mainly as a result of immigration.[106] Most of these immigrants, many of whom were sailors in search of work, were poor and ended up in the hands of the local medical poor relief when they fell ill. The 'professionalising' of the Middelburg hospital coincided with the Reformation and the war against Spain. It shifted those patients suffering from syphilis, leprosy, plague, or insanity to special houses and old people were cared for in separate wards, as a result of which the emphasis in the Gasthuis shifted increasingly on its patients.[107] The Gasthuis employed two physicians and four surgeons by 1681. However, the intake of patients was usually small, apart from in times of crisis such as war. In 1594, there were 23 patients treated in the hospital; in 1664, there were 15 patients; in 1700, 21 patients; in 1701, there were 150 sick soldiers in the hospitals; in 1710, 38 patients; and in 1799, the hospital had to take in 153 ailing prisoners-of-war.[108]

The nursing in the hospitals was carried out under the aegis of a male or female chief housekeeper (*binnenvader* or *binnenmoeder*). They supervised the work of the *zaalknechten* and *zaalmeiden* [male/female headnurses and their assistants (*ziekenoppassers*)] who had to clean and feed the patients.[109] In the second half of the seventeenth century, the Binnengasthuis had a men's ward, a women's ward, a surgical ward (*verbandzaal*), an anatomical dissection room, and a guesthouse, intended for poor travellers and foreigners. A rudimentary sifting of patients into specific categories was made, according to the division of work of physicians and surgeons. Depending on their gender and their illness or injury, the patients were placed either in the men's or women's ward or in the surgical ward, the last being more or less the surgeon's office. The beds were placed alongside the walls, often two or more patients had to share the same bed, which was an excellent way to keep the hospital in business.[110]

The most important hospitals during the seventeenth century were the Binnengasthuis (St. Pieters Hospitaal) in Amsterdam and the Gasthuis in Middelburg. Amsterdam could boast of quite a few other hospitals, such as the Oude Mannen- en Vrouwengasthuis (hospital for the elderly), the Burger- en Aalmoezeniershuis (the Almshouse), the Pesthuis (the Plague House) and the Dolhuis (House for the Insane), whereas various religious communities made their own provisions for the poor and sick in their congregations.[111] Surgeons were usually employed at these hospitals for the care of the inmates.

Strictly speaking, not everyone was admitted to these hospitals. The Binnengasthuis of Amsterdam was primarily meant for the poor burghers (*poorters*, or those with full citizenship), the sailors of the Admiralty and the East India Company, as well as for soldiers. It was also intended for sick travellers who lodged at the hospital's guesthouse (*baaijerd*). However, these rules were not applied very strictly: occasionally, there were more than 700 patients, many of whom did not belong to the 'official' categories.[112] For those who could afford it, there were the private surgical practices. Between 1750 and 1788, there were some 200 to 300 surgeons practising in Amsterdam.[113]

The career of a surgeon

If the knecht had passed his master's examination to the satisfaction of the guild, he could set up a barber's/surgical shop in town. He would then have to invest financially in his surgical shop. The estate left by Master Surgeon Hermen Lubbertsz (Elburg, circa 1546-Hoorn, 1602), who practised in Hoorn, allows us a view of such a surgical shop. Hermen Lubbertsz and his wife fell victim to the plague in 1602. At the time of his death, the inventory of the shop consisted of two shaving chairs, shaving towels, scissors, razors, and combs, lancets, spatulas, spirals, 24 other unspecified surgical instruments, mortars, a pestle, and a plate with weights for the preparation of medicines, (unspecified) surgical books, and a press for the setting of bones.[114]

The investment of time and money in surgical schooling and later on in a shop was rather substantial. Therefore, many a *knecht* did not come that far. Once a *knecht* (journeyman), he could swap masters (*verwandelen*), or go to work in another city or country, which was quite a tradition among German journeymen in their *Wanderschaft*.[115] Though this kind of journeying was not obligatory in the Republic, Dutch surgeons-to-be often switched masters for a number of years in the same city. The *knecht* could also join the army, the navy, the merchant fleet, or seek work as a country surgeon. A country surgeon did not always need to be fully qualified, being able to avoid this because of the lack of local control mechanisms as well as the lack of surgeons in the countryside. In the small villages around Breda, for instance, where surgeons and midwives practised without being organised into any particular group, so many complaints arose about their 'malpractices' that, finally, in 1756, a medical officer for the region (*'s Lands Doctor*) was appointed. His tasks included the examination of all surgeons and midwives practising in the countryside of Breda and the annual inspection of their instruments and medicines.[116]

The country surgeon was sometimes trained from an early age by a local surgeon and, by his master's testimony to his good behaviour, could establish a practice in due time somewhere in the countryside. Research done on seventeenth- and eighteenth-century country surgeons at the province of (nowadays) North Holland showed that only half (40) of the 83 country surgeons were fully qualified, having successfully taken the master's examination at a guild. Fifteen surgeons had been examined by the Admiralty or army, a diploma, which, apparently, did not have quite the status as that of a surgeon's guild. Twenty-eight surgeons appear to have had no papers at all, but relied on their reputation, and were doing quite well by it.[117] Their success could be explained by the fact that the basis of a surgical practice, certainly in the countryside, was the regular shaving of clients. It does appear, however, that in the eighteenth century the percentage of qualified surgeons in the countryside rose.

There was no obstacle to the *knecht* seeking employment in the army and becoming a company surgeon or *veldscheer* (field barber) . The Dutch army (the *Staatse Leger*, the army of the States-General) had been created during the first years of the Dutch Revolt against Spain. In the second half of the seventeenth century, the army had to fight against the French who launched several invasions against the Republic. At first, as far as this was possible, the Dutch army used the existing medical facilities available in the countryside. This meant, for instance, that contracts were drawn up with Dutch towns to admit wounded soldiers (and navy-ratings, as the case might be) into their hospitals.[118]

Prince Maurice of Nassau (1567-1625) employed one physician, two surgeons, and one apothecary on a permanent staff basis. Their task was to advise the army and to assist the company surgeons would the need arise. The companies of his army each had their own *veldscheer* or company surgeon, who was supervised by the permanent medical staff. The *veldscheer* was ranked fairly humbly, being a mere barber or surgical apprentice.[119] They also served the army as barbers.[120]

William III (1650-1702), stadtholder of Holland and Zeeland, Prince of Orange, and King of England and Ireland, introduced field hospitals, which were erected near the battlefield. Wounded soldiers, after preliminary treatment by military surgeons on the spot, were swiftly transported to these field hospitals for further treatment.[121]

Neither the country surgeon nor the veldscheer or a ship's surgeon could establish himself as a master in a Dutch city unless he became a burgher of that city and took the master's examination there. Master surgeon I. Schilham, for instance, was refused permission when he wanted to settle as such in his native province. Born in Zwolle, he had been employed by the East India Company as a ship's surgeon for three voyages; he had even succeeded in passing his master surgeon's examination in Leiden in 1725. The surgeon's guild of Kampen, where Schilham wanted to settle in 1753 as master surgeon, ruled, however, that he had to take the master's examination over again.[122]

Concluding remarks

In short, by 1700, the Dutch Republic provided a professionalised medical system for its inhabitants, although it was largely restricted to the major cities. As elsewhere, the physicians occupied the top echelon of the medical hierarchy. They received their education at a university and were specialised in the diagnosis of internal diseases. The surgeons, who practised day-to-day surgery, were ranked below them. Their education was largely practical and organised in a guild system. Surgical guilds flourished in the sixteenth and seventeenth centuries, during which time the age-old talents of the empirics were incorporated into the professional field of the surgeon. The sixteenth and seventeenth centuries also witnessed a rapid growth in the knowledge of anatomy and pharmacology, but this increased knowledge did not immediately lead to more cures and better health.

There were no radical breakthroughs in surgical practice, which basically remained focused on shaving, the setting of broken bones, the treatment and bandaging of contusions, and the treatment of skin diseases. The surgeons continued to be trained in the tradition of Galen, treating illnesses as 'imbalances' of the body, and as such, these illnesses were the physician's privilege to diagnose and to prescribe their therapies. To cure these illnesses, the body had to be brought back into balance, by purging, bleeding, and clystering. On the other hand, the new discoveries of the sixteenth and seventeenth centuries had shaken Galenism profoundly: through the dissection of human bodies, as practised by Vesalius, it had been proven that Galen's anatomy was not correct. Harvey's demonstration of the circulation of the blood destroyed Galenism even further. Paré criticised the use of cauterisation, the Arabic idea of the influence of astrology on the body of man was given up, and Paracelsus questioned the entire scholastic (Galenistic) tradition in medicine, which led to the question of whether Galenism should remain the basis of medical and surgical practises. The crux of the matter lay in the fact that, for medicine and surgery, there was no clear alternative, which made it all the more painful and difficult to discard the old scholastic traditions.

The surgeons and their guilds were well aware of the critics of the old tradition. The guilds acquired the newest publications in their fields, although these did not as yet provide a new medico-physical system in which what had been learned by observation could be properly explained and interpreted. The Galenistic *Chirurgia Magna* of Guy de Chauliac was still widely read; at the same time, the works of Paracelsus, Galen's most bitter critic, entered the surgical libraries and the *materia chirurgica* of the surgeons. Moreover, technical improvements in surgery elevated the social standing of the profession. Physicians turned to surgery, and some surgeons turned to medicine. Slowly, the twin branches began to grow together.

Our surgeon's tale could be concluded here. However, it took many years before an apprentice became a master surgeon. Many apprentices, therefore, never got as far as taking their master's examination. For those who did not, there remained a couple of choices, among which a country-practice seems to have been quite attractive from what is known about it. Or one could choose to become a *veldscheer*, perhaps a less attractive choice for obvious reasons. We do not know much about the army surgeons, but it appears from literature that they were not fully qualified either (i.e., not having taken a master's examination). Another opportunity for those who had not finished their training was employment at a surgeon's shop in town. At the beginning of the seventeenth century, yet another escape route presented itself when it appears that the *knecht* could take the much 'easier' examination for ship's surgeon, the so-called *zeeproef* (sea examination), after an apprenticeship of only one year.[123] At least both Enkhuizen and Amsterdam provided this possibility. With this certificate in hand, he was deemed qualified enough to become a ship's surgeon and he could then seek a living with the Admiralties or with the merchant fleets of the Republic. Was he really qualified enough? And what would life and practice at sea bring him?

2. The world of the East India Company surgeon

The origins of maritime medicine

One might wonder if there were any differences between surgery practised on land and surgery on board in the age of sail. It could easily be argued that there was not because surgery is surgery wherever it was practised. As we shall see, surgery on board (or maritime medicine) comprised of the medical treatment (including diagnosis and treatment of internal diseases) that a ship's crew received on board and on land in the tropics. The practice of a ship's surgeon was distinct from that of his colleagues in Europe because a ship's surgeon also served as a physician in the treatment of infectious diseases contracted as a result of the unique physical environments of Asia and aboard a ship. The absence of physicians on board did not mean that the physical mishaps that befell the crew on board or in Asia was restricted to the field of surgery. Moreover, the ship's surgeons of the East India Company treated tropical diseases that their European colleagues had no experience with. Therefore, 'maritime medicine' or ship's surgery may be defined as (i) the treatment on board of crew members by specially appointed medical personnel with their own unique surgical degrees (the ship's surgeons), (ii) the surgeons' written records of their experiences with a variety of diseases and injuries on board plus their diagnoses, and (iii) the treatment of (tropical) diseases they encountered in the various settlements abroad.[1]

In England, until 1153, no seaman arriving at a home port on one of the King's ships or on an English merchantman could claim any medical assistance except what was offered by family, friends, hospitals, and the mercy of God. But this was about to change. With the marriage of Henry II (1133-1189), Duke of Normandy, to Eleanor (1122-1204), Duchess of Aquitaine and future mother of the crusader Richard the Lionhearted, in 1154, the Laws of Oléron were adopted in England. Eleanor had been married to Louis VII of France (1120-1180) and had studied the so-called Maritime Assizes of the Kingdom of Jerusalem in Jerusalem in 1149 (where she had accompanied Louis VII on a crusading expedition). Upon her return, she had introduced these rules in her duchy. In the maritime court of the Island of Oléron, an island to the northwest of Bordeaux in the Bay of Biscay, maritime cases were prosecuted and the new rules were enacted over an increasingly broader area. These laws and customs, or, as they were called, the Rolls of Oléron, seem to have been the first code to emerge in the Mediterranean and Western world since Antiquity, and would become a kind of international law. As a whole, they were based, in all likelihood, on the *Lex Rhodia*, a body of regulations governing commercial trade and navigation in the Byzantine Empire, which were promulgated in the seventh century.[2]

In two of its clauses (vi and vii), the Rolls of Oléron stipulated that the treatment of an illness or injury incurred by a crew member while serving on a ship should be paid for by the owner or master of the ship, with the exception of those injuries incurred as a result of disputes among the crew, and venereal diseases. The owner/master should land the ill or injured sailor as soon as possible and provide payment for his care and/or cure.[3] Clearly, a sense of responsibility towards the crew had begun to develop in medieval Europe.[4] The Rolls became the nucleus of a slowly emerging maritime law, not only in England and France but also in Spain, Scotland, the Low Countries, Prussia and Aragon during the Middle Ages. The Ordinance of James I of Aragon of 1258, Article xx, for instance, made full provision for the case of a mariner falling ill or dying while serving on a ship, as does the Ordinance (Article vii) of Peter of Aragon of 1340.[5] There would seem to be sound evidence that, for Western Europe, the tradition of maritime medicine or ship's surgery started with these Rolls.

Naval engagements were rare throughout the Middle Ages, and voyages were still too short to cause any severe deficiency or infectious diseases, therefore, the need for medical treatment on board was still limited. Notwithstanding, as maritime trade slowly increased in Europe, and as ships returning from the Levant were often plague-ridden, the need for hospitals in some ports was so great that the seamen themselves sometimes set them up, the one in Venice established by Gualterius, a ship's surgeon.[6] The appearance of the Black Death in the 1340s led to the introduction of the Venetian 'quarantine' system, which meant that crews of in-bound ships were examined for illness prior to their disembarking. If it was found to be infectious, the crew was not allowed to land for 40 days.[7] The practice quickly became widespread in the Mediterranean world; the length of 40 days, or quarantine, was replicated in the port city of Marseilles in as early as 1383.[8]

Venetian ships trading with Southhampton in the fourteenth century carried a surgeon, but this was not yet the established practice for English ships. The idea prevailed in England was that surgeons were only useful during times of war.[9] However, by 1410, when guns were being supplied to English warships, it was soon found that the stone balls and iron shot that were fired by these cannons could pierce a ship's hull, to say nothing about the effect they could have on men.[10] In 1513, the English war fleet that was sent in to do battle with France had four master surgeons and some surgeons' mates, and, during the 1545 campaign, a rudimentary form of organization had been created to provide warships with surgeons, and even physicians.[11] Nonetheless, most English merchant ships were limited to their home waters or in coastal trade across the Channel which required the Channel to be patrolled by English warships. These warships accompanied the fleet to ensure that the (wool)trade with the European continent could flourish. Under these circumstances, a wounded man could soon be set ashore and the need for ship's surgeons would be obviated.[12] Consequently, there was only a limited demand for surgeons in the English Navy and none for the merchant vessels. At the time, surgeons were not employed the care for the crew but served as the personal attendants of the commanders. The advent of long-distance voyages would change all this, and, taken in conjunction with the Oléron obligation of the owner/master of a vessel to its seafarers, this change of thinking would eventually blossom into full-scale medical services on board.

The medical impact of the Iberian long-distance voyages

As marine design and cartography improved, compass, astrolabe and Jacob's staff were introduced, ships were increasingly able to make long-distance voyages. The exploratory voyages of Bartholomeu Diaz (c. 1450-1500), Christophorus Columbus (1451-1506), Vasco da Gama (1469-1524) and Ferdinand Magellan (c. 1480-1521) laid the foundations for the Spanish-Portuguese trading empire. The main objective of these daring seafarers was to find a sea route to the costly commodities of the East Indies – nutmeg, pepper and cloves – to be found on the Spice Islands in the Moluccan Triangle. Control of this lucrative trade in fine spices had traditionally been in the hands of the Chinese and Malays in the East, the Indians and Arabs in its middle reaches, and the Levantines and Venetians in the West. Now, European seafarers from Spain and Portugal appeared on the scene.[13] Dias rounded the Cape of Torments in 1488 and renamed it the Cape of Good Hope, and in 1498, Vasco da Gama dropped anchor at Calicut in India. In 1511, with the fall of Malacca, the Portuguese reached Java and remained there to control the entire spice route from the Moluccas to the West for most of the sixteenth century.

Columbus, in the service of the Spanish king, discovered the Americas instead of the Spice Islands. He made his first voyage with three ships, each one carrying its own ship's doctor. The ships were lightly manned: 40 on the flagship and 24 on each of the other two ships. The crossing took only 33 days and was, as such, too short to produce scurvy. Columbus lost only one mariner to disease. Following Columbus's first voyage, the Treaty of Tordesillas (1494) divided the non-Christian world between Portugal and Spain: the eastern part of the overseas world fell to Portugal, and the western part to Spain, ratified by a papal blessing presented in Leo X's *Praecelsae Devotionis* bull of 1514.

These discovery voyages began the process of European settlement abroad. This had consequences for the inhabitants of these distant countries where the Europeans traded and settled, for the European traders and settlers themselves, as well as for the crews of the vessels that plied these long-distance routes. When the Spanish came to America, their diseases wrought havoc among the Native

American population. Smallpox and measles were probably the two most devastating illnesses that the Europeans brought along.[14] Smallpox, an infection that usually spreads from victim to victim by airborne bacteria, was an ancient human ailment in Europe, and by that time no longer fatal, until it flared up again in the sixteenth century in the new settlements in Africa and America, where it struck the indigenous populations, leaving fear, dread, and death in its wake.[15]

Some diseases, such as yellow fever and the falciparum form of malaria, which did not exist in Europe, came to the Americas from Africa. The Europeans had never been exposed to tropical malaria, yellow fever and such like and had therefore no resistance to these diseases, which were introduced via the slave trade. The Atlantic slave trade was unique in how it linked the three major disease environments of North Europe, Africa south of the Sahara, and the tropical and subtropical areas of the Americas. Every Guinea ship served as the meeting place of these geographically remote disease environments, their human cargoes became the incubators for diseases such as dysentery, diarrhoea, ophthalmia, malaria, smallpox, yellow fever, scurvy, measles, typhoid fever, hookworm, tapeworm, sleeping sickness, trypanosomiasis, yaws, syphilis, leprosy, and elephantiasis.[16] The most effective defence Africa could throw against the European slave traders was, in short, disease. Until far into the nineteenth century, the Europeans were unable to truly establish any permanent settlements there because they would all soon fall victim to the environment. The Portuguese certainly experienced this in their Asian and African tropical coastal settlements during the sixteenth, seventeenth and eighteenth centuries.

The Portuguese were the first Europeans to arrive in Africa and Asia, and found themselves almost immediately ravaged by attacks of agues, fluxes, poxes, and fevers.[17] They founded a hospital in Mozambique that dates back to as early as 1507.[18] Goa was conquered by Alfonso Albuquerque in 1510 and it became the Portuguese headquarters in the East. There the Royal Hospital was established (exact date unknown), followed by the lepers hospital (St Lazarus, 1529).[19] According to Jan Huijghen van Linschoten (1563-1611), a Dutch traveller and explorer who sailed to Goa in 1583 as a bookkeeper and secretary to the Archbishop of Goa, the most prevalent diseases there were cholera (also called *modexijn* or *mort de chien*), dysentery, and fevers (malaria).[20] Cholera, in particular, remained a fatal disease in the tropical regions. Between 1604 and 1634, some 25,000 soldiers died from cholera and malaria in the Royal Hospital in Goa.[21] Even some two centuries later, in 1782 in Trincomalee (Ceylon), the English naval surgeon Charles Curtis noted that cholera was still a major killer: '… the *mort de chien*, or cramp … had been very frequent and fatal among the seamen, both at the hospital and in some of the ships …'.[22] The strongholds Goa and Mozambique were particularly regarded as graveyards.[23] Likewise, the Dutch would become prone to an early death in eighteenth-century Batavia.

Inevitably, there were also the consequences of long-distance journeys that the seafarers had to endure, as the route to the riches of the East was long and taxing. The first outbreak of sea scurvy was recorded during the Portuguese expedition of Vasco da Gama to India in 1497. His crew may have numbered as many as 170, of whom more than a hundred succumbed to scurvy, so that probably only 55 were to return, although the exact number of survivors is not known.[24] Of Magellan's last expedition, barely 20 members survived the voyage. He had left from Spain with five ships, carrying about 270 men, in 1519. A year later, the crews of the remaining three ships were stricken with scurvy, feeding on rat-fouled biscuits and were reduced to eating the leather off the yardarms. One ship managed to return to Spain in 1522, with only 17 European survivors, although it was laden with spices. During these and later voyages, while revictualling along the route, sailors experienced by a process of trial and error, that citrus fruits and fresh vegetables were antiscorbutics.

Small wonder that surgeons began to be carried along on the Portuguese carracks as a rule rather than an exception and hospitals were founded in Asia. Maritime medicine began to include the diagnosis and treatment of deficiency diseases, such as scurvy and beriberi.[25] These deficiency diseases manifested themselves after an uninterrupted voyage on the high seas lasting three to four months. Furthermore, infection diseases, such as dysentery, typhus, typhoid, pneumonia and venereal diseases, could and did take their toll. Initially, care of the ill on the Portuguese galleons or carracks was one of the responsibilities of the captain and of the priests on board: religious ritual was deemed far more important than medical treatment. A sick member of the crew had to make his confession and have his will written by the scribe; above all it was necessary to have his soul prepared. The presence on board of a surgeon or physician was not standard practice prior to the middle of the sixteenth century, if not later. The pharmacy on board must certainly have been stocked with medicines, but the care of the sick was mainly in the hands of any priests on board because they were specifically charged with this task.[26]

The most important people on board – counts and marquises, viceroys and governors – were accompanied by their own personal surgeon and physician who could be called upon to assist in the care of any sick crewmembers.[27] Later, the galleons were each required to have a qualified physician and a surgeon on board. He carried an amply stocked medical chest provided by the Crown, although a great gap still yawned between theory and practice. Finally, in 1698, a viceroy proposed that the Crown should arrange for two friars of the nursing order of San Juan de Dios to sail on each Indiaman, accompanied by four nursing orderlies to tend to the sick under their supervision, a suggestion which was adopted.[28]

The European population in Goa initially completely ignored European medicine and consulted only Hindu physicians. According to the French traveller, Jean

Baptiste Tavernier, these physicians prescribed the old Hindu panacea of cow's urine three times a day to their patients 'in order to recover their colour, one glass in the morning, one at midday, and one in the evening'.[29] Dalrymple, in his work on eighteenth-century India, is convinced that all 'invaders' eventually adapted themselves to the Indian way of life: 'Over the course of years, the women, the environment and the sheer distance of Goa from Europe all worked on the new arrivals, so that gradually, generation by generation, the conquistadores began abandoning the ways of Portugal and taking instead the customs of India.'[30]

However, most governors and other high officials brought their own doctors with them from Portugal. These Portuguese doctors were nearly always rewarded by being appointed chief physician of the Royal Hospital in Goa. European professionalism soon made its mark: in 1618, the municipal council of Goa decreed that no one could practise medicine or surgery without taking an examination set by the Chief Physician and Surgeon of the Royal Hospital. By then, European medical care had found favour amongst the Portuguese community.[31] Again, to make matters even more confusing, Dalrymple notes that the English factors (traders) in India 'in 1630 ... have almost completely given up using the Western drugs that the [East Indian] Company was in the habit of sending out to Surat, preferring to take the advice of local Mughal doctors'. As William Methwold, the president of the English East Indian Company in Surat from 1633 to 1638, declared 'wee for our parts doe hold that in things indifferent it is safest for an Englishmen to Indianize and, so conforming himselfe in some measure to the diett of the country, the ordinarie phisick of the country will bee the best cure when any sickness shall overtake him'.[32]

For Spain, the voyages of discovery and their consequences on the health of ships' crews led to the founding of universities in Mexico City and of Lima in Peru as early as 1551. Mexico City had a chair of medicine in 1578 and the University of Lima gained one in 1621. The eighteenth-century medical reforms in New Spain changed from care by charity to care by specialized medical professionals, and was considerably boosted by the formalization of surgical training with the founding of the Mexican School of Surgery in 1769. The students attended four-year courses in anatomy, experimental physics, general pathology, surgical pathology and physiology, and during the last two years, they studied chemistry, botany, bandaging, and surgical procedures. This school was modelled upon and subordinate to that of the Surgical School attached to the Cadiz Hospital, which was established in 1748, where anatomical instruction was offered to prospective ship's surgeons.[33]

The English long-distance experience

While the Portuguese and the Spanish were opening up the world, ship design and naval gunnery technology were being transformed in England. The impact of the gun was first experienced with the wounded suffering burn injuries and it was to these wounds that Tudor surgeons directed their chief attentions.[34] At the Battle of Lepanto in 1571, however, these guns, loaded with their trombs (iron balls with hollow centres containing combustibles), proved relatively ineffective. On the *Mary Rose*, one of Henry VIII's navy ships that sank on its maiden voyage in 1545, archaeological findings proved the existence of two small surgeon's cabins on the starboardside of the main deck, as well as a walnut surgical chest and a long, low fourlegged bench.[35] The number of surgeons in Henry's time must have been small and the odds are that some ships had no surgeon at all. However, the larger sixteenth-century vessels that went on longer voyages created the need for ship's surgeons and provided the facilities to accommodate them. By 1585, the English Navy was more or less regularly employing ship's surgeons who also served as barbers.[36]

In Europe, the Armada of 1588 had been a turning point in the regular provision of medical care to mariners in the form of surgeons on board and facilities ashore, at least on the English side.[37] The surgeons for the English Navy were pressed by the Barber-Surgeons Company of London.[38] William Clowes, the chief surgeon in the English fleet against the Armada, published the first textbook on naval surgery in 1588.[39] The Chatham Chest, a benevolent fund for disabled or poor seamen, was founded by Sir Francis Drake and Sir John Hawkins in 1590. Chatham Hospital, licensed in 1594, was especially built for the care of mariners.

At this time, the port of Lisbon was closed to English and Dutch shipping, and merchants from England and the Dutch Republic went in search of the Eastern trade themselves, for which end the Company of Merchants of London trading on the East Indies (or the East India Company, EIC) received its royal charter in 1600, while the Dutch East India Company or *Vereenigde Oost Indische Compagnie* (VOC) received its charter in 1602 to protect its trade in the Indian Ocean and beyond. During the seventeenth century, the Dutch East India Company successfully excluded English and other European competitors from the East Indies, controlling the trade with Asian traders, and established its own commercial monopoly. The EIC settled in India to trade in cotton and silk, indigo, and saltpetre, with spices from South India, where its first hospital was established in Madras in 1664.[40]

The early English trading posts were usually short of surgeons, who died as often as their patients, and it took more than a year before a replacement could arrive from Europe. This shortage led to the employment of Indian physicians (as the Portuguese had initially done), and this became official policy for the EIC in the first half of the seventeenth century. Cogently, it was considered that Indian diseases were best treated with Indian remedies.[41]

The EIC employed a surgeon and his mate who were supplied by the Barber-Surgeon's Company in London, for each ship on a permanent basis.[42] In 1606, surgeons were no longer permitted to serve either on sea or on land before they and their medicine chests had been examined by their employer or the guild; beginning in 1745, each applicant had to be certified at the Surgeons Company Hall in London.[43] Any English apprentice who wanted to be a ship's surgeon paid a certain admission fee to the freedom of the United Company of Barber Surgeons, and then, as a freeman, was subject to all its rules while working under its jurisdiction, although he was, as the English country surgeon, a 'foreign brother'.[44] The majority of English ship's surgeons and surgeons' mates in the Royal Navy were press-ganged, a practice not known in the Dutch Republic.[45]

The Surgeon's Company in London also allowed apprentices to complete their apprenticeship at sea, as mates to full ship's surgeons, the latter supposedly acting in the capacity of masters and supervising the mates' training. No harm would have come of this had it not been for the custom of promoting a mate to full surgeon if the senior surgeon died or deserted. The captain's decision then replaced the surgeon's examination required by the Surgeons' Hall in London, and, over time, this practice came to be regarded as a normal promotion, without considering the relative change in levels of professional responsibility which it must carry ashore, the more so, because the certification in Surgeon's Hall was felt to be inadequate.[46] Thomas Robertson, for instance, a naval surgeon in the period 1793-1828, travelled to London in 1796 to undergo his belated professional examination to confirm his promotion on board from surgeon's mate to ship's surgeon. He noted in his diary that 'The examination at Surgeons' Hall is the first Thursday of every month. The first examination (by the surgeons) I found teasing and inadequate to ascertain ability. The physician's examination is superficial. Four of us went at the same time for that purpose; all, out of compliment and from its being customary, purchased his books.".[47]

Surgeons on the English East Indiamen, for instance, were employed for one or for many voyages as well as for overseas service and this meant that there was a clear need for an official body in London to assess the expertise of candidates and to supply them with the proper equipment. In 1612, this need was met by the EIC merchants who established a stock company, appointing John Woodall (1556-1643) as their first surgeon-general.[48] Woodall subsequently published an influential guide especially for those surgeons who had completed their apprenticeship, called *The Surgeon's Mate* in 1617.

Woodall's duties were defined in 1621: (i) to be in daily attendance in his office and in the shipyards; (ii) to appoint a deputy to carry out his duties at the Company's chief anchorages in the Thames; (iii) to supply the ship's surgeons and train them in the use of the contents of the medical chests which he was to furnish; (iv) to trim the hair of the Company's employees in the shipyards every six weeks; and (v) to report the unfit among these employees.[49] In short, his function was a mixture of medical examiner, provider of medical services, clerk and hairdresser. By

1620, all of Woodall's medical chests were viewed by two fellows from the College of Physicians. Shortly thereafter, the Society of Apothecaries secured the right to supply the medicines. Under Woodall's guidance, the EIC eventually provided a central body which required its surgeons to submit reports, thus establishing a repository of medical experience, and laid down a scale of equipment that surgeons would be required to take to sea.

The seafaring activities of the Dutch

The development of a Dutch overseas' empire was a direct consequence of the expansion of Dutch trade. During its war with Spain, the Republic had managed to maintain its trade and extend it to all of Europe and, after the turn of the century, as far as East Asia, to which end the VOC was founded in 1602. By replacing Antwerp as the principal warehouse and trading centre of Europe, Amsterdam and the lesser ports of Holland and Zeeland became the main European suppliers of grain and naval supplies from the Baltic, to which they shipped manufactured goods and wines from southern Europe. The bulk of Germany's exports were now shipped down the Rhine, as Dutch ports also replaced the Hanseatic towns of northern Germany. The bulk of French exports were carried on Dutch ships, and even Spain and Portugal depended on the Dutch for the transport of grain and naval stores. During the seventeenth century, the Dutch assumed a major role in supplying grain and other northern commodities to the countries of the Mediterranean and also became the principal importers of spices and other luxury goods from the East. Shipping clearly played an important role in this rise to power and became a significant source of employment in a country with a population of barely two million people (Table T2.1).

Table T2.1: Estimation of people employed in the Dutch seafaring industries[50]

	1680	*1725*	*1770*
Admiralties	3500	3500	2000
Merchant marine (including trade in the West Indies)	22500	22000	21000
VOC	15000	23000	29000
Whaling	9000	9000	6000
Herring fishing	5000	2500	2000
Total	55000	60000	60000

The Dutch shipping industries included fishing, whaling, the merchant navy (including trade on West Africa and the West Indies), the Admiralties (navy), the trade on the East and West Indies, and associated industries ashore, such as salting and shipbuilding. The Dutch fishing industry concentrated on herring, which was usually caught off the coasts of England and Scotland, in the vicinity of relatively known shores.[51] No surgeons were employed on the fishing fleets, but it is highly probable that the skipper of a fishing vessel had a small medical chest at his disposal in case of emergencies. The ship owner was responsible for surgical costs incurred for treating any of his crew injured on board.[52] As early as 1613, there was a possibility to insure oneself against the hazards of life on board, in the form of the *bentcontract*, which insured against accidents on board, as well as against damage caused by pirates, and if a member of the crew drowned, his next-of-kin received some kind of (pecuniary) assistance.[53]

Around 1610, the race for whale (or train) oil started. The larger Dutch whaling ships had a surgeon on board, as did the North German whalers.[54] Obviously, in the icy climate in which the whalers worked, there was less fear of infectious diseases than in the tropics, as many bacteria and viruses thrive only in a warm climate. The risks mainly involved the dangerous work of harpooning, when whalers would incorrectly use their harpoons and knives, which could lead to ugly wounds, but which should have been no problem for properly educated surgeons. At any rate, every whaler had a medicine chest on board, the so-called *lapdoos*, and the master of the ship, in the absence of a surgeon, assumed these duties.[55]

The merchant navy undertook hauls to and from the Baltic and short trips to England, as well as trade further afield in the Mediterranean, West Africa, and the West Indies. The last was organized by the *West Indische Compagnie* (West Indian Company, or WIC) and the *Middelburgsche Commercie Compagnie* (Middelburg Commerce Company, or MCC). The WIC and MCC employed a surgeon, or even several surgeons on board, not only for the crews but also to make sure that the slaves bought on the African West Coast arrived at their destination in good condition.

The medical facilities in the Dutch navy had their origins in the fifteenth century when the Netherlands were still part and parcel of the Habsburg empire. Then, when a naval fleet was assembled, a surgeon was usually employed as a personal servant to the admiral. When Philip II of Spain (1527-98) equipped a 'Dutch' fleet, a surgeon was employed for the benefit of the mariners.[56] Occasionally, a ship was assigned to serve as a hospital ship, as in 1556 when the *St. Jehan* served as such.[57] Ships fighting under William of Orange (1533-1584), leader of the revolt of the Netherlands against Spanish rule, also carried surgeons.[58] The organization of the navy of the Dutch Republic was decentralized in five Admiralties (those of Amsterdam, Rotterdam, Middelburg, Hoorn and Enkhuizen, and Dokkum/Harlingen), and, consequently, medical care was not unified. Each Admiralty had its own medical advisor, a surgeon-general. Master Andries Herls, for instance, was the surgeon-general of the Middelburg Admiralty in 1602; his tasks were to treat wounded sailors and to go wherever the admiral thought he might be needed. Although ship's surgeons were employed on every ship, it was only in 1667 that the Admiralty of Amsterdam stipulated that everyone was to receive free treatment from the (ship's) surgeon and his mate(s) for common diseases and accidents resulting from routine work on board or from enemy action.[59] As in England where the Navy's health-care system was based on that of the EIC, the medical facilities of the Dutch Admiralties were modelled on the pattern provided by the Company, where free treatment by the surgeon had been a rule from the very beginning, with the exception of the consequences from bouts of *Bacchus* and *Venus*. Injuries as a result of quarrels and venereal diseases were not to be treated by the ship's surgeons at the expense of the Company or by the Admiralties.

At around the time that the First Anglo-Dutch War (1652-1654) broke out, physicians were appointed by the Admiralties to verify the contents of a surgeon's medicine chest and his skills. Grand fleets were regularly accompanied by the physician and surgeon-general of the various Admiralties who acted both as a kind of supervisor of the ship's surgeons and as an adviser to the war council regarding cases of contagious diseases and the treatment of the wounded. The patients were usually sent ashore to local hospitals, as there were no naval hospitals in the Republic.[60] By the end of the seventeenth century, the Admiralties of Amsterdam, Rotterdam and Middelburg each employed a surgeon-general, later to be assisted by a physician, at their headquarters.

The Company's medical service

As early as the 1590s, groups of merchants in various Dutch towns established companies to discover the trading routes to the East Indies. The government-sponsored merger of these private companies led to the foundation of the Company in 1602. Its organization was decentralized (as was the Republic itself and its navy) to the cities where, prior to the 1602 charter, private companies had existed independently. The offices in these cities (Amsterdam, Delft, Enkhuizen, Hoorn, Middelburg, and Rotterdam) were now called 'chambers' (*kamers*). The representatives of these chambers met in a central body known as the *Heeren XVII* or the 'Seventeen Gentlemen' (Gentlemen XVII), in which Amsterdam and Middelburg exerted a dominant influence.

From the very inception of the Company, the Gentlemen XVII were convinced that the investment in and overhead incurred by employing ship's surgeons, the provision of surgical instruments and well-stocked medical chests were of vital importance to the survival of the crews and to the overall success of the Company. This conviction was based on the experiences of Portugal and Spain, intelligence of which, of course, had reached the Republic,[61] and on the tradition of responsibility towards one's crews which, over the centuries, had emerged from the foundations laid by the Oléron laws and strengthened by the ideology of the Reformation: the treatment of the sick seafarers on Company vessels was considered the responsibility of the Company as a social God-fearing duty, except for injuries resulting from quarrels amongst the crew and illnesses resulting from venereal diseases. Every year, the Company would dispatch numerous vessels, each one manned by 100 to 300 hands, including crew, soldiers and the rare passenger, all of whom would encounter a variety of climates and diseases during their long voyages.

As a rule, the Company would employ one ship's surgeon with two mates on each East Indiaman, following more or less the hierarchy of surgeons and apprentices ashore: the master surgeon would be the senior surgeon or first surgeon (*oppermeester*, *opperchirurgijn* or *opperbarbier*), with his on-land apprentice serving as the surgeon's mate (*ondermeester* or *onderchirurgijn* or *onderbarbier*), and the pupil serving as the third surgeon (*derde meester*). Their monthly salaries did not change much over the two centuries that the Company existed. The first surgeon earned between 32 and 50 Dutch guilders per month, the surgeon's mate between 24 and 28 Dutch guilders, and the third surgeon between 14 and 18 Dutch guilders.[62] This consistent wage rate throughout two centuries was germane to all those who sailed on Company ships (i.e., sailors and soldiers).[63]

The Company employed a medical staff in Amsterdam and Zeeland. In Amsterdam, for instance, the tasks of the Chamber's physician were of a supervisory and advisory nature: he had to check and supervise the Chamber's pharmacy (located in the East India House); he had to examine the knowledge and skills of surgeons applying for employment with the Company; he also examined Company employees who fell ill, and advised his superiors on the 'compensation money' to be allocated to these patients, as the Company paid allowances in cases of permanent disability on the basis of the physician's report.[64] The Company pharmacist of the Amsterdam Chamber prepared all of the medicines necessary for the forts, the trading posts and *comptoiren* (settlements) in Asia. The Surgeon-Examiner of the Amsterdam Chamber joined the physician and the *Heeren van het pakhuis* (i.e., the chamber's officials overseeing the storehouses) to aid in the examination of candidates for surgical vacancies on board.[65]

Besides employing surgeons on the Company vessels and providing a bureaucratic medical structure at the chambers, the Company charter also included the right to found settlements in Asia, in which hospital-based health care would figure prominently.

Employment qualifications

Specialized trained surgeons were what the Company's ships needed for its long sea voyages. Candidates in some towns were offered the opportunity to take the

Zeeproef or 'surgeon's sea examination', which required a shorter preparation period than for the *Huisproef* (i.e., 'master's examination'). The senior members of the surgeons, guilds served as the examiners of the candidates for the *Zeeproef*. The municipal archives of Amsterdam and Enkhuizen provide ample evidence of this practice. The fees for the sea examination were considerably lower than those for the master's examination: for example, Gerrit de Graaf of Enkhuizen paid 16 Dutch guilders for his master's examination in 1759, while Jan Bruel, Jan Hendrik Blok, Pieter Dekker and Christiaan de Wolf only paid six guilders for their sea examinations in 1776, in 1778, 1780 and 1787 respectively.[66] Moreover, it seems that the duties of a ship's surgeon were supposedly of a more limited scope than those of a master surgeon ashore as the body of theoretical and practical knowledge that one needed to pass the sea examination was smaller. That has been the usual interpretation by historians of the Dutch East India Company.[67]

The *Zeeproef* included a theoretical part with questions about: '*accidenten als ter zee meestendeels voorvallen als van allerhande fracturen, dislocatiën, geschooten wonden, contusien, verbrandtheijd, gangraenatione ende diergelijke*', meaning that the candidate was examined on his knowledge of accidents that commonly occurred aboard such as fractures, dislocations, wounds caused by guns, contusions, burns, gangrene and other similar ailments and how to treat them. This did not diverge greatly from the master's examination. The practical part of the *Zeeproef* consisted of the proper way to sharpen lancets and perform venasection (bloodletting), for which the candidate had to know the anatomy of veins, and was very much the same as that of the barber-surgeon's examination (the phlebotomy test). These requirements were stipulated in the 1636 Ordinance of the Council of Physicians and Surgeons of Enkhuizen.[68] The ship's surgeon apparently did not have to know about unnatural growths, ulcers, open sores, their treatment, and complicated operations, knowledge which was necessary for the master's examination. The ordinance went on to stipulate that every ship's surgeon had to have his skills examined prior to his employment on one of the Admiralties' ships or a merchant ship.[69]

Those who successfully passed the ship's surgeon's examination were not licensed to practice ashore but could obtain the rank of full or first surgeon on board. The candidate could take the ship's surgeon's examination if he had completed his three-year apprenticeship (*leerknecht*), as well as a one-year journeymanship (*knecht*). The time the candidate had served on board as a surgeon's mate (*onderbarbier*) was considered the equivalent of a journeymanship.[70] A minimum of a two-year journeymanship was required to take the *Huisproef*, which licensed the surgeon to practise both on shore and on board, at least in Enkhuizen.

Although no such ordinance has been found in the archives of Amsterdam, nor, for that matter, in those of the Republic's other port cities (Rotterdam, Hoorn, Middelburg and Delft (Delfshaven), where the Admiralties and the East and West India Companies all had offices), this particular sea examination was, in all probability, offered there as well. In Amsterdam, the surgeons guild not only differentiated between a master's examination and a ship's surgeon's examination but also within the latter, making a distinction for surgeon's duties on ships exceeding 360 tons and those below that size: for instance, Benjamin Miseroy tried his minor sea examination (*Zeeproef Klein Reglement*) on 16 March, 1787. He succeeded and was licensed to practise on ships smaller than 360 tons, whereas Simon Gastman sat for the major sea examination (*Zeeproef Groot Reglement*) in 1779 but failed.[71] Gerrit Jansz. Sluijs, who had started as a pupil (*leerknecht*) on 7 July, 1777, passed his minor sea examination on 5 April, 1785.[72] Presumably, the idea was that on smaller ships, the crew was commensurably smaller and therefore the frequency of accidents would be fewer and these would be less drastic.

Indeed, the policy pursued by the Dutch East India Company from the inception and confirmed in 1686 was that the size of the vessel determined the size of her medical staff. The line of thinking was probably that the bigger the vessel, the larger the crew, the more medical aid was necessary: three surgeons (that is, one full surgeon with two assistants) staffed the largest ships which measured over 140 feet in length. During times of war when there was a consequent shortage of surgeons, only one first surgeon (*oppermeester*) and one surgeon's mate (*ondermeester*) were allocated to a vessel of this length, one *oppermeester* and *derde meester* to ships between 120 and 130 feet, and only one surgeon's mate was allocated to vessels smaller than that.[73] The surgeons had to sign on for at least five years. Clearly, a system of training and examination for those surgeons attracted to 'maritime medicine' existed in the Dutch Republic and was already quite well developed by 1636 when Enkhuizen formalized its criteria for maritime medical service.

In the Swedish East India Company in the eighteenth century, the ship's surgeons were not examined by a medical board but had an interview with a committee in order to prove their professional competence as potential ship's surgeons.[74] This was an exception. Most other European ship's surgeons on East Indiamen were examined or certified before employment, like their counterparts on Dutch vessels. At least in Amsterdam, Enkhuizen, and Middelburg, it was a prerequisite to have passed the sea examination before the interview took place. This practice was probably also prevalent in the other chambers. As we have already seen, criteria set for the sea examination were undoubtedly of a lower standard than those of the examination for master surgeon ashore, as the practical training was shorter than that required of the master surgeon and there was no examination on extensive anatomy, the trepanning of a skull, or on amputation.

The most apparent reason for this would appear to have been a presumed lack of surgeons willing to serve at sea. The Enkhuizen Ordinance (1636) was formulated in the first half of the seventeenth century, a period of a rapid commercial expansion in the Republic, transforming the young state into a centre of world commerce, a status which it was to hold for more than a century.[75] At the beginning of this period, surely there was no shortage of labour in the Dutch Republic, not least because of a great influx of émigré populations, including many skilled persons. The Ordinance itself gives some clue to the reason why it was formulated. It states that owing to disputes among the physicians and surgeons of Enkhuizen, the medical organization of the town had been reduced to such a sorry plight, that the officials of the town wanted to sort out the fragmented chaos.[76] Ship's surgeons were included. In all probability, the new rules were not seen by the city officials as a lowering of standards, but as a means of improving efficiency, and the city officials must have thought that the criteria set for the sea examination, were those needed for service on board a ship. It would seem that the expanding trade and growing economy of the Republic, in which Enkhuizen certainly participated during the first half of the seventeenth century, resulted in a professionalization of the discipline of medicine and the craft of surgery which until then had lagged behind and were still fragmented.

The professional standards of a Company surgeon were thus guaranteed, and in all probability did not diverge greatly from those surgeons educated in the smaller towns of the Republic. Besides his master surgeon's examination or sea examination, the candidate was required to pass an extra examination presided over by the chamber's physician, its surgeon-examiner, and members of the chamber's committee who were responsible for personnel.[77] In Middelburg (Zeeland Chamber), this requirement was made effective as early as 1610.[78] It applied only to full surgeons and surgeon's mates, but not invariably to the third surgeons (*derde meesters*). In Amsterdam, the *derde meester* too had to be examined from 1681.[79] Furthermore, in the first half of the eighteenth century, the Admiralty of Amsterdam asked the city surgeon ('municipal officer of health') Abraham Titsing to instruct the ship's surgeons during wintertime.[80] The municipal authorities of Rotterdam made the *Zeeproef* obligatory in 1717 before a surgeon could be employed by the merchant fleet,[81] and from 1770 there was special instruction to ship's surgeons given by the city physicians Patijn and De Monchy.[82] When a candidate was interviewed by the other chambers, which did not employ a medical staff, the candidate ship's surgeon had to submit papers proving his competence and was examined by surgeons from the city with which the chamber had made an arrangement.

Although a stringent requirement, the ship's surgeon's examination did not do much to elevate his status. People tended not to rate the quality of a ship's surgeon's 'craft' highly. For instance, some considerably experienced ship's surgeons who wanted to turn to surgery ashore in the port city of Flushing (Vlissingen) and who required to become a member of the surgeon's guild were invariably rejected, and forbidden to treat patients other than those among their own crew. This has been seen as a confirmation of the low professional competence of the ship's surgeon.[83] However, it is much more likely that the master surgeons of Flushing were afraid of the competition offered by these ship's surgeons newly arrived in their town, and tried to protect their business.

Some years later, in 1719, the authorities of Flushing decided to examine the competence of these ship's surgeons and to view the surgeon's medical chests before sailing, a task performed by Flushing's city physician Dr. Willem Derrix and the city surgeon, Hendrik de Bruas.[84] This regulation, presented under the guise of quality control, may have also been a protective measure, not of quality but of the interests of the local surgeons. The surgeon's examination by the Company personnel staff was made obligatory for each chamber in 1751, at which time the Gentlemen XVII ruled that all the Company's officers (including *derde meesters*) should pass an examination before being accepted as employees.[85]

As in other East India companies, it sometimes came to pass that a Company *derde meester* was rapidly promoted to full surgeon on board because of the untimely deaths of his superiors. If this happened outward-bound, the *derde meester* was certified at the Cape of Good Hope by the chief surgeon of the Cape's hospital and some first surgeons of other vessels at anchor there. For instance, the surgeon's mate on the *Herstelde Leeuw*, Hendrik Belde, was promoted to chief surgeon as his superior had to remain in the hospital at the Cape in 1719. The third surgeon, Cornelis Bogaard, was promoted to surgeon's mate, and the sailor Johannes Glasenhap was made third surgeon.[86] These promoted surgeons never received the full wage usually attached to the function, as the promotion had to be certified by the authorities in Batavia. Only then, would they be paid commensurably. In Batavia, the medical authorities in Batavia Castle joined by those of the Batavia Hospital would certify these promotions or refuse to acknowledge them. If homeward bound, the ship's surgeon was certified in the Republic. Nevertheless, until such time, he acted without certification in a certain surgical rank with all the corresponding responsibilities, sometimes an impossible task. One surgeon's mate noted in his journal that 'one surgeon's mate had already died here on board, and as the first surgeon is now very sick, and as the number of patients is so great, it is a sheer impossibility for me to keep a surgeons log'.[87]

This organization of medical personnel also applied to non-Dutch surgeons who offered their services to the Company. Charles-Ghislain Wilmet, born in Gembloux (Belgium, Austrian Netherlands), wrote to his family on 11 March, 1779, to confirm his safe arrival in Rotterdam at the home of a colleague (Master Surgeon Van Putten, in the Breestraat in Rotterdam). He asked his family to send him his surgical and medical books, because he had offered his services to the Company a few days before. After the Company officials had scrutinized his certificates, he was subsequently examined by the physician of the Rotterdam Chamber of the Company, a test which he apparently passed with flying colours as he was subsequently employed as first surgeon on the *Rotterdam* at a monthly wage of 36 Dutch guilders and a bonus of 500 guilders on the successful conclusion of the voyage.[88]

In the first half of the eighteenth century, the first surgeon acquired the right to his own cabin among those of the officers. During the seventeenth century, the surgeon could not have taken the cabin for granted, although he did mess at the captain's table.[89] The seventeenth-century ship's surgeon Nicolaas de Graaff tells us that those who messed with the captain on board were the merchant, the bookkeeper, the clerk, the commander of the soldiers, the minister (*ziekentrooster*), and the chief surgeon, though the latter slept in the gun room.[90] The second surgeon and the third surgeon also shared a sleeping place separated by a piece of canvas in the gun room.[91] The senior surgeon on board slung his hammock in the gun room until 1739, when a new instruction for surgeons was issued in which the first surgeon was allocated his own cabin and bunk.[92] This instruction probably formalized an already existing custom; at any rate, his high social status on board was thus guaranteed.

Ship's surgeon's duties

Until the Company's first General Instruction (*Artikelbrief*) was drawn up for all employees in 1634, nothing specific was laid down regarding the duties of the ship's surgeons, on whose shoulders rested the whole burden of medical care in Asia. Only four of the 122 articles in this *Artikelbrief* dealt with ship's hygiene and medicine, merely formalizing methods and procedures that had been in use since earlier times.[93] These consisted of cleaning the ship and providing special food for the patients. As a result of the high mortality rates during the period 1690-1695, the Gentlemen XVII issued an instruction in 1695, which essentially formalized the duties of a Company ship's surgeon. These consisted of (i) upon embarking, to prepare the dressings, cottons, compresses, bandages, and splints immediately, using the *lapdoos* (literally, the rag box, the same *lapdoos* used by whalers and introduced by the Company in 1682) in contrast to the big medical chest used during the voyage. Because the crew often had to wait a long time on board ship before departure was possible, this *lapdoos* also included some basic medicinal drugs; (ii) to hold surgery (a consultation hour) in the morning and in the evening at the main mast; (iii) to visit the ill and wounded twice a day, thrice a day for more serious cases; (iv) to regularly clean and wash bed-ridden patients; (v) to record all cases in a daily surgeon's log (*chirurgijns journaal* or surgeon's journal); and (vi) to purify the air between the decks by means of boiling and sprinkling vinegar as well as by the occasional burning of powder.[94] This instruction was not to change much throughout the eighteenth century.

In contrast to the EIC, where even Surgeon-General John Woodall was required to shave EIC employees, nothing was officially laid down for the surgeons of the Dutch Company regarding this task. The general assumption among historians is that the Company surgeons also served as barbers aboard Company ships as a matter of routine. It was so routine, in fact, that nothing about this service is found in the Company archives.[95] In his thesis, the maritime historian H. Ketting mentions one example of a *provoost* (provost) demanding to be shaved by a surgeon. However, this example occurred during the *tweede schipvaart*, even before the Dutch Company was formed, and proves rather thin as evidence that the Company surgeons shaved crew members as a matter of routine. On the contrary, shaving was not one of the assigned tasks of a Company surgeon. He may have shaved his fellow seafarers occasionally when he had the time to do so, but then he was probably paid by the customers' own pockets. Of the *circa* 90 lists of surgeons' possessions found in the Company's financial records in the archives in The Hague (inventories made up after their demise on board), there were only nine surgeons who possessed shaving gear (consisting mostly of razors, that is, knives used specifically for shaving, in Dutch, *scheermessen*).[96]

Table T2.2: Possession of razors

Name surgeon	*Rank*	*Date of death*	*Shaving instruments*	*Source NA*
W. Belkol	First surgeon	24/7/1729	14 razors	VOC 6378
C. Brauns	First surgeon	20/6/1769	2 razors	VOC 6524
J.W. Stilzer	First surgeon	31/10/1770	2 razors	VOC 14.489
Chr.G. Jager	First surgeon	19/2/1789	6 shaving basins	VOC 14.813
W. Meijer	Surgeon's mate	1/11/1719	4 razors and 1 scissor	VOC 5742
H. van der Kemp	Surgeon's mate	6/11/1719	5 razors	VOC 14.139
J. van Melligem	Third surgeon	7/4/1721	4 dozen razors	VOC 5767
N. Lameij	Third surgeon	10/7/1745	7 razors	VOC 14.433
P. Josse	Third surgeon	21/9/1762	1 shaving basin	VOC 6401

The Company's surgeons must have considered the barbering aspect of their profession far beneath them, as did their colleagues ashore, even though shaving services ashore often filled the money-bag. It may well have been the same on board. However, if as a general rule they did not possess any shaving gear, how were they even able to shave their clients on board? Next to that, these clients would have had to pay for it, which, with the exception of the officers, not every member of the company on board was in a position to do. Moreover, to shave a crew of two to three hundred men on a regular basis would be quite a time-consuming business, time the ship's surgeon could have ill afforded. It is far more likely that the Company seafarers, as soon as they reached the Cape of Good Hope, Batavia, or a home port, would have gone to the barber ashore, if they had any money in their pockets!

Medical chest and treatment

The Company surgeon was provided, as part of the ship's surgeon's instruments, with a medical chest containing potions and herbs with their curative properties noted on prescribed lists. During a voyage (at the Cape and in Batavia) and at its end, the surgeon had to do an inventory of medicinal supplies he had used. A Chamber official then drew up an official declaration of the surgeon's inventory statement. This is how the 'accountant' of the Company stores in Hoorn declared that Johannes Verwoert, senior surgeon of the *Aurich* had accounted satisfactorily for his use of medicines upon his return in 1784.[97]

In Amsterdam, it was the chamber's own pharmacist who provided the medical supplies with the assistance of the *Gasthuis*.[98] Among the smaller Chambers, this task was delegated to local pharmacies. During the two centuries of the Company's existence, the contents of the chests remained more or less the same, consisting of some 130 different 'potent/curing' ingredients, from which the surgeon could choose to prepare his prescriptions. They were divided into various kinds of plasters (*emplastra*), ointments (*unguenta*), oils (*olea*), opium derivations in the form of pills (*opiata in massam pilularum redacta*), purgatives (*laxativa*), roots (*radices*), honey preparations (*mellitta*), waters (*aquae*), marmalades (*conservae*), powders (*pulveres*), herbs (*herbae*), flowers (*flores*), bark, fruits, woods and seeds (*cortices, fructus, ligna, semina*), concentrated juices, gums, and resins (*succi condensati, gummi, resinae*). The chests also contained ingredients such as mercury, laurel, vinegar, turpentine and juniper, necessary for the preparation of plasters, as well as sulphur, sulphuric acid, anti-diarrhoea preparations, ground carrots, barks, and animal parts (like pig's feet, crab's eyes, deer antlers, and Spanish fly).[99]

Armed with these ingredients, the surgeons were able to concoct an endless array of medicines. A lead plaster, for example, consisted of a boiled mixture of oil, lard, and lead. The plaster called *De ranis cum 4 drup: merc.* was made of boiled frogs and lead monoxide plus some drops of mercury. Soap plasters were made of wax, colophony, turpentine, ammonia, and saffron.[100] Prescriptions made of a combination of *radix ipecacuanhae* (also called 'vomiting root' or 'dysentery root') and *cremor tartari* or *cremtart* (cream of tartar, a crystallized red tartaric acid made from grapes) were used on patients suffering from a 'slimy stomach' and was used as a purgative. A dose of *radix jalappe* (root of the Mexican *Ipomoea purga Hayne* with a laxative effect) and *cremtart* as indication of purging was given to patients suffering from oedema. A mixture of *flor cammonil* (flowers of the camomile plant), *sapon venet* (Venetian soap), *sal comun* (common salt), and *cogin aqua marin* (boiled sea water) was considered an efficacious *lavement* or enema, particularly for weak patients. The contents of the medical chests of the ships sailing from the other East India Company's ports did not diverge greatly, which is not surprising as the medical knowledge of the time was pretty much agreed upon.[101] Besides his medicines, the surgeon was also authorized to provide a higher quality of food (as served to the officers) for the ill, including French or Spanish wines, butter, sugar, syrup, honey, smoked ox-tongue, ham, meat, extra cheese, biscuits, Turkish beans (corn), raisins, saffron, spices, carrots, onions, and turnips.

It is known that the orphanage and the poorhouse in Middelburg provided quite a few third – sometimes second – surgeons to the Company. These orphaned ship's surgeons-to-be were provided a sea chest, which usually contained some clothes, surgical books, and lancets. Furthermore, it appears that these orphans who trained to be surgeons usually took an impressive supply of 'spirits' along with them. Jan Kakelaar, for instance, took along some 50 bottles of white wine and 12 bottles of Dutch gin (*jenever*) on his first voyage as third surgeon for the chamber of Zeeland at the age of 14. Although it has sometimes been suggested that these 'spirits' were needed as antiseptics and anaesthetics, it is far more likely that the alcohol was meant for private trading, as we will see in chapter 6.[102]

The *lapdoos* was introduced in 1682 at a meeting of the Gentlemen XVII as a measure to combat the theft of medicines from the big medicine chests. Many a surgeon apparently sold these medicines and then replaced the stolen goods with poor substitutes.[103] This was also a common practice in the French East India Company until, as a countermeasure, the medical chests were kept under the control of the master of the ship until the vessel had set sail.[104] The Dutch Company soon followed suit after the Delft Chamber proposed that the big medical chest should, in the future, be locked up in the presence of the ship's surgeon and the keys kept by the master of the ship, only to be opened after the ship had sailed and in the presence of both the master and a clerk.[105] The *lapdoos* was used mainly while the ship was still in harbour and comprised only some small quantities of basic medicines and some linen.

The Company provided a quantity of old linen to serve as dressings, although most ship's surgeons were careful not to depend on what was provided by the Company and usually took along some linen of their own. This linen had been completely teased and frayed until it came unravelled or wispy. All of the dressings, compresses and *cataplasma* (poultices) were made from this linen. Dressings were rarely 'dry' as they were usually soaked in a curative concoction of herbs, honey, wine, and sometimes plasters made of mushrooms, and other potent ingredients were put beneath it.[106]

Bloodletting, among the various treatments employed by the ship's surgeons, appears to have been one of the most common. A patient with a fever (*febris biliosa*, *febris continua*) or any other internal complaints was usually bled. An oral medication, usually a laxative, often followed. Laxatives were not only prescribed when a patient was constipated, but also when he suffered from diarrhoea, oedema, fevers, or abdominal pains. The surgeon also used non-oral medications such as enemas or *lavements*. A *lavement*, apart from being a synonym for an enema, was also a dressing for open, suppurating or gangrenial wounds. Another weapon in his armoury was *vesicatoria*, plasters used to produce a blister. These plasters were usually made from Spanish fly and were applied to those parts of the body where the surgeon suspected an excess amount of evil body fluids had accumulated. After some six hours, a blister developed, which was lanced after two to three days so that these fluids could be drained. These therapies were (still) based on Galen's humoral-pathological notions that conjectured that the human body's balance could only be re-established with the purging of evil humours.[107]

There were no fixed rules regarding the placement of the big medical chest or, for that matter, the patients themselves. For example, Nicolaas de Graaff, who made no less than 16 voyages as ship's surgeon in the seventeenth century and early eighteenth century, usually placed his patients near the cable tier.[108] Senior surgeon Johannes den Engelsman initially placed his chest against the bulkheads of the foremost cabin.[109] When the Company ship the *Walvis* arrived in the roadstead of the Siam River near Bangkok in August 1655, it had to prepare for battle immediately as it found the enemy, three Portuguese vessels, that were already anchored there. Ship's surgeon Gijsbert Heeck was immediately ordered to transfer his patients, plus chests and boxes to the hold.[110] The lack of adequate accommodation for the patients on board was a universal complaint on the overcrowded vessels of the various European East Indian companies. The usual operating theatre in the English Navy ships was the cockpit, situated on the orlop deck just before one reaches the mastergunner's cabin, and which was illuminated by lanterns. Here, the medical chest was usually kept and where operations were carried out. A sick bay would be constructed when needed: the space between two guns, or any space between decks, which was sometimes made over into a sort of apartment by means of a canvas partition.[111]

Instruments

Though the Company supplied medicines according to prescribed lists, it did not provide instruments. The Gentlemen XVII in 1630, had explicitly stated that the ship's surgeon was expected to have his own set.[112] Apart from the two months' of advanced salary which each Company employee (on board and in Asia) received, the ship's surgeon was allowed a third month's advance to buy his instruments. Apparently, this was usually not enough because in 1656, the Gentlemen XVII decided that each chamber should have surgical instruments and materials in stock, which a surgeon bound for Asia could then buy or rent.[113]

These instruments included pieces of pasteboard (thick, stiff paper), small skeins of silk used for stitching, clyster pipes for bladders, pig's bladders, sponges, leather skins, mortar and pestle, syringes and nozzles, drinking mugs and oil bottles, pewter cups used for cupping blood or other liquids from the body, funnels, kettles, suppository spoons, pans for the making of decoctions (boiling down of herbs), spatulae, hammers, needles, linen and the like.[114] Not included were scalpels, lancets and shaving gear. The Company's surgeons were expected to own their own lancets.

Usually, those instruments borrowed from the Company stock were needed in connection with the dispensing of medicines, although shaving basins figured as well. The latter, could also serve a variety of other purposes, however, and, as no razors were ever borrowed, they probably did. The *pakhuismeester* ('manager of the stores') of the Company in Zeeland declared that senior surgeon Pieter Hooijkaas on the *Petronella Alida* had returned some borrowed instruments, such as an alembic, a large and a small pan, a large and a small syringe, and scales with some weights to the Company.[115] In 1732, the senior surgeon Johannes Winkelaar returned the following instruments: 1 alembic; 1 suppository spoon, 1 small pan with its lid, 1 mortar and pestle, 1 shaving basin, 1 funnel, 1 *gangebecken* (a basin of which the size and function is unknown), 1 large and 1 small syringe (*seringa*), 2 saws, 5 jars, 2 small lancets (*vlijmaatjes*), a one-pint jug, a half-pint jug, 1 small scale with weights, 1 small mortar and 1 sieve.[116] Petrus Wilhelmes Callenfels, who had been chief surgeon on the *Willem de Vijfde*, had borrowed the following: 1 alembic, 2 small pans, 1 mortar and pounder, 2 basins (*gangbekkens*), 1 large syringe (*spuijt*), 1 small box with scales and weights, 2 sieves, 3 trusses (*breukbanden*), 2 shaving basins, 6 jars, a one-pint beaker, a half-pint jug, 3 mugs, 1 stone mortar and a wooden pestle, 1 mortar of stone and pounder to pound serpentine, 1 iron spoon.[117] Dingenis van den Abeele, chief surgeon on the *Velzen*, returned the following instruments in 1767: 1 alembic made of copper, 2 copper pans, 1 mortar and pestle of copper, 1 copper shaving basin, 1 box with scales and weights, 1 tin syringe, 2 tin syringes for wounds (*tinnen wondspuiten*), 1 pewter basin (*tinnen gangbekken*); 6 tin mugs, 2 tin jugs, a 150-cl tin jug, a 75–cl tin jug, 1 tin funnel, 1 iron suppository spoon, 1 sieve, 3 old trusses, 1 medical chest, and 1 iron lock.[118]

The particular instruments provided by the Company differed from those provided by the Admiralties, whose lists were far more extensive: a November 1792 list includes some of the most essential instruments that surgeon-majors in the service of the Dutch Admiralty needed. It included straight and curved scissors, razors, scalpels, bistouries, lancets, probes, amputation pincers, amputation saw, trocars, catheters, trepan-instruments, tourniquets, artery forceps, needles, and hooks. Moreover, shaving was also a required task of the Admiralties' surgeon.

Surgeon's log

According to the 1695 instruction, the Company ship's surgeon was obliged to keep a so-called surgeon's log or journal. As no guidelines were laid down about the contents of this journal, there is no uniformity in them to be found. The journals consisted of blank pages until the surgeon wrote in it. Some surgeons only penned down the number of patients, others the consumption of medicines, and yet others truly embraced the task wholeheartedly and noted the patient's name, symptoms, diagnosis, and treatment. Fifty-two journals covering the period of 1695-1700 are kept in the Company archive in The Hague. For the eighteenth century, this number is even fewer; for the period 1764 to 1786 some 15 full-scale surgeon's logs exist, although an extensive search in the *Overgekomen Brieven en Papieren* ('Letters and Documents sent from Batavia to the Republic') may produce more. There is strong reason to suppose that, as so very few journals have survived, the 1695 instruction was no longer stringently enforced anymore after the first five years. As the ship's surgeons had to report at the Cape of Good Hope, there are numerous reports of ship's surgeons to be found there in the state archives.[119]

These journals and reports provide a general impression of the ship's surgeon's practice. He started his mornings with the preparation of plasters and wicks, compresses and splints, bandages and medicines for internal use, after which he administered them to his patients. He then held the *Verband* (surgery) at the main mast and attended to any dressings. Having done so, he distributed the food and made his rounds. Moreover, he was also on call for patients at any hour of the day or night.

The ship's surgeon's patients

Generally speaking, the seventeenth century did not present any serious recruitment problems for the Company. The majority of the seafarers were recruits from the Republic, particularly from the seaports and countryside areas in the Dutch maritime provinces (Friesland, Holland and Zeeland), even though the general populace of these regions basically considered employment in the Indian companies, either the East or the West (and for the Admiralties), a disgrace. It was often seen as the last desperate opportunity to earn a living in some way.[120]

Population growth in the Dutch Republic began to stagnate in the 1650s, and even declined in Holland and Friesland, precisely during a period when trade was expanding in Asia. This meant that the Company encountered – sometimes severe – manning problems during the eighteenth century. Another consequence of this was that the already considerable number of non-Dutch nationals in the service of the Company grew, sometimes reaching more than half of the vessel's entire crew. In order to secure sufficient numbers of soldiers and sailors for the Dutch East Indiamen and for service in Asia, a class of crimps nicknamed *zielverkoopers* or 'soul sellers' emerged in the ports of the Republic. The crimps offered to provide board, lodgings and work to the men who had come to the ports seeking employment. These crimps provided the men with lodgings, which often left much to be desired, in return for an obligation (*transportbrief*) until they sailed out on the next Company ship. As C.R. Boxer wrote: 'Obviously, men who were confined in such quarters for any length of time came aboard their ships in no condition to resist the onset of infectious or contagious diseases, even if they were lucky enough not to have contracted one already. Ship or jail fever was usually introduced on board by the infected clothing of the contaminated recruits provided by the crimps.'[121] The reputation of the crimps was known far and wide, and prospective sailors in Germany were warned against them.[122]

It has been argued that the general level of skills and the general health status of those recruited by the Company declined steadily during the eighteenth century.[123] This was particularly true, it is said, of the soldiers the Company employed who proved to be flea- and lice-ridden, causing diseases (often typhus) to break out among the prospective 'crews' even before the ships sailed. This problem navies and merchant fleets all over Europe experienced. Crews were suffering from epidemic diseases on a scale greater than ever before. According to the Dutch maritime historian J.R. Bruijn, there were instances when entire Dutch, English, and French naval squadrons were immobilized by disease.[124]

The ever deepening dearth of specific nautical skills and experience of the Company's crews in the eighteenth century reflected their positions on society's ladder. Among them were a number of vagabonds, outlaws, fugitives, the destitute, orphans, and adventurers attracted by the lure of travel and possible lucrative rewards. Thus, it is impossible to foster any illusions about the state of health of these men, particularly when it is borne in mind that these recruits, crimped by brokers and having become indebted to the Company for an advance on their pay, were often put up for months in the boarding-houses run by these brokers. When they finally did manage to board a vessel, they often had to wait for a favourable wind to make their departure. The fact that there were hundreds to thousands of these undernourished, weakened, infested with lice, meant that the Company's surgeons faced a terrible challenge even prior to setting sail.[125]

Living conditions on board

Not only were many of the men in bad health when they boarded, the accommodation on the ships left much to be desired, to say the least. They slept on the orlop, between the cannon. Ventilation was minimal on this lowest deck. The hammocks of sometimes 300 or more men (on a ship measuring 160 feet long and 40 feet wide) hung right next to one another. Fresh air was provided by the open portholes, of which all but one remained closed in bad weather. Living conditions in the orlop especially in the more tropical areas must have been pretty intolerable – certainly from our point of view – because of the heat, vermin, overcrowding, and stench.

The diet on board, although copious, was, out of sheer necessity, often poor in vitamins. It consisted of dried and salted products, such as biscuits, groats, peas, beans, as well as meat and dried fish, mostly prepared in water or fat.[126] Water and provisions for approximately a year were brought on board and stored in the stuffy and foul-smelling hold, which did not exactly improve the quality of the primitively preserved provisions. Preserving food in those times was basically limited to the drying of fruit and the salting of fish. In the early morning, barley porridge was served, to which some dried prunes or raisins were added, and then diluted with water, beer, or wine. Sometimes, live cattle, pigs, and fowl were brought on board. These animals would then be slaughtered during the course of the voyage.

At noon and in the early evenings, meals were composed of boiled green or grey peas, or beans, served in a butter sauce of gravy and some fish, meat, or bacon. Bread was distributed weekly, beer daily, and a considerable amount of cheese was handed out upon boarding; onions were added around 1742 and *sauerkraut* containing vitamin C circa 1760.[127] As such, the diet was not significantly different from that found on the vessels of other European East India companies. The food was often devoid of the nutrition to be found in fresh fruit and vegetables. The Cape of Good Hope provided the very much needed revictualling in terms of vegetables and water.

Clothes were often sopping wet from the rain, the sea spray, and the water that seeped in through the hull. The stomachs of crew members were often upset from eating rotten food, or drinking water that turned green and putrid after a few weeks of being stored in casks. Mattresses and clothing swarmed with lice and other bugs. The combination of poor diet and substandard sleeping and living quarters plus the climate put a severe strain on the physical resilience of the crew. Outbreaks of plague, dysentery, or fever could decimate a crew within a few short days. Such was the experience of the senior surgeon Johannes den Engelsman from Middelburg in Zeeland in 1772.

In that year, Den Engelsman, a fairly experienced traveller, undertook his fourth voyage to Asia. He sailed on board the *Bleijswijk* in November 1772, earning a wage of 36 guilders a month. A month into the voyage, while on the roadstead of Ile d'Aix near Rochefort in France on 17 December, 1772, he wrote a letter to his friend the physician Servaas van de Coppello describing how he had just experienced a very sad month. Den Engelsman, described how as soon as the *Bleijswijk* had entered the English Channel, she had encountered extremely stormy weather (rain, hail, and mist), which meant that the hatches had to remain battened down from 18 November until 10 December. Moreover, since the ship was loaded down with cargo, four to five feet of water seeped into the hull, leaving most of the men on board sleeping in wet clothing and bedding. He described how there was nothing left aboard, that was not already rotten or damaged. Moreover, to add to the physical misery, the crew was plagued by disease, particularly the *febris maligna* or *continua* or *putricia*. The misery was only further exacerbated when 12 sailors were swept overboard and drowned. But that was not the end of their plight because all three masts broke during the storms and were lost to the sea as well. The special beds (*britsen*) for the patients were also damaged by the storms, and all of the sea chests were lost overboard; crew members were seen swimming between decks to try to save their belongings, which led to the further drowning of another 19 men. Finally, his medical chest, which was usually fastened to the bulkhead of the foremost cabin, alongside the companion-way to the pumps, had been moved because of all the activity surrounding the pumping and was subsequently so damaged that its contents were also lost. His patients, who numbered some 70 to 75, were dying on a daily basis. In total some 100 men lost their lives. On 12 December, the *Bleijswijk* anchored near the Ile d'Aix to purchase new masts at Rochefort. Den Engelsman asked his friend and colleague to send him a new medical chest and some new linen as he had to bandage some twenty-six patients every day.[128] Johannes den Engelsman returned to the Republic in 1775, and stood ready to be employed for a fifth voyage that same year.

Mortality

During the seventeenth century, the overall mortality rate on the outward bound Dutch East Indiamen was 6.7 per cent, rising in the eighteenth century to 7.3 per cent. In the period 1690-1700, it was slightly over nine per cent and during the period 1770-1780 it was nearly 12 per cent (Table T2.3). However, within these two ten-year periods, the years 1690-1695 yielded a mortality rate of 20 per cent, and, in the years 1770-1775, it rose to 23 per cent.[129]

Table T2.3: Company personnel outward-bound to Asia and their mortality rates [130]

Period	*Voyagers*	*Deaths %*	*Vessels*	*Period*	*Voyagers*	*Deaths %*	*Vessels*
1595-1602	5300	?	66	1700-1710	49000	5.4%	281
1602-1610	8500	?	76	1710-1720	59900	4.6%	310
1610-1620	19000	?	117	1720-1730	71700	6.0%	382
1620-1630	23700	?	141	1730-1740	74300	8.2%	375
1630-1640	28,900?	?	157	1740-1750	73100	10.2%	314
1640-1650	33,100?	?	165	1750-1760	80500	5.5%	290
1650-1660	40,200?	4.2%	205	1760-1770	85500	6.2%	292
1660-1670	40900	6.4%	238	1770-1780	75500	11.9%	290
1670-1680	42700	6.2%	238	1780-1790	61900	6.2%	298
1680-1690	37800	7.0%	204	1790-1795	22900	3.8%	119
1690-1700	43000	9.2%	235				

It has been suggested that, during the period 1690-1695, the Company's crews were infected by the Rickettsia virus, the typhus host, which is passed onto humans via lice found on clothes. The isolated community on board, which was forced into its cramped quarters, formed a natural breeding ground for endemic infections. A situation of potential danger prevailed, which was further exacerbated by a rapid sequence of climate changes, a lack of healthy food and (fresh) water, and contact with foreign disease environments.[131] Given the physical circumstances of long-distance sea travel (and bearing in mind that it was only in the nineteenth century that the causes of and cures for most infectious diseases were discovered), it is surprising that the Dutch East Indiamen crews only began encountering severe health problems after 1690.

The homeward-bound voyages had fewer fatalities perhaps because the voyage was a bit shorter, especially the Batavia – Cape of Good Hope stretch, which took some three months. A death rate of 2 to 4 per cent was not unusual (Table T2.4). The homeward-bound ships carried considerably fewer people, whose physical constitution may have been toughened by their time spent in the tropics, or, perhaps, the weak had already passed away. No detailed data are available on the Cape of Good Hope – Republic part of the voyage, but it is presumed that mortality rates on this part of the voyage were also low.[132]

Table T2.4: Mortality rate Asia-Cape of Good Hope

Period	*Mortality Asia-Cape in %*	*Period*	*Mortality Asia-Cape in %*
1690-1700	2.1	1750-1760	3.3
1700-1710	2.1	1760-1770	3.4
1710-1720	1.9	1770-1780	4.8
1720-1730	2.7	1780-1790	6.2
1730-1740	3.7	1790-1795	8.6
1740-1750	4.2		

Dysentery

Besides the treatment of simple fractures and dislocations (for which they had been trained and employed), the surgeons also had to treat a number of diseases, that were often fatal. One of the most virulent was dysentery, which the English called 'bloody flux', the Swedish 'röda lopp', 'blodgang' by the Danish, and 'rode loop' by the Dutch. It is an infectious intestinal imflammation caused by *bacilli* or amoeba. Its symptoms are abdominal pain and straining, and diarrhoea with stools that often contain blood and mucus. Dysentery is commonly contracted when people are crowded together, especially in tropical climates, and only have access to the most primitive of sanitary facilities. The sanitary facilities on board were clean in themselves when under sail (they were located at the head of the vessel, continually sprayed by waves), but not so when the ship was lying in a quiet roadstead under a burning sun. Nor were they always used. Dysentery is transmitted by way of contaminated drinking water, and is highly contagious within 'closed' and crowded communities such as a ship's crew. A surgeon's curative intervention was limited to prescribing tea, rhubarb, and *tinctura catechu.* Individual isolation on a ship was almost impossible.[133]

The provision of drinking fluids on board was quite problematic. Beer was handed out daily, but after a couple of weeks it became undrinkable and the men were then dependent on the water, which was stored in casks. However, the quality of the water deteriorated quickly. In 1620, the Amsterdam Chamber's physician, Dr Aegidius Snoek, invented a method to distil fresh water from salt water. However, there was strong opposition to the introduction of the apparatus among the Chamber's directors, because of the amount of space needed for the wood it used to burn as fuel. It was improved in 1690 which made it more space-efficient and soon after, the Amsterdam directors approved its use. Between 1702 and 1707, these cauldrons were to be placed on every ship for the heating and evaporation of seawater. Scurvy grass was often added to the fresh water the apparatus produced. There were several drawbacks, however, which caused the experiment to fail: the cauldrons heightened the risk of fire on board; they gave off an unbearable amount of heat, especially in the tropics; the storage of the wood remained a problem; and the stoking of the cauldrons was arduous work.[134] The whole process was simply not efficient enough. On the ships which did install these distilling machines, however, dysentery was rare.

Scurvy

Another typical disease of long sea voyages was scurvy. John Woodall, Surgeon-General of the EIC, recorded the symptoms of scurvy in *The Surgeon's Mate* (1617) as follows: '... a general laziness and evil disposition of all the faculties and parts of the body .... Their eyes of a leady colour, or like dark violets. Great swelling in the face, legs, and over all the body ... swellings of the gums, rottenness of the same, with the issuing of much filthy blood and other stinking corruption thence ...'.

The cause of scurvy, a deficiency of Vitamin C, was not discovered until the twentieth century, but the knowledge that citrus fruit and fresh vegetables could prevent the disease had been fairly common among seafarers for generations. The problem was that it was presumed that fruit was only one of many remedies. Many attributed the value of citrus fruits to their astringency and recommended vinegar and bitters as suitable substitutes. The standard antiscorbutic at that time was elixir of vitriol, which consisted of oil of vitriol, spirits of wine, sugar, cinnamon, ginger and other spices. The prevailing general medical opinion was that the principal cause of mortality on board was the foul air, though, in the eyes of many ship's surgeons of the time, it was 'the laziness of the crew' that caused scurvy because their body fluids required the individual crew members to exercise, and in failing to do so, the fluids would begin to rot and cause scurvy.

Sources of vitamin C seldom figured in the diet provided on board. Oranges and lemons were not easy to preserve, and although the juice of lemons was taken along on Dutch East Indiamen, this was in small, inevitably insufficient quantities. Ship's surgeon Jan van Riebeeck, claiming the Cape of Good Hope on behalf of the Dutch Republic in 1652, built a victualling station there so that Company vessels could take on fresh supplies, and patients suffering from scurvy and other ailments could recover in a hospital on dry land. Company ships would eventually end up staying here as long as a month on the outward-bound journey.

It seems that especially on English ships, for reasons that remain unclear, scurvy was one of the most malignant of all maritime diseases in the eighteenth century.[135] During the naval expedition of 1740-1744 led by Commodore George Anson and commissioned to attack the Spaniards on the South American coasts, 1,300 of 1,995 crew-members on five ships apparently died of scurvy.[136] The news of the incredibly high mortality rate on Anson's voyage inspired the Scottish naval surgeon James Lind, to perform possibly the first controlled clinical science study of scurvy. Cruising the English Channel in 1747, while serving on the man-of-war the *Salisbury*, Lind used some of the scurvy-stricken sailors as his 'guinea-pigs'. Twelve men, with similar symptoms, were confined and given the same diet: gruel with sugar for breakfast, broth with mutton or pudding for dinner, barley and raisins, rice and currants for supper. He divided his subjects into six pairs, giving each a different prospective remedy every day for a fortnight. The antiscorbutics tested were a quart of hard cider; drops of elixir of vitriol; two spoonfuls of vinegar three times a day; half a pint of sea water; a paste of garlic, mustard seed, balsam of Peru, dried radish, and myrrh-resin; and to the lucky pair, two oranges and one lemon. The patients given a daily lemon improved after six days, at which time Lind ran out of fruit and they switched to elixir of vitriol. At the end of the two weeks they were the healthiest of the subjects, followed by the men who drank hard cider. There was no noticeable improvement in the others. He published his findings in a 400-page *Treatise of the Scurvy* in 1753, in which he unfortunately concluded that a damp climate and an unhappy disposition caused scurvy. Nevertheless, he recommended that fresh citrus fruit and lemon juice be included in the sailor's diet. Lind's recommendations were not adopted by the English Navy until 1795; thereafter, scurvy became a rare affliction.[137] The remedy was implemented so late because of the persistence of the old Galenical regimen, which prevailed over the evidence of empirical experience until 1795. Lind's study was translated into Dutch by the Middelburg physician P. de Wind in 1760.

Although scurvy was not as severe among the crews of the East India Companies as in the English Navy, they still suffered regularly from scurvy. The French East India Company was founded in 1664 by Jean-Baptiste Colbert and its activities in the seventeenth century remained limited to the sending of one or two vessels per year around the Cape of Good Hope, headed east. But after 1720, maritime traffic increased and in 1750, the French began sending approximately a dozen vessels a year to the Indian Ocean.[138] The French East Indiamen carried surgeons on a regular basis, because in 1681 Colbert had ordered that every merchantman with a crew of more than 20 should have a surgeon with a medical chest. This surgeon was, like his English and Dutch counterparts, fully examined before he was hired.[139] The French usually revictualled at the Isle of Bourbon, which they had colonized in the late seventeenth century, and later at the Ile de France, which was colonized in 1735. Mortality rates on the French East India merchantmen during the period 1725-1770 seem to have averaged nearly 14 per cent, though an accurate estimate of mortality is difficult to arrive at due to a lack of sources. In 1750 this rate began to decrease as the use of proper antiscorbutics in the form of lemon juice was greatly increased.[140]

In the Swedish East India Company, established in 1731, mortality rates from scurvy were incredibly low, with only two deaths from scurvy being recorded during the period 1733-1767.[141] This can only be explained by the fact that the Swedes had been using lemon juice on a regular basis since 1743, plus *sauerkraut*, which remained relatively fresh until a ship's arrival in Canton (China). In the Atlantic, the Swedes spent a week or more at St. Helena for revictualling, although, like the French, they preferred Ascension, as the English had already established themselves in St Helena and supplies and drinking water were free in Ascension. A significant difference between the Swedes and the English, French, and Dutch East Indiamen was that the Swedes did not regularly transport large numbers of troops destined for garrison duty in the colonies. This had beneficial repercussions on the living conditions on board; the men were simply less liable to fall victim to the infection of typhus and the crew's quarters were generally less cramped.[142] Hence, the number of men on board, between 100 and 150, was much lower than those carried by the Dutch and English vessels. Another contrast was that scurvy on the Swedish vessels occurred mainly on the return voyage, because the food stocks they had brought along for the entire voyage (a roundtrip could take anywhere from 16 to 30 months) had lost their freshness.[143] It is therefore surprising that the mortality rate in the Swedish company in the period 1731-1766 averaged as high as 12.2 per cent.[144] For this, no explanation has been found.

Beriberi

Beriberi, now known as vitamin B1 deficiency, is, like scurvy, a nutritional disorder caused by a deficiency of, in this case, vitamin B1 (thiamine). It usually struck when (white) rice was introduced into the diet on board on the homeward-bound voyage. In East Asian countries, where polished white rice is a dietary staple, beriberi has been known for more than a thousand years. Vitamin B1 is plentiful in many different foods but is lost during processing, particularly in the milling of grains. It was first described by the Company physician Dr J. Bontius (in 1631) and by Dr N. Tulp (in 1651). In the British Royal Navy, it was recognized as a disease distinct from scurvy in 1897.[145] No detailed data are available on beriberi related mortality rates on board, though a ship's surgeon did recognize it as early as 1665 when senior surgeon Gijsbert Heeck mentions it three times in his journal of this third voyage for the Company. He travelled, *inter alia*, to Siam (Thailand) on the aforementioned *Walvis* where he noted that the crew suffered from beriberi.[146] Later that year, Heeck replaced the Surgeon-General (*Hoofd der Chirurgie*), Petrus Andreas, in Batavia, who had retired to his estate outside Batavia because he was suffering from beriberi.[147] The last time Heeck mentions beriberi is when Portuguese prisoners on his ship (captured in Goa) suffered from it.[148]

Fevers and typhus

Fevers and typhus are often mentioned as the causes for the high mortality rates on board. Typhus is caused by the *Rickettsia* micro-organism and is transmitted from person to person via body lice. The bacteria grow in the cells of the louse and are excreted in the insect's faeces. Humans are commonly infected by scratching a louse bite, thus rubbing the infected faeces of the insect into an open wound. The disease is often associated with people crowded together in filthy conditions and occurs during times of war and famine, in prison camps and jails, on ships, and in concentration camps. Devastating epidemics of typhus occurred intermittently throughout Europe in the seventeenth, eighteenth and nineteenth centuries. It was this disease that particularly affected the crews of the Dutch East Indiamen in the eighteenth century. It has been suggested that it was mostly the soldiers from Germany who carried these infected body lice in their clothes, thereby spreading the disease on board, as a result of which the years 1690-1695 and 1770-1775 were disastrous in terms of health on board Company ships.[149]

Malaria

A possible cause of the extremely high mortality rates in Asia among Company employees was somewhat vaguely called the 'unhealthiness of Batavia', especially after 1733.[150] The historian Dr P.H. van der Brug in his admirable dissertation, elaborates on an old and almost forgotten idea, which he derives from M.L. van Breemen (physician in the public health service of Batavia) and A.L.J. Sunier (director of the Batavian fisheries) in 1917, that malaria was the main cause of the unhealthiness of Batavia, where it was prevalent as a result of the proximity of fishponds along the coast. Van der Brug traces this idea back to the beginning of the construction of these fishponds near Batavia from 1733, which became the breeding grounds of the mosquitoes that carry the *plasmodium falciparum* parasite, which causes the severest and most malign form of malaria.[151]

It is estimated that malaria was 'born' some 3,000 to 10,000 years ago.[152] Dr Frank Livingstone, an American anthropologist, in an article in *Science* in 1958, proposed that the emergence of malaria might be connected to the introduction of agriculture. He argued that sunlit pools, left in patches of forest cleared for farming were perfect breeding grounds for the mosquitoes that carry the disease. He also hypothesized that the increasing number of people who lived nearby the tilled fields provided an abundance of convenient hosts.[153]

The same thing occurred in the West Indies, where malaria produced fevers that were dangerous for Europeans, particularly after the rapid expansion of shipping in the eighteenth century, which brought new people who had no immunity to the disease to the region. More European soldiers in the Caribbean died of malaria than in actual fighting, with some estimating that as many as 90 per cent of all military fatalities were attributable to malaria and yellow fever.[154] In Batavia, malaria was endemic long before 1733 and the construction of the first fishponds, and was also, for that matter, prevalent in certain areas of the Dutch Republic, but that form of malaria was a benign one (*plasmodium vivax*). In contrast, the form of malaria which struck Batavia in 1733 was the much more aggressive, malignant variety. The ponds provided the perfect environment for the locally extant Anapheles type.

Van der Brug substantiates this idea by noting that Batavia's hospitals were always overcrowded after 1733, and the bulk of the patients consisted of new arrivals from the Republic who were not immune to malaria. Before 1733, the mortality rate of Company personnel (soldiers and sailors) hovered around 21 per cent, while after 1733 it rose to 39 per cent,[155] whereas the mortality rate among the (more or less) permanent inhabitants of Batavia did not rise after 1733. Consequently, the inhabitants must have been immune to the disease which struck Batavia in 1733, an immunity that was denied the newly arriving Company personnel. The victims were indeed mainly new arrivals from abroad, since mortality dropped significantly in 1782-1783 and after 1795 – two periods when the flow of new personnel from the Republic was temporarily stopped during several of the Republic's wars with England. Furthermore, Van der Brug states that the initial period after arrival in Asia was when Company employees were most at risk, and that disease and death struck especially around January and August, when the rainy seasons brought great increases in the *Anopheles* mosquito population, which, of course, greater increased the risk of malaria. After personnel became acclimated to their new environments, the risk of infection decreased,[156] which was also the case in the West Indies, where European soldiers who survived a year's service stood a three times greater chance of survival than newcomers.[157]

Other East India companies

Apart from the Dutch, English, French, and Swedish companies, there were three more European actors trading in Asia. One of these was the Danish East India Company, established in 1616, and reorganized in 1732 as the Danish Asiatic Company. Each winter, this Company would outfit one or two outward-bound and two homeward-bound ships.[158] As in the other companies, the most frequent cause of death on board was illness, but rarely scurvy.[159] The Ostend East India Company was founded in 1722. Only some twenty company vessels were sent out in the period until 1732, mainly to Canton and Bengal. In general, the mortality rates on the Ostend ships were low and averaged circa 8 per cent.[160] Lastly, the Prussian Company undertook six voyages to Canton in the period 1751 to 1756. The medical practice on its ships was organized along the same lines as those of the other East Indian companies. Two to three surgeons worked on every merchantman. Not much is known about the health on board these Prussian East Indiamen; it very much depended on the revictualling stops along the route. During this Company's first voyage, the first revictualling stop was in Java; as a result of this stop, mortality rates were quite high on the outward-bound journey. The second voyage took on fresh victuals on one of Cape Verde's islands, as a result of which no members of the crew died on the outward-bound journey.[161]

Some speculations on treatment and causes of diseases

We will conclude this chapter with a few ideas about the causes and the treatments of diseases that were developed by physicians and surgeons in the service of the East India Companies. In the first half of the sixteenth century, little was known about tropical diseases in Europe. The first known European to write on the subject was Garcia d'Orta of Portugal, the most distinguished European physician in the East in the sixteenth century. His *Coloquios dos simples, e drogas he cousas mediçinais da India ...*, or 'Colloquies on the drugs of India' , printed in Goa in 1563, was the earliest book on medicine in India, and the first European work on tropical medicine.[162] His example was followed by many others. The Dutch physician, Dr Jacobus de Bondt, or Bontius (1592-1631), left the Republic in 1627 for Asia and wrote his *De Medicina Indorum* in 1631, in which he described beriberi amongst other diseases.[163] Upon his arrival in Asia, Bontius immediately read the works of both Garcia d'Orta and Christophorus à Costa to acquaint himself with the plants and herbs of Asia.[164] Dr. Willem ten Rhijne (1649-1706), a school friend and fellow student of Joannes Groenevelt, who arrived in Asia in 1674, published his findings on Asiatic leprosy in *Verhandelingen van de Asiase melaatsheid* or 'Treatise on Asiatic Leprosy' (Amsterdam, 1687) as well as his earlier pioneering study on tea in Jacob Breyn's *Exoticarum plantarum centuria primai* in 1678, and his *De Acupunctura*, the first detailed treatise on acupuncture to appear in Western Europe. The Dutch ship's surgeon Wouter Schouten, born in 1649, wrote the first description of Madura foot (a chronic, progressive local infection caused by fungi or bacteria) in his *Aanmerkelijke Voyagie, gedaan door Wouter Schouten naar Oost-Indien* (1676) or 'Remarkable Voyage made by Wouter Schouten to the East Indies'. Perhaps the best known, is Rumphius (1627-1702), the 'Blind Seer' (*blinde ziener*) of Amboina. German in origin, Georg Everhard Rumph, or Rumphius, of Hanau in Hessen, first took employment with the Company in 1652. Though neither medically schooled nor indeed employed in a medical capacity by the Company, his twice lost thrice recovered lifework *Herbarii Rumphi*, a description of the plants of Amboina, is a work of exceptional quality, in which he also provided a preventive against beriberi: *katjang idjoe* which is still in use today.[165]

The recurrent eighteenth-century health crises led the ship's surgeons to speculate – sometimes rather wildly – on the causes of the diseases. The Dutch

Company surgeons Claas Lembroek (surgeon on the *Buis*) and Willem Blenke (surgeon on the *Noordwijkerhout*) were convinced that scurvy was caused by the distribution of inadequate water rations (*kleine rantsoenering*).[166] Although it loomed large, scurvy was not a major problem on the Company's vessels. The major problem was fevers, unknown fevers with an often fatal outcome. Anthonij Sas, surgeon's mate on the *Steenhoven*, in 1734, wrote that these fevers were the result of the salty, hard food which caused the blood to circulate too strongly as well as arousing an enormous thirst, which, in its turn, resulted in too much drinking with the consequences being constipation, pleurisy, and fevers. The changes in climate putatively led to changes in the balance of human body fluids, factors that surgeons also took into account.[167] Jacobus Cartier, chief surgeon on the *d'Jonge Wilhelm*, noted in 1732 that the fevers were caused by (i) the changing climate; (ii) the beer on board; (iii) the water on the island of St. Jago; (iv) the presence of soldiers who were not used to the sea; and (v) soldiers who had destroyed their physical health before boarding through indulging in 'Baggus or Venus'.[168] This opinion was shared by Jan Cats, surgeon on the *Barbestein*, and Jan Dirksen van der Baan, surgeon on the *Westcappel*.[169] Adriaan Vink (surgeon on the *Opperdoes*) and Jan Elleputte (surgeon on the *Zorgewijk*) added the long period spent in the doldrums to those already mentioned.[170] Most surgeons attributed these diseases to laziness and indolence.[171]

In 1736, the Company asked the advice of the most famous medical faculty at that time, that of Leiden University, where Professor Boerhaave held a chair.[172] The advice produced by Boerhaave's staff, however, was less than useful: it summarized the medical views of the time, underlining the significance of a surgeon's log. It noted that diseases in the northern seas were likely to be caused by cold and scorbutic ailments, while those in the tropics were probably caused by the heat, the rotten food, and the water on board.[173]

During the 1770s, discussions regarding the rising mortality rates on Company ships was no longer confined to just surgeons; it had become a national issue. Scientific societies awarded prizes for those who discovered cures for the diseases found on ships; but the solutions ended up being of little value.[174] In 1772, the esteemed city physician Dr S. de Monchy explained that fevers were caused by rotten fluids in crew members' bodies, an explanation that was widely accepted.[175]

Concluding remarks

Maritime medical treatment was laid down in the Oléron Laws. These introduced a new element in the care of crew members, namely that in cases of illness, the master/owner of the ship was responsible for their care while they were in the service of the ship. With the expansion of the Spanish and Portuguese overseas empires, ship's surgeons became more common on board. When the north-western

European countries began setting out on their own expeditions to the East and West, ship's surgeons sailed on board as a matter of course. Medical chests were taken along, which were stocked according to the prevailing medical ideas of the time: a mixture of old and new, of Galen and Paracelsus, although the purpose of every ingredient was to restore the physical balance of the patient by exorcising the evil fluids from the body through purging, expelling and sweating. The supplanting of Galen's ideas occurred gradually, and, at first, it was deemed unnecessary. Indeed, during the greater part of the seventeenth century, no severe health problems were encountered on any of the whaling, merchant, or East India ships. They were adequately served by a surgeon armed with his *materia chirurgica* who could provide his version of first aid. It was thereby forgotten that a voyage to Asia was longer and inevitably more prone to 'strange' illnesses and deficiency diseases, although these were only encountered on a major scale toward the end of the seventeenth century, when the Company had to enlist crew members who were less physically robust. However, the Company surgeons were well informed. The new diseases they encountered in Asia quickly became part of their medical knowledge. In fact, Gijsbert Heeck was quick to recognize beriberi, only some 20 years after the first description had been made by Bontius.

During the second half of the eighteenth century, (ship's) surgeon schools began to be established in Europe. In Denmark and in Spain, for instance, these schools issued licences that had the same amount of status as those obtained upon completion of a medical degree at an university. In Rotterdam in the Dutch Republic, a 'school' for ship's surgeons was founded under the leadership of Patijn and De Monchy, the city's physicians, although this school did not survive for long and its status never reached that of those in Denmark and Spain.

The Company's surgeons were never subjected to the 'degrading' task of their profession, that of shaving, which certainly was a common part of the job descriptions of their colleagues at the Republic' Admiralties, as well as of their English colleagues. The Company stood for professionalism, which was displayed in the special measures taken with regard to the sick on board. First, the ship's surgeon was fully examined before being employed; second, beginning in 1695, he had to maintain a medical log; third, provisions were made for the care of the sick on board in a separate sickbay, however small it might have been; fourth, instructions were issued to provide order and cleanliness on board; and, fifth, interest was shown in pharmacopoeia and in diet. These regulations, however, could not prevent the eighteenth century being disastrous for the Company in terms of health. The ship's surgeons' tasks no doubt became incredibly difficult during this period. They, along with their patients, often ended up drawing the short end of the straw. Did their employer take any notice of their plight?

3. The medical service of the Dutch East India Company

As seen in the previous chapter (table T2.3), hundreds of people boarded vessels that the Company outfitted every year for voyages to Asia. Men not only needed to sail the ships but also to populate and defend the trading settlements (*factorijen* or *comptoiren*) the Company had founded or conquered. Although every East Indiaman since 1652 had anchored halfway along the route to Asia at the Cape of Good Hope, the centre of activities in the tropics was Batavia, the city that Governor-General J.P. Coen had founded in 1619, which provided the Company with a seat of government and a shipping rendezvous. In Batavia, houses, schools, warehouses, churches, workshops, a prison and, indeed, hospitals were built. And, similar to other European trading companies, such as the EIC in India, the Company realized that military strength would guarantee its trading interests. Therefore, the Company's expansion into Asia and its concomitant transition from a trading company to a territorial power in the eighteenth century necessitated the transport of increasingly larger numbers of employees, especially soldiers. In the decade 1610-1620, 19,000 people sailed to Asia. This number increased to 40,000 in the decade 1650-1660, and climbed even higher, to 85,000 per decade a century later.

The administration of the trading settlements comprised much more than mere bookkeeping and commercial activities. The Company's initially tasks included the supervision of all the subjects who lived in its territories, the maintenance of relations with Asian rulers, the development and management of trade, and the maintenance of the military apparatus. The Company favoured the introduction of Dutch settlers into Batavia. Such had been the policy of the first Governors-General of the settlement who had also encouraged intra-Asian trade and the conquest of important trading posts. The Banda Islands were conquered in 1621, Malacca fell to the Company in 1641, and, as mentioned above, the settlement at Cape of Good Hope (Cape Town) was founded in 1652 by the Dutch surgeon Jan van Riebeeck. Amboina was taken in 1655, Ceylon became a Dutch possession in 1663, Makassar in 1667, Ternate in 1677, and, along the coast of India, in Formosa, and even in Japan, agreements with local rulers were concluded and trading posts were built, some of which were doomed to a brief existence. The Company became a major power with its own fleet, an army and territorial possessions far larger than those of its country of origin.

Provisions for the ill among Company personnel were made in each settlement, ranging from a room or two within the local fort to a fully staffed hospital. The Dutch personnel in the Asian settlements preferred their own kind of doctor and did not seek, as the Portuguese and British had done, the help of indigenous healers. Throughout the Company territory, hospitals were mainly staffed by ship's surgeons and stocked with medicines provided by the Amsterdam Chamber of the Company.[1] This concern for the health of its employees was a direct consequence of the primary aim of the Company as well as of its Calvinist background. One of the principles of the Protestant Reformation was that, within a Christian community, and the Company should be seen as such in the settlements, individuals (that is, Company personnel) had a right to charitable assistance (which went hand in hand with one's obligations to assist others).[2] Before the Reformation, charity was largely based on the donations provided by wealthy and pious (Catholic) Christians. Now, certainly in Asia, the charitable institutions were immediately incorporated within the framework of the Company; their incomes were structured and dependent upon tax revenues and levies as well as profits generated by the Company. Charity thus became channelled. Moreover, the primary aim of the Company was to make a profit. In order to achieve this, the Company's personnel were a most valuable natural tool in need of protection, in order for it to be able to maximize its productivity.[3]

By the end of the eighteenth century, the Company could boast of its own hospitals, great or small, in the settlements of Amboina, Banda, Batavia, Bengal, Cape of Good Hope, Ceylon, Cheribon, Coromandel, Houghly, Macassar, Malabar, Malacca, Padang, Palembang, Persia, Suratta, and Ternate. In terms of personnel and patient figuring in these hospitals, Batavia was the largest, followed by the Cape of Good Hope, and Colombo (Ceylon).

A rather fine-tuned organisation had to be established in order to make countless decisions regarding a wide variety of medical problems, which affected the staffing and stocking of the Company's vessels, the trading posts and the hospitals. It also had to deal with devastating illnesses which broke out on board and those which were endemic in the East. The care of its sick and ailing employees on the high seas or in Company settlements, which included the management of the hospitals overseas, was also the Company's responsibility. This chapter investigates the establishment and functioning of this organisation. How did it develop and function? Who made the medical decisions and formulated medical policy, if any? If it was specified, how effective was this policy? How were health-care problems dealt with, bearing in mind that most of the diseases that the medical staff had to treat were, at the time, still incurable?[4] The emphasis will be on Asia, where the Company set up its own hospitals, and, more particularly, on Batavia, because the administrative structure, contrary to the situation in the Republic itself, was centralised there at its Asian headquarters. We will start with a brief description of the medical arrangements made by the Company in Europe.

The Company and its medical staff in the Dutch Republic

Company management structure rested on two pillars, a decentralised structure of chambers in the Dutch Republic (Amsterdam, Middelburg, Enkhuizen, Hoorn, Rotterdam, and Delft) with their seventeen representatives gathered into a central management board (the Gentlemen XVII), and a centralised structure in Asia: the Council of the Indies in Batavia with its subordinate overseas factories, which extended from the Cape of Good Hope in South Africa to Deshima in Japan. If approved by the Gentlemen XVII, regulations laid down in the Chambers became policy for the entire Company. Amsterdam asserted a dominant influence in the decision-making process because its representatives constituted a near majority.

The Gentlemen XVII met thrice, and later twice annually for several weeks. At their meetings, they worked their way through a formal agenda, which was made known beforehand, so that the chambers could instruct their delegates accordingly. There was a broad range of subjects as well as some trivia that was covered during these meetings. The items discussed varied from the kind of goods to be purchased in Asia, increasing profits, the number of troops to be shipped out, to the smaller issues such as the drunkenness of one staff member and a request by someone to have his wife and children accompany him to Asia. They also discussed the issue of the provision of necessary medicines on board and in Asia. Important time-consuming items were studied in advance of the board meeting by smaller sub-committees, which drew up draft resolutions that were generally accepted. These subcommittees consisted of members drawn from each chamber, so that the chambers were all fully informed and involved. Once again, Amsterdam had the largest numbers of delegates, and it was usually involved in the preparation of draft resolutions well in advance of the meetings. The minutes of the meetings clearly reveal that the topics that were discussed – although not necessarily decided upon immediately – were often drawn up by the Amsterdam Chamber. As a consequence, the directors of the Amsterdam Chamber exerted a dominant influence on the Company's decision-making processes in the Republic.

Like the other chambers, Amsterdam had its own working committees. Subjects relating to medical care and its primary dispensers were delegated to the *Heeren van het Pakhuis* ('Gentlemen of the Warehouse') during the first 150-year period of the Company's existence. For unknown reasons, after 1750, they were usually referred to as the *Heeren van de Commercie* ('Gentlemen of Commerce'). These committees supervised, in both Amsterdam and in Zeeland, a medical staff, consisting of a physician, a surgeon-examiner, and, in Amsterdam, a pharmacist. The medical staff of the Amsterdam Chamber found quarters in the East India House, and the pharmacy was located here as well. It was the task of the medical staff in Amsterdam and Zeeland, as well as of their supervising committees, to interview the ship's surgeons before they were hired. Each chamber had the authority to determine whether or not to employ a medical staff for its employees.

If not, as was the case in the smaller offices in Enkhuizen, Hoorn, Rotterdam and Delft, the applicant for the post of ship's surgeon, if unknown to the chamber, had to provide references confirming his medical credentials and was also examined on his professional expertise by members of the Chamber's board and a local physician or surgeon. An additional surgical sea examination (*Zeeproef*) could be demanded as a minimum requirement before a ship's surgeon was actually hired. The smaller chambers depended on local pharmacies for the provisions necessary for their medical chests.

The Amsterdam Chamber's physician was entrusted with the following tasks according to his job descriptions in 1669 and 1708: (i) checking the pharmacist's bills and counter-signing these with the pharmacist for payment; (ii) checking deliveries to the pharmacy; (iii) testing the knowledge and skills of surgeons applying for jobs on board and overseas in Asia; (iv) examining the medical chests of hired surgeons; (v) examining sick employees in Amsterdam; and (vi) reporting on patients who had become unfit to work during their service with the Company (this was necessary because the Company paid permanent disability allowances based on physician's reports).[5] There was usually enough time left for him to combine these tasks with other pursuits, such as a private practice or a prominent position at the university. Dr Joan de Vrij, for instance, physician of the Amsterdam Chamber in 1669, also acted as burgomaster of Gouda, some 60 kilometres from Amsterdam, which was, at the time, not exactly next door.[6] The physician drew an annual stipend of 500 Dutch guilders from the Company, a sum which did not increase throughout the course of the Company's existence.

During the Company's early years, the Amsterdam physician sought local advice about medicines from several barbers. At the time, the medical chests were provisioned for the entire voyage, both outward- and homeward-bound. However, after a pharmacy had been founded at the Amsterdam Chamber in June 1612, a pharmacist was employed.[7] As the Company began to move into Asia, the pharmacist's responsibilities increased by so much that he was allowed to hire an assistant to do the drying, pounding and preparation of medicines.[8] The pharmacist's tasks were many and varied. He had to be at the East India House from 8 a.m. till noon every day, but on busy days he worked there until the evening. Moreover, it was essential to his work to keep the furnace burning. Furthermore, he had to advise the *Heeren van het Pakhuis* on the pharmacy's needs and to await their instructions regarding how, where and from whom he could buy the ingredients necessary for his medicines, because he was not authorised to sell or buy anything himself. After purchasing the ingredients, he was responsible for checking the quality of these ingredients. He also had to allow the physician to check anything he had personally prepared. He was also required to submit any bills and orders to the physician for his signature. He was advised to buy as cheaply as possible and to inform his superiors (the *Heeren van het Pakhuis*) if he noticed anything suspicious. He was under strict orders to not accept gifts of any kind. He was expected to keep all of his medicines in the East India House and not at home. His most important job was to personally prepare all of the medicines needed in the Asian forts and trading posts. He also had to buy the drugs needed for Batavia, the Cape of Good Hope, and Ceylon. It was he who prepared the surgeons' medical chests according to the official *Pharmacopeia Amstelodamensis.* He was obliged to swear an oath of loyalty on the clauses containing these stipulations. Lastly, he was not allowed to run his own pharmacy in the city.[9] His duties increased so much that he had no time for a private practice. This is reflected in his income which increased steadily from an annual 300 guilders in 1615 to 1,200 guilders in 1780.

Table T3.1: Wages of the Amsterdam Chamber medical staff in Dutch guilders[10]

Year	*Pharmacist*	*Physician*	*Surgeon*	*Year*	*Pharmacist*	*Physician*	*Surgeon*
1615	300.00	<500.00	<200.00	1720	>800.00	500.00	>200.00
1630	400.00	<500.00	<200.00	1735	>800.00		>200.00
1645	500.00	500.00	200.00	1750	1000.00		>200.00
1660	600.00	500.00	200.00	1765	1000.00		>200.00
1675	600.00	500.00	200.00	1780	1200.00		>200.00
1690	>800.00	500.00	200.00	1795			>200.00
1705	>800.00	500.00	>200.00				

The obligations of the Amsterdam Chamber's surgeon-examiner (or, 'examiner of full surgeons and surgeon's mates') were also pretty detailed. In concert with the chamber's physician and in the presence of the members of the *Pakhuis* committee, he had to examine the surgeon candidates before they were employed to work on the ships and in the settlements. He was expected to check the ship's surgeons' medical chests. It was also his duty to examine employees who fell ill while in the service of the Company and to report on them to his *Pakhuis* committee superiors. He also had to be ready to advise them as well. Like the pharmacist, he was forbidden to accept any gifts, regardless of the circumstances. He was also forbidden to trade in products of Asia. He was prohibited from allowing the full, second (surgeon's mate or *ondermeester*) and third surgeons (*derde meester*) to purchase their instruments from anywhere else other than from the chamber's stock. Lastly, he had to swear an oath of allegiance to the Company.[11] Like the physician, the surgeon-examiner had other sources of income. Master surgeon H. Hartman, the chamber's surgeon-examiner during the period 1638-1658, received an annual income of 200 guilders from the Company and an additional 400 guilders a year for providing the same services simultaneously to the Amsterdam Admiralty.[12] Jan Coenderdingh, surgeon-examiner for the Amsterdam Chamber during the period 1680-1706, was also a City Surgeon (*chirurgicus civilis* or 'municipal officer of health') from 1660-1706.[13]

The chief tasks of the pharmacist, physician, and surgeon-examiner, in short, were characteristically those of provision, supervision, and examination. Furthermore, the physician and the surgeon-examiner provided a kind of 'after-care' for those employees who returned home as invalids as a result of injury. If an employee lost the use of an eye, hand, arm or leg in the course of his work and, after a careful examination, it was determined his claim was valid he would be entitled to receive a compensatory payment from his employer ranging from between 400 to 1,200 guilders.[14] In 1772, for instance, the committee *Heeren van de Commercie* received a request for financial support from five sailors who had been disabled during their employment to the Company. The sailors supported their request with documents provided by the captain of their ship, the ship's surgeon who had treated them, and Company officials at the Cape of Good Hope.[15] Having carefully examined the patients, the surgeon-examiner declared them incapacitated. The *Heeren van de Commercie* therefore advised that four of them were to be entitled to a sum in accordance with the gravity of their injuries, and that the fifth man should be given a job ashore.[16] Another example was that of Piet Pieterse, a sailor on board the *Leijden* in 1790, who became disabled as a result of injuries sustained in a storm. Dislodged by the heavy swell and force of the winds, while he was working on deck, the chests stowed on the deck of the ship shifted and pinned him down, seriously injuring his legs, which had not yet healed by the time he applied to the *Heeren van de Commercie* for financial assistance. The surgeon-examiner, however, did not think that his injuries would lead to permanent incapacitation. Therefore, he was sent to the *Gasthuis* in Amsterdam for treatment, which was paid for by his employer.[17]

The assessment of financial compensation for those who were definitely disabled in the Company's service, was decided upon as early as 1611. The Company, as mentioned earlier, never paid for injuries sustained in brawls or for the treatment of diseases resulting from sexual intercourse (*Bacchus* and *Venus*). Surgeon Justus Jenning Benraath, for instance, complained to the authorities at the Cape of Good Hope settlement that he had not been paid by the patients he had treated in the hospital for *morbus gallicus*. Benraath claimed that it was customary to pay the surgeon-in-charge a sum of ten rixdollars for each such patient. The Political Council of the Cape thereupon decided to pay him eight rixdollars, even though these patients were each charged ten rixdollars, which was taken out of their wages.[18]

The Company also took care of its employees when they were struck down by disease within the Republic. In November 1771, the Amsterdam Chamber received reports submitted by the commander on the island of Texel and Den Helder's city surgeon about the numbers of patients awaiting their departure on three Company vessels, namely the *Huis ter Meije*, the *Honkoop*, and the *Groenendaal*, all part of the autumn fleet. The *Heeren van de Commercie* of the Amsterdam Chamber decided more surgeons were needed there. Meanwhile, the Amsterdam Chamber's board sent a hulk from Amsterdam to Texel to serve as a hospital ship[19] and the *Heeren van de Commercie* asked the governors of West Friesland and the Noorderkwartier for permission to use De Schans fortress on Texel to accept their patients. By that time, the disease had spread to eight vessels and since most of the patients were crew members, part of the fleet was unable to set sail.[20] The commander at Texel blamed the crimps for delivering injured and undernourished troops. In April 1772, the Gentlemen XVII convened to discuss the partial failure of the departure of the fleet the previous autumn. They decided that those members of the crew who had been unable to work until they had fully recovered and subsequently remained behind to convalesce, were nevertheless entitled to receive their wages from the moment their ships had sailed. Moreover, the Company paid for their clothes and food provided during their illness. Some patients were admitted to the *St. Pieters Gasthuis* in Amsterdam, the costs of which were paid by the Company.[21]

The Company's medical policy

During the seventeenth century, the chambers made fairly arbitrary decisions regarding medical care, which were usually based on a few basic premises. Ship's surgeons were needed for the Company's vessels and in Asia. The skills of these surgeons had been examined locally in conformity with the decision of the local chamber. The Company ensured that medicines were taken on board in medical chests. It provided monetary compensation for employees injured while on the job, although every case had to be assessed before payment could be made. The Company employed a medical staff in the Amsterdam and Zeeland Chambers; when the smaller Chambers needed medical services, they farmed these out.

There does not seem to have been much discussion about long-term planning nor was there much attention paid to future developments. For instance, medical matters raised during Amsterdam Chamber meetings were primarily concerned with vacancies that needed to be filled. Only 10 of the 40 resolutions retrieved from the seventeenth century dealt with larger issues with long-term implications, such as the job descriptions for pharmacist, physician, and surgeon-examiner of the Chamber. Apparently, there seems to have been a consensus among the chambers regarding the salaries for ship's surgeons, the medicines that should be included in medical chests, the manner of treating ailing crew members, and on the instruments to be used. In short, since there were no major medical crises during the seventeenth century, there was no real need for any extraordinary measures or changes to existing structures, organisational mechanisms, rules, and general habits.

This complacency received a rude awakening during the period 1689 to 1695, when the mortality rates on board the outward-bound ships rose to 20 per cent, caused, in all probability, by typhus (also referred to as jail fever or ship fever).[22] This compelled the Gentlemen XVII to consult the Amsterdam physician, pharmacist, and surgeon-examiner and thereupon issue the *Ordre en Instructie* of 1695, which outlined the duties of the ship's surgeon in great detail. The *Ordre* basically stated, albeit wrongly in hindsight, that scurvy was the main disease on board and thus, more and better medicines to combat this illness were needed on board. The captains of the ships were required to ensure that their ships were swabbed regularly and that the ship's surgeons examined patients at least twice a day, and kept a 'journal' (log) of the patients' diseases. This important ordinance did not change structurally throughout the eighteenth century, even though equally high mortality rates were experienced during the period 1730-1780.[23] The eighteenth century was characterised by relatively 'healthy' interludes that alternated with periods ravaged by serious and lethal diseases, which sometimes broke out even before setting sail for the East.

The eighteenth century challenged the skills of the administrators and medical staff of the Company. The increasing numbers of people shipped from the Republic imposed an extraordinary strain on the Company's organisation. The insidiously rising mortality rates, the enormous waste of employees' lives on board and in the tropics, and the increasing reluctance of many an eighteenth-century Dutchman to work for the Company meant increased personnel shortages, which the Company resolved by recruiting foreigners, especially Germans. The Company directors complained that ship's surgeons were also difficult to recruit, with their dearth being increasingly felt after 1740.[24] The Gentlemen XVII, who had maintained a more or less passive role with respect to health care during the seventeenth century, were forced to assume a more active role after 1695.

One incentive used to attract more surgeons was to offer better employment conditions. The Gentlemen XVII discussed higher wages for the ship's surgeons or a larger allowance of goods that surgeons were permitted to bring home from Asia. In 1742, the directors offered a full surgeon a premium of 500 guilders for every return voyage, and in 1783, the ship's surgeons were even offered a premium of five guilders for every man they brought back to the Republic alive.[25] This might have seemed like an adequate solution but the Gentlemen XVII basically feared that offering more money would not be enough to deal with the scarcity of surgeons. Further steps were necessary and, by issuing new instructions, the directors sought to define the ship's surgeons' duties in a way that would allow them to deal with disease on board more effectively.[26] In 1751, it was decided by the Gentlemen XVII that every surgeon (and surgeon's mates and third surgeons) had to be examined before employment.[27] This decision applied to all of the Chambers.

The Chambers were unable to cope with the eighteenth-century health crises among their employees either on board or in Asia. The Amsterdam Chamber basically remained occupied with the filling of medical vacancies and revising the *pharmacopeia* up to the late 1760s. However, the issue of the quality of medicines provided by the Company remained a steady item on the agenda of Gentlemen XVII meetings from 1705 until the end of the century. As we saw in chapter 2, the *pharmacopeia* was sent to the leading medical expert at the time, Professor Herman Boerhaave, at the medical faculty of Leiden University, in 1736 with a request for comments and revisions at the behest of the Gentlemen XVII. Boerhaave's subsequent advice, however, did not lead to many changes in the Company's medical/surgical practice.[28] The historian C.R. Boxer even noted, perhaps a bit bizarrely, that Professor Boerhaave's advice actually hampered medical developments on board for more than a century.[29] The high mortality rates later in the eighteenth century attracted the attention of the entire Republic's scientific community, becoming national front page news. Scientific societies, as mentioned earlier, even offered prizes to those who discovered a cure for the prevailing diseases found on board.[30]

The considerable human losses sustained during voyages in the eighteenth century were matched by rising mortality rates in Batavia itself, and even on the vessels anchored off Texel, in the Meuse, and in Zeeland waiting to sail. Sometimes, even the Dutch population at home was affected. Virtually the entire staff of Middelburg's *Gasthuis* died as the result of the admission of 37 sailors from the *Woestduijn*, who were suffering from contagious, febrile diseases, at the end of January 1770. The *Gasthuis* assistant, Michael Bremer, died on 10 February, the servants Pieter Ernste and Johanna Cappellen on 16 February; the chief housekeeper Johanna van Hoeke on 18 February; the assistant Valentijn Kamelaar on 19 February; the assistant Frans Brusteijn on 5 March; the wife of the male housekeeper on 6 March; and the hospital's physician on 21 April, 1770![31]

In 1773, constructive, concerted action was taken by the Chambers of Amsterdam, Zeeland, Hoorn, and Delft. They sought to establish the true nature and cure of these devastating diseases.[32] The Amsterdam physician, Dr C.J. de Famars, sent a letter to the directors of the Amsterdam Chamber in July 1773, in which he stated that he, along with the Zeeland, Delft, and Hoorn Chambers, shared the common view that the problems were caused by overcrowding on the ships, the enfeebled condition of many of the crew and troops, and the general lack of cleanliness on board, which was further exacerbated by the long waits prior to the vessels' departure when the vessels lay windbound.[33] Dr De Famars suggested possible solutions, such as becoming more selective in their hiring practises. The *Heeren van de Commercie* of the Zeeland chamber objected, arguing that they had no choice with respect to the physical condition and professional quality of its crews and troops. The practice was 'to take what you can get' because the Company needed more and more people in Asia. It was clearly impossible to refuse any one person willing to work for the Company. The Zeeland Chamber, indeed, had more problems than the other chambers in filling vacancies on its vessels.

Although, in 1774, the Gentlemen XVII ordered that overcrowding on board was to be avoided, the chambers could not actually enforce this.[34] Another suggestion was made by Dr De Famars, who recommended that the sick be separated from the healthy, but this was considered too expensive, as was his suggestion that the crew be deloused and given new clothes immediately prior to embarking. Patently, the long waits could not be avoided because they were beholden to weather conditions and the locations of the harbours; vessels had to wait for the necessary north-easterly winds to set sail.

Hospital ships

After 1771, it became more customary to send the Amsterdam hulk to the Nieuwe Diep (between Texel and Den Helder) each year, to serve as a hospital ship to isolate the sick from the healthy. It was not only Amsterdam's ships, but also those from the Hoorn and Enkhuizen Chambers, which used the hulk as such, since Texel was the point of departure for the ships of these Chambers too. The Admiralties also found the Amsterdam hulk quite convenient, and began using this hulk as a hospital ship in 1779.[35] Zeeland made its own arrangements for the sick, where, in 1787, the Chamber employed no less than four surgeons to care for employees who had fallen ill on board before setting sail.[36] Twelve years earlier, the Zeeland Chamber had asked the Gentlemen XVII for financial help to construct a special hospital in the Rammekens fort, where these patients could be adequately cared for. However, the Gentlemen XVII – disappointingly – were unwilling to give them the financial support they needed.[37] In response, the Zeeland Chamber bought an old merchant ship, the *Suzanna Helena*, that from then on served as a hospital ship, that lay anchored in Flushing.[38] The use of these hospital ships was a common occurrence in Europe during this period, and it inspired an anonymous poet to pen the following impromptu verse upon hearing a sentinel calling: 'All's Well' on a hospital ship:

In yonder ship 'tis strange to tell
Each night they call out 'All is Well',
Though sick and sad doth there abound,
Some with consumption, some with wound,
And other evils far too long
Thus to describe in transient song
Then why do they bawl with ruffian-note
And strain the lungs and stretch the throat
When all's not well, we clearly know?
If well above, they're sick below.[39]

In short, the Company tried to alleviate some of the health problems at home by passing the ill on to the *gasthuizen*, by composing a small first aid kit, and requiring that surgeon's keep a log on their ships (in 1695), by providing a hospital ship off Texel and one near Rammekens, by using one small building as a hospital on Texel, and by updating the *pharmacopeia*. The home-based staff included two physicians (in Amsterdam and Zeeland), two to five full surgeons, one pharmacist with his assistants, and – upon occasion – a few extra local surgeons. This medical staff did not have any decision-making powers at the level of the central board, but acted as an executive, advisory and examining body. The recommendations they made were usually not well received, particularly if money was involved. The ultimate decisions were made by the higher ups, the Gentlemen XVII, who, in the eighteenth century began seeking medical advice elsewhere, such as at the University of Leiden. Unlike the situation overseas, the home-based staff did not have Company-owned hospitals at its disposal, but had to farm out the patients to reception-centres such as the hulk or the Zeeland *Suzanna Helena* or to local *gasthuizen*. The organisation was largely autonomous, in the sense that decisions, at first, were left up entirely to the chambers themselves. However, over time and because of the issues at stake, decisions became increasingly complex and difficult, and the Gentlemen XVII were forced to become more involved.

Medical provisions in Asia: A 'modern' institution?

It was quite a different matter in Asia. There, the Company built, owned, and administered its own hospitals. The *Hoge Regering* ('High Government'), with its seat in Batavia, consisted of the Governor-General and the Council of the Indies (*Raad van Indië*). It ruled over all of the possessions, trading settlements, and the ships, as well as exercising jurisdiction over the Company personnel. The High Government was only responsible to the Gentlemen XVII. The Indies Council consisted of the Governor-General, who served as chairman, and six members, each of whom had a specific judicial, military, commercial, or medical function.[40]

The Council had already decided as early as 1632 that one of its members should be responsible for the medical chests and all matters related to medicines and surgery in Asia.[41] Although a simple guild structure was set up in both Batavia and in Colombo, it had little autonomy, while the overseas surgeons were not part of an 'Asian' surgical guild.[42]

Historian R. Raben's statement that many Europeans in Asia preferred consulting a Malay or Indian Muslim doctor proves rather thin given his unique example of Isaac Jansz, a Batavian Mardijker (Asian Christian) who, indeed, did see an Asian doctor when he became severely ill.[43] Only those Europeans who had actually settled in the Indies – like the English and Portuguese in India – to some extent adopted to the Asian way of life and the culture of the land. However, when Company employees fell ill overseas, they depended on the Company's medical facilities. In Asia, caring for the sick was a dire necessity: as the majority of the Company's employees were comprised of a floating population, arriving or leaving with the fleets, the sailors and troops had neither permanent housing nor kith and kin to turn to in times of illness and therefore had to rely on the Company for help. And even if they did have friends living in the Dutch settlements in Asia willing to offer hospitality, the Company did not stimulate this; indeed, after careful consideration, it actually forbade its servants to seek such succour.[44] The Company suspected its employees of faking illness during their stay in Asia – they were generally considered a lazy bunch, *luie gasten* – and, as it continued to pay at least half the salary of any employees who were indisposed, the Company preferred to spend its money building a hospital where an employee's behaviour could at least be monitored and his disease, hopefully, quickly cured.

This was not an uncommon argument. As in Europe, a certain element of 'social control' of the poor probably served as a (perhaps unconscious) factor that underlies the establishment of the pre-modern hospital.[45] Professor Roy Porter elaborated on this theme when he borrowed French historian Braudel's concept of the 'gift-relationship':[46]which states that 'he who gives dominates', to describe the pre-modern hospitals as nothing more than paternalism institutionalised.[47] Among historians, it has more or less been agreed upon that hospitals served the social interests of those who founded and supported them, be this the church or the state, lay or medical.[48] Spain, for instance, established naval hospitals both at home and in Cuba, while the Order de San Juan de Dios served the Spanish mariners in hospitals in Central and South America and in the Philippines.[49] Cortes built the first hospital for the Indian and Spanish poor in Mexico City in 1521, and, by the end of the seventeenth century, there were over 150 hospitals in New Spain. Pertinently, these hospitals were church-run and seen as a means of converting Indians to Christianity.[50] The English East India Company built hospitals at its settlements as this effectively prevented – as it was said – the sick from 'indulgence in their favourite vice, debauchery'.[51] As such, the founding of the Asian hospitals was a mixture of need and social control. However, from the very outset, the Company hospitals in Asia, though partly inspired by a traditional and suspicious view of their patients, were mainly founded to heal the sick – a quantum leap forward compared to conditions found in Europe. After all, in Europe it was only the late eighteenth century that saw the old 'hospital' radically transformed into the (modern concept of the) *Krankenhaus* institution or infirmary.[52] Moreover, the administration of the Asian hospitals was controlled by the Company, in itself a sign of institutional progress and the rationalisation of management.

The hospitals in Asia were built to cure the ill and the injured. They were called hospitals instead of *Gasthuizen* right from the start and were set up and financed by the Company, not by wealthy patrons, and certainly not by the church. They served the Company's needs and were 'professional', rather than charitable, institutions (with the possible exception of some religious institutions in the larger settlements). Patients always paid for their admission to the hospital, with at least half, sometimes with their complete month's salary.

The head of surgery

It was Jan Pieterszn. Coen, one of the first Governors-General of the Indies, who ordered the construction of a new stronghold in Batavia in 1619. This Castle (*Kasteel*) would serve as his headquarters and was located alongside the existing small wooden fortress at Jacatra. All of the Company's employees were housed in this Castle, with a chief surgeon and a physician among them. The first surgeon we know of was Pellegrom Pietersz, then still called 'barber', a term that would become obsolete in Batavia after 1630 when referring to a surgeon. Although Pellegrom Pietersz may have been called upon to shave the Company's employees, his main duties concerned the patients, mainly soldiers and sailors from the newly arrived ships and those arriving from other settlements who, in the absence of local medical care, had been shipped to Batavia.[53] Pellegrom occasionally used the old fortress as a hospital to house the ill and the injured. He remarked that his patients frequently suffered from ulcers.[54] Permanently disabled patients ('incurables') were usually sent back home, a practice that prevailed throughout the Company's existence.

As already mentioned in the previous chapter, to supervise the overseas surgeons and to set up a health-care organisation, the Gentlemen XVII sent the physician Jacob de Bondt (Leiden 1592 – Batavia 1631), or, as he is usually called, Dr Bontius, to Batavia in 1627 as physician, chemist, and supervisor of all (if still few) of the Company's medical personnel in Asia, and, as such, he became (the first) Head of Surgery in Asia.[55] Prior to 1627, the Company's overseas surgeons were not answerable to anyone else for their professional performance. The ship's surgeons were formally under the command of the ship's captain. Like every other Company employee, they swore an oath of obedience to the Company upon their embarkation. In the absence of surgical knowledge and a medical bureaucracy in Asia, neither the settlements' governors nor the ship's captains were able to sufficiently supervise or correct the surgeons professionally, leaving them a free hand with respect to their methods of treatments they chose to follow. Until the Company's first General Instruction (*Artikelbrief*) was formally drawn up in 1634 for all of its employees nothing specific was stipulated regarding the duties of the ship's surgeons, on whose shoulders rested the complete medical care in Asia, and, until 1695, there were but few specific regulations that governed the activities of the captain and the surgeon on board with respect to those who fell ill on the vessels.

Cogently, as the Company's trading territory expanded into largely unknown Asian countries in which the Company's employees might possibly succumb to any one of many tropical diseases, the ship's surgeons, who were forbidden to practise internal medicine in the Republic, were called upon to treat diseases as if they were indeed physicians. Moreover, these ship's surgeons were not united in a guild. As we saw in the previous chapter, guilds in the Dutch Republic (and in Europe) served as a quality control organisation that ensured that the art or trade (i.e., services provided) met certain standards. They also offered schooling and examinations to further ensure their standards. The only institution that could ensure the quality of the surgeons in Asia was the Company itself. As we will see, the Company did offer a system of schooling, examinations and promotion, and no other authority was valid.[56] Bontius' arrival marked the onset of a structured medical health service system overseas.

Bontius, who had a strong personal interest in tropical medicine[57], advised the Council of the Indies on medical matters and headed the surgeon's and chemist's shop in the Castle as well as overseeing the medical services in Asia; he decided which ship's surgeons were posted on which vessel or to which settlement. After Bontius died it proved increasingly difficult to find physicians willing to work for the Company in Asia and thus the Batavia Castle's senior surgeon often assumed the position of Head of Surgery. This Head of Surgery has ever since then supervised the entire Asian medical services. And, as medicines began being shipped from the Republic to Batavia and stored in a special room ('the Dispensary'), Batavia, already the administration and trading centre of the Company, became the hub of its medical-care system in Asia, from where directives, medicines, instruments, and surgeons were sent to the other settlements.

The City Hospital of Batavia (*Binnenhospitaal*)

During Batavia's first turbulent years, the city was repeatedly attacked and besieged by the English, the Bantamese and the Javanese. According to the 1622 Resolution of the Council, the old fort of Jacatra served as a hospital, where Hendrik Goch served as its chief surgeon.[58] The bamboo fort was destroyed and rebuilt several times until it was finally totally reconstructed in brick in 1639-40. During numerous battles and during the reconstruction process, an unused ship in the roadstead was used as a hospital ship, or patients were sometimes evacuated to the small island of Onrust, three miles north of Batavia.[59]

The Council of the Indies, in its administration of the hospital, duplicated the model used back home, where *Gasthuizen* were managed by a board of *regenten* (trustees and/or wardens). In Asia, two types of *regent* existed, namely the *buitenregent* (trustee), who was responsible for the general management and bookkeeping, but worked and lived outside the institution, and the *binnenregent* (warden or superintendent), who worked and lived at the institution and who was responsible for the daily management and administration, which included the administration of patients, the keeping of the hospital's daily journal (with a copy to the Castle in order to halve or suspend the patient's wages), the regulation of the food and beverages purchased and consumed, and to supervise the personnel. This warden was generally not qualified in any medical or surgical capacity. Though the German Hendrik Goch of Düsseldorf was employed as the hospital's senior surgeon in 1622, it was Adriaan Bouwens (born in Delft), a 'layman', who acted as the hospital's warden and manager. Bouwens' successors were Van de Voorde, Pieter Louwers, Johannes Roemers, and, in 1638, Hendrik Martijn, none of them surgeons and none of them competent. Even then, the Council of the Indies closely monitored the development of the hospital. A member of this Council (the *fiscaal* Abraham Webrigh, neither a surgeon nor a physician) drafted the first hospital rules in 1638, which consisted mainly of disciplinary measures to counter drunkenness and fighting among the patients, who, apparently, were (seen as) an unruly crowd. As such, these regulations serve a traditional document in which correct behaviour was deemed more important than recovery from illness.

The 1638 instruction mentions the presence of a warden (then called *schafmeester*, or foodmaster), and a *huisvader* ('housefather') with overseers (*binnenvaders*) to assist the warden.[60] The main duty of Hendrik Martijn (the warden) was the provision of food for the patients, as it had been for his predecessors. During this early period, the authority of the hospital wardens rarely extended beyond control of the domestic staff and the purchase of food and other household provisions. In all probability, they were not selected for their presumed technical competence. The overseers' duties consisted of domestic chores and preventing fights among the patients. Clinical care, as we know it today, was not provided.[61]

In 1639-40, a new brick hospital was constructed, within Batavia's city walls. In time, it became known as the *Binnenhospitaal* or City Hospital. On this occasion, a new committee of trustees was set up to manage the Hospital, as the Council of the Indies was more concerned about the number of patients arriving from the Republic. This committee consisted of a member of the Council of the Indies (Cornelis Witsen), a captain (Johannes Landuis), and the first surgeon of the Castle, Jan Hille (the Head of Surgery and appointed warden of the hospital). Together, they drew up the 1642 regulations for the hospital, which clearly betrays Jan Hille's influence: it strikes a different, more medical, tone although it still mentions numerous disciplinary measures regarding unruly patients. However, the committee was now required to make the weekly rounds, accompanying the hospital's warden and surgeons to check whether the needs of the patients were being met.[62] The 1642 instruction also insisted that all sick Company soldiers, sailors, and petty officers should go to this hospital exclusively for treatment in case of illness.[63] The trustees and warden continued to meet regularly for the next 150 years or so, and because both a member of the Council of the Indies and a surgeon were included, a strong administrative and medical/surgical input was guaranteed, which allowed decisions to be made and acted upon quickly.

Keeping pace with the growth of Batavia and the Company trade for the remainder of the seventeenth century, this hospital expanded not only in physical size but also in terms of numbers of employees and patients. Ship's surgeons, newly arrived from the Republic, were stationed there, to assist the warden (who now was either a senior surgeon or a physician) and to improve their knowledge and gain some practical experience. The ship's surgeon, Nicolaas de Graaff made five voyages to Asia – in 1639, 1644, 1668, 1676 and in 1683 – and at one time was posted at the Castle surgeon's shop to assist the chief surgeon, Jan van Rostok. De Graaf witnessed the growth of the City Hospital as it was transformed into an institution with some 200 to 300 patients in its care. The City Hospital was further expanded at the end of the seventeenth century, when it was enclosed by high walls and enlarged to include extra wards that could accommodate as many as 600 patients.[64] The hospital was by then divided into separate wards: the *Middenhuis* ('Middle House') was reserved for the most dangerously ill; the *Grote Huis* ('Big House') was allocated for emergency injuries, operations, and its ambulant (not bed-ridden) patients. There was a special beriberi ward that also accommodated those who were permanently incapacitated, and included a laboratory or 'distillery'. And lastly, there was a building reserved for patients with chronic ulcerations, which continued to be a common, although nasty disease. By 1700, Batavia's hospital had been transformed into a general hospital with specialised wards.

The medical personnel eventually included a physician, two full surgeons (including the warden) and four surgeon's mates (*ondermeesters*), a pharmacist, a dresser (*verbandmeester*), and an 'operator' (*operateur*). This medical staff was supplemented by a parson (*ziekentrooster*), a bookkeeper, a treasurer, several overseers (*ziekenvaders*) and attendants (*oppassers*), and a number of servants and slaves (who had to clean and assist the patients).[65] One of the tasks of the physician, or, in his absence, of the hospital's senior surgeon, was to visit the Company vessels (on Sunday and Wednesday) lying in the roadstead to see if there were any sick people on these vessels. If there were, the hospital boat would pick these patients up.[66] The dresser was an assistant to the full surgeons at the patient's bedside and in the operating theatre. He performed minor surgical procedures and changed dressings in the surgical wards. Moreover, the dresser visited the medical wards at the request of the physician and/or full surgeons in order to perform bloodletting and other similar minor operations.[67] Some 60 years later, in circa 1760, these special wards of the Hospital included not only a laboratory, but also a *Salvatiekamer* (casualty department), a *Middenhuis* ('wards'), a *Verband* ('dressing-station'), a *Nieuw Middelhuis* ('new wards'), and a *Persihuis* ('dysentery ward').[68]

The surgeons in Batavia

According to Pieter van Dam, advocate-general to the Company, who wrote a history of the Company at the end of the seventeenth century, the following surgeons were at work in Batavia around 1700:[69]

Table T3.2: Number of Company surgeons in Batavia around 1700

*Binnen*hospitaal	2 first ship's surgeons, 1 physician, 4 surgeon's mates; 1 dresser	*Rotterdam Gate*	1 first ship's surgeon and 1 surgeon's mate
Roadstead	1 first ship's surgeon: the *visitateur ter rheede*	*East Outer Gates*	1 first ship's surgeon and 3 surgeon's mates
Ambachts quarter (also New Gate)	1 first ship's surgeon; 3 surgeon's mates	*West Outer Gates*	1 first ship's surgeon and 3 surgeon's mates
Isle of Onrust	1 first ship's surgeon and 3 surgeon's mates	*Kruitmolen* (Gunpowder works)	1 surgeon
Castle	1 first ship's surgeon, 1 chemist, 1 physician, 1 laboratory assistant, 6 surgeon's mates, 1 druggist	*Bacassin*	1 surgeon's mate
Wharf and Vierkant	1 first ship's surgeon, 2 surgeon's mates	*Tanjonpoura*	1 surgeon
Diest and Utrecht gate	1 first ship's surgeon, 1 surgeon's mate	*Cornelis buitenwacht* (outer guards)	1 first ship's surgeon and 1 surgeon's mate
Tangerang and Sampura	1 first ship's surgeon and 1 surgeon's mate	*Pantichiallangs*	1 surgeon's mate
Orphanage	1 surgeon	*Batavia's poor*	1 City Surgeon

There were some 50-odd surgeons employed by the Company in and around Batavia. They were stationed at the various gates and districts of the city, in the *Binnenhospitaal*, at the wharf and at the gunpowder mill (*Kruitmolen*), to care for the Company's servants working there. At the Castle, besides the hospital, there was also a second medical centre where one chief surgeon worked in his surgeon's shop, assisted by six surgeon's mates, one clerk, one chemist and one laboratory assistant (*laborant*).[70]

By 1700, some 70,000 people were living in and around Batavia, of whom only 6,000 were European. Those who arrived in Batavia found a bustling city, home to many different population groups of which the Chinese and the *Mardijkers* (a free Christian group of Asian/Portuguese descent) were the major ones. Other inhabitants of Batavia included Amboinese, Balinese, Bengalis, Buginese, Ceylonese, Maccassarese, Malays, Timorese, and the Europeans (the Company's employees and free-settled ex-employees: *burghers*).[71] By the end of the eighteenth century, Batavia and its immediate surroundings (the *kampongs*) totalled more than 150,000 inhabitants, of whom less than 6,000 were European, many of them soldiers.[72]

Although, demographically speaking, Batavia was a Chinese city, the Company tried to create a European society in an Asian setting. Many Dutch institutions were represented in which a member's significance was measured by his rank in the Company's hierarchy. A grammar school was established to educate the European children, and a Dutch Reformed and a Lutheran church were founded for the spiritual guidance of Company employees. The town also had an orphanage and a poorhouse. The administrative bodies that governed these institutions were copies of those found in the cities of the Republic such as a board of aldermen, wardens for the orphanage, while the bailiff and his men maintained public order.[73] The rules of rank and status were closely observed and grew all the more important as Batavian society became more bureaucratic.[74] All Company officials were subordinate to the hierarchy in Batavia. Principal among the employees of the factories (*factorijen*, i.e. settlements) were the merchants.[75] The word 'merchant' referred not only to a professional occupation, but it managed to accrue so much importance that it became its own social rank. Consequently, it was essential here to acquire the rank of 'merchant' as soon as possible, as most employees, such as surgeons, carpenters, military personnel, cooks, and the like did not have any rank at all.

Surgeons did not enjoy *a priori* the rank of merchant, though some medical/surgical functions did acquire this blissful status in the course of time. However, the Batavian surgeons did climb socially so that by 1752, as a result of the nature and composition of the chief surgeon's work at the City Hospital, it had generally been recognised that the division in status and profession between physician and surgeon could no longer be maintained. The surgeons practised as physicians, treating internal diseases, the logical solution to the great number of patients and the scarcity of available physicians. By 1683, it was already customary to call the full surgeon a 'practitioner' (*praktizijn*) or doctor, and the superintendent/warden of the *Binnenhospitaal* was officially indeed called a *praktizijn*.[76] This status became officially recognised in 1752, when the Indies Council elevated full surgeons in Batavia's City Hospital to *praktizijn*, with the stipulation that because they were also treating *interna*, they no longer wanted to be referred to as 'surgeon', which sounded inferior and was paid less.[77]

At Batavia Castle

When the Company fleet arrived in Batavia, its ship's surgeons were met by the Castle's chief surgeon (in his capacity as *visitateur ter rheede*, or, literally, 'examiner of the roadstead'), to whom they had to account for the treatment of their patients and the use of medicines during the voyage. The chief surgeon examined their logs and arranged transport to the hospital for patients on board. In Batavia Castle, decisions were made where the ship's surgeons would be stationed next: in Batavia hospital, at one of the other settlements, on an intra-Asian ship, or on a homeward-bound vessel. It was at the Castle where the ship's surgeons were provided with medicines-chests and instruments.[78]

As most physicians were unwilling to work for the Company in Asia plus the Company's custom to promoting these physicians to higher, purely administrative functions, the Castle's chief surgeon responsibilities increased and were upgraded and he was often appointed as the Head of Surgery. His surgeon's shop became an out-patient clinic (including first aid) for Castle employees and inhabitants. He examined junior surgeons seeking promotion, and he became responsible for the preparation, storage, and distribution of medicines throughout Asia. But as the growth of trade and a growing population with ever more garrisons, trading posts, and hospitals meant an increased demand for medicine, the chief surgeon's workload gradually assumed alarming proportions.

Medicines in Batavia

Chemical medicines were made in the laboratory, at least after 1665. Pellegrom Pietersz, the chief surgeon of the Castle, was already demanding the urgent attention of the Amsterdam Chamber as early as 1620, as he thought that the medical chests of the ship's surgeons and of the Castle were badly stocked.[79] At the time, the medical chests used to be filled all at once for both the outward- and homeward-bound voyages. With a central port of call, however, the surgeons refilled their chests in Batavia, before returning to the Republic or travelling onwards, and Batavia Castle became the storehouse and dispensary for both medicines and instruments.[80] Cogently, this chemist's shop also provided medicines for all of the factories and settlements throughout Asia. These outer settlements placed monthly orders, which were collected in Batavia and sent home. The Amsterdam Chamber was responsible for ensuring that these orders were followed up and delivered to Batavia, from where they were distributed to their allocated destinations.

After chief surgeon Pieter van Berthem's demise in 1667, the Council of the Indies reorganised the provision of medicines and decided to set up a pharmaceutical centre for Batavia. The Council contracted the pharmacist H. Cruijs to manage a semi-privatised Hospital Pharmacy, stocked with medicines and/or raw ingredients bought from the Castle.[81] Cruijs sold his medicines to the hospital but also to the (free) population of Batavia and, moreover, to the chemist shop in the Castle. He had to swear a special oath, as did the pharmacists in the Republic, in which he and his assistant guaranteed the quality of their products, in contrast to the lab assistants and chemists working in the Castle who swore only the Company's standard employee oath of allegiance.[82]

In 1667, the dispensary in the Hospital began being called the 'City Apothecary' (*Stads Apotheek*) and the chemist's shop in the Castle, the 'Dispensary' (*Medicinale Winkel*). The *Medicinale Winkel* was placed under the supervision of the chief merchants of the Castle, one of whom was the Director-General of the Council of the Indies, as the raw medicinal materials stored in the Castle were now part of the business.[83] Although an interest in local medicines emerged, initially among the surgeons and physicians and later also among the higher administrative echelons of the Company, their use was (at first) not promoted; during the seventeenth century, Dutch-made medicines were used to more or less general satisfaction.

In 1667, Andreas Cleijer was appointed chief of the Dispensary in the Castle to succeed Pieter van Berthem. Cleijer re-established Bontius's job description, which combined the three most important medical jobs, which also included Castle physician and Head of Surgery. Moreover, in 1676, he also added managing the City Apothecary to his already impressive number of functions. Even though a committee audited both the City Apothecary and the Dispensary semi-annually, Cleijer managed to accrue a debt of 30,000 guilders before he left for Japan in 1682. The Council of the Indies in an ordinance in 1682, thus decided to separate the supervision of the Castle Dispensary from the Castle's physician in order to reassert its influence over its administrators. This ordinance effectively transferred the function of Dispensary manager to the chief surgeon.[84] The City Apothecary remained contracted out to prevent a repeat of Cleijer's practices. [85]

By 1729, the Castle's chief surgeon still served as the manager of the Dispensary, but was now also appointed the position of 'First Administrator of the Dispensary' or Surgeon-General when he combined this function with serving as Head of Surgery (in the absence of a Castle physician) and Examiner of the

Roadstead. By elevating his rank to that of Chief Merchant, the Council of the Indies had come to recognise his impressive workload. A second administrator (a 'layman' with the rank of merchant, but not a pharmacist, surgeon, or physician) was assigned to the Dispensary to assist in the administration of medicines.

Because many medicines, which were mixed according to the *Amstelodamensis Pharmacopeia*, often arrived in a dubious state due to the wear and tear of travel, the Council of the Indies, in 1744, ordered surgeons throughout Asia to submit a list of local medicines. A medicines committee was appointed that same year, consisting of the Head of Surgery, the first practitioner of the *Binnenhospitaal*, and the Chief Surgeon of the Castle.[86] This committee compiled the Batavian *pharmacopeia*, which was published in 1746. The medicines it named were to be used exclusively by burghers and patients in the City Hospital. The medicines needed on board or at the trading posts outside Batavia continued to be prepared mainly in Amsterdam or in Batavia's Dispensary.[87] Many complaints by ship's surgeons about the low quality of the medical chests began to pour in. So many that the Council of the Indies decided in 1752 to again reorganise the supervisory function of the administration of the Dispensary. The second administrator (Merchant Reiner Harmensz.) would henceforth be responsible for its management and administration. The first administrator (Head of Surgery), Dr H. van Santen (also Batavia's pharmacist at the City Apothecary) would be accountable for the supervision of surgery and thereby lost his lucrative Dispensary manager position.[88] The merchant Reiner Harmensz. was to pay an annual sum from revenues to Dr van Santen because the Head of Surgery was no longer directly involved in the selling of dispensed medicines or raw ingredients. With this reorganisation, the Council of the Indies attempted, once again, to avoid any conflicts of interest and embezzlement.

Failed attempts at schooling

Surgical training was offered in the Castle. This was largely practical and, sadly enough, never standardised or formalised. Nonetheless, from its very inception, the surgery of the chief surgeon of the Castle served as a surgeon's 'school' with the chief surgeon acting as a teacher and examiner of surgeons prior to their promotion.[89] For instance, in the 1630s, Christiaan Hasendonk, Caspar Jansen, and Jessebert Lanre received three years schooling in the Castle after which they were employed as surgeons.[90] In 1639, Jan Harmens was trained as a surgeon and was examined by Horst, the chief surgeon of the Castle.[91] In 1653, the Council of the Indies decided that the examination should be taken in the presence of several senior surgeons, the Head of Surgery, and two Castle merchants.[92] A few years later, this rule was also applied to the burgher surgeons in Batavia. The Ordinance for Surgeons issued by the Council of the Indies in 1664 stated that no European was permitted to open a private dispensary or surgery practise unless he was a 'Registered Government Surgeon'. Certification depended on whether the applicant passed the examination.[93]

Schooling was not provided on a fixed and regular basis, but was offered on an ad hoc basis in a series of courses. An anatomy course was established in 1673, for which an anatomy theatre was equipped at the New Gate of Batavia.[94] Dr Willem ten Rhijne lectured on anatomy there and in 1679 Dr Louis de Keijser taught the surgeons of Batavia hospital. These courses and lessons were always subject to the 'needs of the time', defined by criteria that included the prevalence of disease, and the quality and quantity of available surgeons. As soon as the urgent need for schooling ebbed away, the courses and lectures followed suit. In the eighteenth century, when mortality rates among employees rose to unheard-of levels, the Council of the Indies tried once again to raise the surgeons' competence and to further find a solution of their relative scarcity by ordering lectures on anatomy and surgery, which occurred in 1745 and 1779. All surgeon's mates and third surgeons in Batavia had to attend. Meanwhile, (orphaned) Batavian youngsters were placed in the hospital to train them as surgeons.[95] The German surgeon Joan George Badenhausen, according to his will of 1758, served as their instructor (*informator der leerlingen van de Chirurgie*) at the *Chirurgie*.[96] These lessons, however, proved to have no great impact. In 1779, the Council decided that by first mail to the Republic the dearth of skilled physicians, surgeons (and also of midwives) in the Indies should be brought to the attention of the Gentlemen XVII, who were urgently requested to send out able physicians, surgeons, and midwives as soon as possible.[97]

City Surgeon and City Physician

The City Hospital and the Castle were medical centres established for the exclusive use of Company personnel. However, the Company saw to it that medical aid was also provided for the non-Company population of Batavia. The function of City Surgeon (*stadschirurgijn*) was established in 1646, and was a clear copy of that office in the Republic.[98] The City Surgeon was paid by the municipality of Batavia and, as such, responsible to the College of Aldermen, which, in its turn, was accountable to the Council of the Indies. The City Surgeon had to treat the ill and poor among the non-Company population. In addition, he served as a surgeon on behalf of the court of justice in cases of brawls and autopsies, and he was also responsible for the care of sick prisoners. Furthermore, he sheltered poor patients in his home as the accommodations in the City Hospital were restricted to Company personnel. If other (non-Company) surgeons gave first aid in cases of injuries resulting from fights, these surgeons reported immediately to him, while he himself reported the incident to the College of Aldermen.

In 1690, his responsibilities became more specifically defined: the City Surgeon treated all poor, free natives, burghers, and *Mardijkers*. His work for the court of justice included performing autopsies concerning drownings and murders. He was allowed to charge fees when he treated defendants. He had to treat other sick prisoners for free. The Dispensary supplied his linen and medicines. As the number of patients lodged in his house increased, it was decided to build two separate rooms in the Poor House and Orphanage, one for the treatment of sick Christians and one for sick non-Christians.[99]

The first mention of a City Physician (*stadsdokter*) occurred in 1651, when Petrus Meijer was appointed. He supervised the City Surgeon, the Castle's surgery and Dispensary.[100] An accurate description of his tasks was first found in 1745, when an additional City Physician was employed owing to the increased workload.[101] His duties then included – besides the supervision of the City Surgeon – free medical service to the Poor House and Orphanage, the Prison, the Chinese Hospital, public societies, and patients with moderate to insubstantial incomes (be they Company employees or free burghers). The physician obtained his medicines freely from the Dispensary at the Castle. His status was equal to that of a merchant and ranked next to that of a first practitioner (*eerste practizijn*) at the Hospital. He took his oath of allegiance in the presence of the Board of Aldermen and drew his stipend from the municipality and from Chinese Funds.[102] A year later, his status was elevated to the equivalent of the Head of Surgery and Chief Merchant. For this appointment, he took his oath in the presence of the Councillor of Justice.

The position of a second City Physician was abolished in 1750 (though re-instated again in the period 1754-1761, because of the endemic diseases that ravaged Batavia); by then he had already been acting superintendent (formerly warden) of the City Hospital for three years.[103] In 1757, the City Physician was again promoted in status and salary to a rank equal to that of Alderman, with an annual salary of 800 *rijksdaalders* (1 *rijksdaalder*, or rixdollar, being, in Batavia, sixty five-cent pieces; a guilder was twenty five-cent pieces).[104] With the death of the chief City Physician came a vacancy that was left open until, in 1769, this position was abolished.[105] His duties were henceforth taken over by the City Surgeon for a commensurate increase in salary. The period 1773-1779 saw the reintroduction of a City Physician, Dr Samuel Christiaan Kriel, in Batavia to deal with the high mortality rates in town.

The Poor House and Orphanage (the Parish Relief Board)

The Parish Relief Board was established in 1626 and after it had acquired a small fortune in the early 1630s, its board decided to spend more on the care of native orphans, the poor, elderly sick, and manumitted slaves. It also ran a small hospital.[106] The Parish Relief Board was primarily created for those who were no longer able to work (*impotente lieden*).[107] A married couple, who were responsible to the Board of Deacons, managed the facility on a daily basis.[108] Its revenues consisted essentially of money collected (*collectes*) and fines, but, in the long run, this proved insufficient to cope with the growing stream of emancipated slaves who were too poor to care for themselves and who increasingly burdened the City and the Parish Relief Board registers.[109] As noted above, the City Surgeon, too, faced the problem of increasing numbers of ill people lodging in his home at his expense. A new arrangement, whereby the Parish Relief Board made accommodations for the patients treated by the City Surgeon, further burdened the Board with even greater expenses. Two years later, in 1692, a more satisfying solution was found: the Parish Relief Board appointed its own surgeon as the City Surgeon's workload showed no sign of abating.[110] Furthermore, the Poor House also provided accommodations for psychiatric patients: in Asia, it was Company practice to 'liberate' (that is 'to set free') the mentally ill employees, and these patients were thrust on the Parish Relief Board's doorstep as their salaries ceased to be paid by the Company once they had been discharged.[111] The Poor House and Orphanage were both examples of a more traditional *gasthuis*.

The Lepers' Hospital

Leprosy was first observed in Batavia by Bontius who wrote about it in his *De Medicina Indorum* (Leiden, 1642), but it spread among the Batavian population only after 1655, perhaps owing to the increasing number of prisoners of war and the progressive influx of Chinese into Batavia.[112] As in Europe, the authorities took measures to isolate the lepers from the general population, not because of any medical or hygienic considerations but prompted more by traditional religious and social beliefs. Accordingly, the rules of the Lepers' Hospital, built west of Batavia at Angké in 1666, were more concerned with segregation, discipline, and order than with medical treatment.[113] Management was organised along lines like that of the other medical institutions. The Aldermen nominated two trustees, one a Company servant, the other a burgher; an overseer (warden) for the daily management of the Lepers' Hospital assisted the two trustees.[114] A decade later, fearing that the river would be polluted by lepers, the Council of the Indies decided to move this hospital to the island of Purmerend in the roadstead of Batavia.[115]

The Council of the Indies initially appealed to every suspected leper within the jurisdiction of the Company to have themselves examined by the supervisor of the Company hospital. If they were diagnosed with leprosy, the patients were sent to the Lepers' Hospital. Not unexpectedly, this appeal met with a general lack of enthusiasm. Therefore, in 1681, the Council of Aldermen, under whose responsibility the Lepers' Hospital fell, installed a committee of three physicians and two surgeons to screen the population for leprosy ('Leprosy Inspectors'), which was increased to six members in 1722 as leprosy continued to spread.[116] The government, apparently at a loss of what to do, recruited a local, indigenous, physician, a certain Care Jagera, from Maccassar, with the express aim of curing the leper patients. This was a total failure as far as combating the spread of leprosy was concerned.[117] Following the removal of the hospital to the island of Purmerend, a third trustee was appointed, who was actually the warden of the Lepers' Hospital. He lived there on the island of Purmerend as the distance between Batavia and the island prevented regular, effective hospital inspections by the trustees. The other two trustees, who lived in the city, were responsible for the administration of the finances of the Lepers' Hospital and were accountable to the Aldermen.[118] As they were empowered to punish the inmates in cases of 'improper behaviour' (for instance, a refusal to pray) by confining them to a diet of water and rice and flogging them in a darkened room, their role was not only managerial and administrative but also judicial and penal. As the disease continued to spread, the nature of the lepers' house slowly changed.[119] At the beginning of the eighteenth century, the Aldermen replaced the warden with a supervisor who had to be a first-class surgeon. The surgeon had to live on the island, never leave it without the trustees' permission, and to visit the patients twice a week.[120] Two surgeon's mates (*ondermeesters*) assisted him. During the seventeenth century, the Batavian *leprosarium* may have been, like the Parish Relief Board, a more traditional institution. The isolation and control of lepers was the prime motive for its founding. The strength of its staff was gradually reduced in the course of the eighteenth century as the prevalence of leprosy dwindled and, to no smaller degree, in response to austerity measures. In 1790, the lepers' house was turned into a general hospital, as its beds were urgently needed for other types of patients.[121]

Chinese Hospital

The Batavian Chinese were members of the Chinese intra-Asian trade network, though many of them were also employed in menial jobs for the Company. Because of the progressive influx of Chinese, the Council of the Indies soon felt the need to develop structures in which institutional ties were forged between the Chinese and the Dutch.[122] Governor-General Coen appointed Su Ming-Kong as the head or captain of the Chinese citizens in 1619, and instructed him to settle all civil affairs among his countrymen.[123] Captain Bencon, as he became known, became a member of the board of Aldermen. He represented the Chinese in their dealings with the Dutch authorities. Some twenty captains held this office until 1800.[124]

As there were so many Chinese in the Company's employ, the Council of the Indies established the position of a special Chinese Doctor. Gnot Hay was the first to act as such in 1635. His duties were to visit and treat the Company's poor Chinese employees who fell ill during the course of their work.[125] Because there were many poor and ill Chinese not employed by the Company, a hospital was built.[126] This hospital was constructed of bamboo and located on the Rhinocerosgracht off the Utrecht Street, but it soon ran into financial difficulties as fund-raising activities yielded insufficient revenue. To compensate, taxes were levied on Chinese funerals,[127] on wayang performances 'with which the Chinese waste their money without purpose', and on Chinese weddings.[128] Although a Chinese overseer managed the hospital, the Council of the Indies had decided that a Dutchman would manage the hospital by the time that the hospital was rebuilt using brick (1666-1667).[129] The Chinese hospital, in 1690 also began serving as an asylum for Chinese suffering from psychiatric problems. In 1753, when Muslim patients began being admitted, it was converted into a 'general' hospital for non-Europeans, paid for by taxes raised from among the Chinese and Muslim populations.[130]

To conclude, we have argued in this brief survey of the medical services of Batavia during the seventeenth century that the Indies' Council created a health-care system according to the needs of the time. Some components of this organisation were entirely traditional, for instance, the Parish Relief Board (Poor House and Orphanage) and the Lepers' Hospital. Others, such as the *Binnen*Hospital, were well in advance of then current practices in Europe and might rightly have been called 'modern'. The Council founded these institutions on its own initiative, more or less autonomously of the Company directors in the Dutch Republic. It is only when problems arose, such as a shortage of surgeons, that it appealed to the Gentlemen XVII for guidance. The Council often intervened directly in the affairs of the medical service institutions of Batavia. It participated on every board, was fully involved in the decision-making process, and constantly tried to improve the administrative structure in order to provide medical care of the highest possible quality.

Medical provisions at the other settlements

By 1700, Batavia could boast, as we have seen, of a number of hospitals and of some 50 surgeons who served the medical and surgical needs of its population. These 50 men were not the only surgeons working in Asia, however. Their professional counterparts worked on the (intra-Asiatic) fleet and in the other settlements.

Table T3.3: Company personnel in Asia during the eighteenth century [131]

Category	*1700*	*1753*	*1780*
Management, Trade & Justice	1026	1731	1506
Church	95	172	148
Health Care	205	378	308
Crafts	1266	2253	1650
Sailors	1375	3314	2881
Soldiers	8923	11040	9173
Divers	201	503	643
Asiatic personnel	723	1724	-
Seafaring personnel on the ships	3913	3054	1285
Total	18117	24879	18452

The data presented in table T3.3 show that the number of military personnel in Asia amounted to *circa* 50 per cent of the entire personnel during the eighteenth century. Comparatively speaking, the medical staff in Asia (excluding the Cape of Good Hope) was rather insignificant, only consisting of 1 per cent of the total number of Company personnel in Asia in 1700, and grew almost imperceptibly to a mere 2 per cent in 1780. The other settlements in Asia were equipped with wards or rooms in forts or fortifications, which were sometimes called hospitals. Bantam, for instance, possessed a small hospital, which could care for 12 sick Company employees daily. In Ceylon, eight hospitals were established: in Colombo (for 300 patients); in Jaffna (for 100 to 150 patients); in Galle (100 to 150 patients); in Trincomalee (60 to 80 patients); and there were smaller ones in Kalpitya, in Batticaloa, Mattara, and in Mannar.[132] In Bengal, a hospital was constructed in Chinsurah along the Houghly River in 1728.[133]

Not every settlement had a hospital, for instance, those in Siam, Japan and Persia, but a number of ship's surgeons did end up practising there at the local 'factory' for the benefit of the Company personnel. Furthermore, ship's surgeons were hired for the vessels engaged in intra-Asiatic trade, and on the outward- and homeward-bound ships. The most distant settlement was that of the artificial island of Deshima in the harbour of Nagasaki, Japan. In 1641, the Portuguese were expelled from Japan, and by then the English had abandoned their attempts to break into the Japanese market. The Dutch, however, were allowed to stay, but were ordered to move their trading post from Hirado to the tiny island of Deshima in Nagasaki Bay. From 1641 until the arrival of the Americans in 1853, the strictly controlled Dutch post on Deshima was Japan's sole window on the Western world. Though Deshima did not have a hospital, the settlement employed a surgeon, a surgeon's mate, and sometimes even an apothecary since 1623.

The Cape of Good Hope and Ceylon

Jan van Riebeeck, himself a surgeon and the founder of the Dutch settlement at the Cape of Good Hope, made sure that a hospital was built there in 1652. It started out with canvas tents but was completed in brick in 1656, and could accommodate some 500 to 750 patients. This hospital at first employed one full surgeon, Adriaen de Jager, who had accompanied Van Riebeeck to South Africa, as well as a surgeon's mate.[134] The management of the hospital was entrusted to *regenten*, members of the local government (Political Council or *Politieke Raad*) and their wives. The wives were responsible for the diet of the patients, the operation of the kitchen and the supervision of the hospital attendants and slaves.[135] This arrangement proved to be unsatisfactory in the eighteenth century, and the management was reorganised and the wives were removed from their positions. As in Batavia, the Cape also possessed a Dispensary, where medicines sent from the Republic were stored. However, there were no known committees responsible for overseeing the convalescence of patients. Contrary to the practice in Batavia, the hospital managers did not actively intervene in the affairs of the hospital.

At the beginning of the eighteenth century, the hospital employed one senior surgeon, assisted by one *ziekenvader*. This *ziekenvader* was responsible for the food and beverage supplies. In 1717, there were seven surgeons employed in the hospital, besides several assistants, a cook and his mate, an assistant to the pox ward, a carpenter, and 13 slaves to tend to the patients. In 1769, the size of its staff had expanded to 77, but in 1792 the staff had declined to only 42, of whom thirteen were surgeons. The surgeons at the Cape, like in Batavia, were eventually designated as doctors or *practizijns*.[136]

It is at the Cape that we mostly encounter the practice of recruiting soldiers for the surgical profession.[137] Because of the demise of surgeons at the hospital of the Cape or on board the vessels, which were on their way to the obligatory stop at the Cape, it was there that any vacancies were filled. When the chief surgeon of the visiting vessel the *Zonderhoef* died in 1717, both his mate and a surgeon's mate from the Cape's hospital, Jan Daniel Butner (born in Halle, Saxony, 1690), sought the promotion to his function. Butner had arrived as a soldier at the Cape in 1712, but as soon as he arrived, he was placed in the hospital as a surgeon's mate. The chief surgeon of the Cape hospital and the chief surgeons of those vessels lying at the roadstead examined the candidates and found that the surgeon's mate of the vessel *Zonderhoef* was incompetent. Accordingly, Jan Daniel Butner was placed as the senior surgeon on this vessel, on the provision that Batavia would certify the promotion.[138] It is likely that Butner had received surgical training in Halle, but was not employed as such by the Company Chambers in the Republic. Although no actual proof as yet has been found of the practise of employing German surgeons initially (by the Chambers in the Republic) as soldiers, there is every indication that this did, indeed, happen. What other explanation could there be for the transfer of the German soldier Fredrik Wervel to Colombo as an apothecary, for which function a certain expertise was required?[139]

Another large and important hospital was the one built in Colombo in Ceylon. The Dutch had confiscated Colombo from the Portuguese in 1656, but they decided not to use the existing Portuguese hospital. They preferred to build a new one to accommodate 200 patients, which later (in 1786) was extended to offer accommodations for 300 patients. In Colombo, the hospital was run by a warden (neither a physician nor a surgeon) responsible for the purchase of provisions and supplying meals to the patients. The personnel included two senior surgeons, three surgeon's mates, and three *derde meesters*, augmented by five assistants. The most famous of the Colombo surgeons was the German physician (!) Paulus Hermanus (Halle 1640 – Leiden 1695), who worked in the hospital from 1672 to 1679. He collected plants and sent these to Leiden University, as a reward for which he was offered the botany chair in 1680. The book *Insulae Ceyloniae thesaurus medicus laboratorim Ceylonicum* by Swedish physician Hermanus Nicolaas Grimm (1641-1711), who worked for Paulus Hermann in Colombo, contains pharmaceutical preparations, the ingredients of which were found in Ceylon, and were used by the local population and the doctors of Ceylon.[140] The non-medical personnel consisted of a cook, a porter, a laundryman, and several slaves.[141]

The crisis of the eighteenth century

The end of the seventeenth century was marked, as we have seen, by an extremely high mortality rates on the outward-bound East Indiamen. The Council of the Indies did not react immediately to these frightening death rates. It seems that the Council did not take these issues too seriously as they did not pose problems for business in Asia. At the turn of the century, the most urgent medical item on its agenda was the building of the lepers' house on the island of Purmerend, off the coast of Batavia. Apparently, the high mortality rates during the years 1690-95 did not have any grave consequences for Batavia. Besides, a volcanic eruption was the focus of the Council's attention in most of their meetings. The volcano Salak erupted in 1699, blocking and polluting Batavia's water supply, the Tjiliwong River. This eruption was compounded by the city being enclosed by walls, canals and houses, and which has long been blamed for the change in Batavia's healthy climate, and effectively transforming Batavia into an eighteenth-century graveyard.[142]

P.H. van der Brug examined the high Batavian mortality rates in his Leiden dissertation of 1994.[143] He states that prior to 1733 the benign vivax-malaria was the dominant type in Batavia. Most of its permanent inhabitants had acquired some resistance; not so the Company servants, as they were a floating population. However, the number of malaria victims among them was fairly low before 1733, indicating a low level of transmission of the malignant *falciparum* malaria as a result of a dearth of breeding places for larvae of the malarial mosquitoes, which are the vectors of this disease. After 1733, the malaria in Batavia was characterised by a high level of transmission and by the frequent occurrence of the malignant form. The mortality rates in Batavia rose accordingly from 19 percent to 29 percent (table T3.4). Van der Brug believes that the cause of this epidemic was the construction of waterworks (the digging of fishponds) near Batavia's coast. These created stagnant salt-water pools and a great deal of vegetation, thereby recreating ideal conditions for the propagation of malignant malaria.[144] It would seem that these fishponds after 1733 were the main cause of the increase mortality rates by malaria among Company personnel, mainly new arrivals from Europe who had had no chance to acquire an immunity. But this trend did not repeat itself among local inhabitants, who, it is assumed, must have been immune to the disease which struck Batavia in 1733.

Table T3.4: Mortality in Batavia 1714-1744[145]

Period	*New Arrivals in Batavia*	*Total Deaths in Batavia (and as % of new arrivals)*	*Mortality in Binnenhospitaal (and as % of total deaths and new arrivals)*	*Average mortality per annum (in absolute numbers)*
1714-1719	23816	2,814 (12%)	2,466 (88%) (10%)	493
1719-1724	30205	3,745 (12%)	3,411 (91%) (11%)	682
1724-1729	25092	4,285 (17%)	3,930 (92%) (16%)	786
1729-1734	23574	4,371 (19%)	3,974 (91%) (17%)	795
1734-1739	30569	8,851 (29%)	8,286 (94%) (27%)	1659
1739-1744	23628	6,106 (26%)	5,562 (91%) (24%)	1112

Table T3.4 presents the mortality rates in terms of total numbers and percentages in Batavia in relation to the total number of new arrivals in Batavia. These new arrivals went to the City Hospital when they became ill; the patients in the City Hospital consisted solely of Company employees. As this table shows, the mortality rates of Batavia as a whole consisted mainly of fatalities in the City Hospital, meaning that the victims came from among the floating population. These mortality figures in Batavia emerged as a major subject of discussion during the meetings of the Council of the Indies. Its ordinances indicate that mortality rates in Batavia rose significantly after 1730, noting, for instance, that, in 1731, the City Hospital had treated more than 700 inpatients, *nota bene* a few years before the digging of the waterworks.[146] The addition of two members of the Council of the Indies to the board of trustees of the hospitals as supervisors in 1731, as well as a general fasting and days of prayer in 1733 and in 1735 did, alas, not yield the desired results.[147] A small hospital was built to accommodate some 100 patients on the island of *Edam* (off the coast of Batavia), supplementing the accommodations on the island of *Onrust*.[148] By 1741, circa 800 patients were being treated daily in the *Binnenhospitaal*, most of whom were suffering from malignant fevers.[149] By employing a physician and a second dresser in 1743, the managers of the *Binnenhospitaal* tried to stem the tide patients.[150] At that time, there were already five chief or full surgeons employed there. In 1752, the medical staff of the *Binnen*Hospital had grown to a superintendent (who was a physician[151]), five – soon six – practitioners (originally chief surgeons), and two dressers (also originally chief surgeons), who were being trained to be practitioners.[152] They were supported by three surgeon's mates and three indigenous *derde meesters*, as well as some European servants and indigenous slaves. In 1766, the servants of the City Hospital consisted of one cook's mate, one carpenter, one cooper (*kuiper*), one bed maker (*beddemaker*), one provost (*provoost*), one *pluimgraaf* (caretaker of cattle and poultry), one porter of the Watergate (*portier van de Waterpoort*), one water carrier (*waterhaler*), one *smeerboer*,[153] ten overseers (*ziekenvaders*), one clerk, and one laundryman (*wasser*). They received the assistance of 56 boys and 31 slaves.[154] These servants and slaves distributed meals to patients, worked in the kitchens, cleaned the wards and buildings, transported the patients within the hospital, and cut the grass needed to feed the cows.[155]

The Outer Hospital (*Buitenhospitaal*)

To lighten the workload of the *Binnenhospitaal*, the Council decided to purchase a large garden with some buildings at the small settlement of Noordwijk, on which a hospital was built in 1743, the so-called *Buiten*Hospital or 'Outer' Hospital.[156] This *Buitenhospitaal* was primarily meant for scurvy patients and convalescents. It soon became a financial burden for the Council of the Indies, however. In 1751, Governor-

General J. Mossel asked of the Head of Surgery, the practitioners and the dressers of the City Hospital to assess whether the Outer Hospital was still a useful facility. They were unanimous in their affirmation, in fact, they thought the City Hospital too small to lodge the number of crew members who arrived ill. It had become impossible – so they said – to separate the patients in the *Binnenhospitaal* according to their diseases. The air on the island of Edam was considered unhealthy for treatment and convalescence. Therefore, the Governor-General decided to maintain the *Buitenhospitaal*, where the patients suffering from scurvy and dysentery, and convalescents from the City Hospital could be kept separated.[157]

Tjipannas Spa (*1744-1761*)

In addition to the Outer Hospital, yet another infirmary was constructed in 1744. During an exploratory tour through the Preanger area, behind the Salak and Gedeh volcanoes, Governor-General Van Imhoff discovered the hot springs of Tjipannas along the way to Tjiandjur. The local population informed the party that the springs had curative properties. Van Imhoff had a road built through the forest, the water sampled, and a small establishment constructed near the spring to accommodate personnel who fell ill. Within a year, a chief surgeon was appointed to manage this hospital. In 1745, everything was in working order, and supervision was placed in the hands of a hospital board of trustees, which became known as Tjipannas Spa ('The Hot Bath of Tjipannas', *Het Warme Bad*).[158]

Tjipannas Spa was initially intended for the benefit of Company employees thought to be incurably ill. These patients had been 'freed' from their Company contracts (and thus became a burden to the Parish Relief Board). Another method to save on expenses was to send these patients back to Europe, where they became dependent on the charity of the almshouses in the Republic. Experience, however, revealed that, miraculously, quite a number of these 'incurable patients' became almost immediately well enough to again work for the Company, to end up in the *Binnenhospitaal* in Batavia once more! They had probably been victims of the crimps in the Republic who had sent them back to Asia under an assumed name. This bolstered the strong impression held by the Indies Council that an increasing number of personnel pretended to be chronically ill in order to be repatriated. Therefore, the Council decided that genuinely incurable patients were to be sent to the Poor House in Semarang; those who were seriously ill but curable were to go to Tjipannas; and, finally, the wealthier among the incurable patients were to be sent back to Europe on the promise that they would never set foot in the East Indies again.[159]

During its nearly 20 years of existence, the Tjipannas Spa was managed by chief surgeon Jan de Put, who served as its superintendent. He was assisted by a warden, a gate keeper, a laundryman (*mantri*), a carpenter and 45 coolies.[160] The Spa was built to accommodate a maximum of 30 patients. Despite the Company's annual contributions, Tjipannas showed financial losses at the end of every year. The Council of the Indies, in its attempts to cut expenses, began to doubt whether a continuation of the Spa would serve any useful purpose. Surgeon De Put reported to the Council that, despite the advantages of Tjipannas (such as healthy mountain air and hot, highly beneficial, mineral water), its main disadvantage was that patients had to endure a journey of eight days by ox-drawn carts over a muddy, mountainous trail to reach the spa. Maintaining adequate food supplies over the 80-kilometre trek was also problematic. Conscious of these difficulties, Governor-General Van der Parra decided to close the Spa in 1761.[161] Perhaps the Tjipannas Spa should not actually be characterised as a hospital, at least not in the Batavian sense of the word. It was primarily a *Kurort*, a place of convalescence for patients.

The Moorish Hospital (*1751-1785*)

The last hospital to be built in Batavia during the Company period was the Moorish Hospital, which was erected in 1751 as a reception centre for Muslim sailors.[162] In the Moorish Hospital, as it came to be called (*het Moorse Ziekenhuis*), Muslim physicians treated the patients. These patients were admitted only after having undergone a medical examination by the chief surgeon of the Castle; the diagnoses by ship's surgeons on the ships were not always accepted. Based on the chief surgeon's examination, the genuinely ill were referred to the superintendent of the Moorish Hospital. Those Muslim servants who were employed ashore were first examined by the *oppermeester* in the area where they worked. Admissions were entitled to normal provisions (food, clothing and medication) but had their salary withheld during their hospital stays. Ward rounds were to be made twice daily by the superintendent of the hospital, a senior surgeon, assisted by two *ondermeesters*, and a Muslim physician who was assisted by two other Muslim physicians of lesser rank. The accountant and the commissioner of the hospital were Europeans; the cook and the orderlies were chosen from among the convalescents. In 1752, the position of the Muslim practitioner was abolished on the pretext that the Muslim sailors on board preferred European surgeons and medicines. In 1753, some Muslim patients were also sent to the Chinese Hospital. The commensurate reduction in expenses was partly used to increase the remuneration paid to the superintendent. The Moorish hospital closed down in 1785, due to the high maintenance costs and the fact that too few patients sought to be admitted there. Patients were henceforth sent to the *Buitenhospitaal*.[163]

Proposals for improving Batavia's health

By 1744, the trustees of the *Binnenhospitaal* and *Buitenhospitaal* of Batavia fused into one management board under the auspices of Governor-General Van Imhoff (1743-1750).[164] The board consisted of one member of the Council of the Indies and six highly qualified Company employees, while the City Hospital's bookkeeper acted as clerk.[165] For once, there was no surgeon or physician on the committee but they were summoned after every meeting and interrogated about their work. Diseases continued to ravage Batavia and the hospitals were permanently overcrowded: there were *circa* 800 patients in the City Hospital in 1756,[166] which rose steadily to the astonishing total number of over 2,000 admissions in the City Hospital and Outer Hospital in 1767. This caused angry recriminations from the Gentlemen XVII.[167] The Governor-General reported that all possible measures were being taken to ameliorate the situation in Batavia. Such measures consisted of cutting back the thick undergrowth; diverting water from stagnant pools back to the sea; prohibiting all unnecessary digging, and, when diseases appeared, the immediate cessation of all groundwork; burning of all offal; removing all lime kilns to a place further away from town; improving the sanitary conditions of drains and gutters; encouraging the planting of trees, lopping them at a considerable height from the ground; constructing large reservoirs along the river into town, both as a precaution against droughts and as a means of purifying the water by allowing the sediment to settle before being used for drinking purposes; replacing the permanent damp wooden floors in the houses with brick floors and the double windows with windows that could be opened; removing all obstacles in the creeks to allow water to rush through freely; allowing faeces to be thrown into the river only in fixed places and at fixed times; placing the soldiers' sentry boxes under shady trees or under bamboo shelters; prohibiting the burning of spices, which was considered very unhealthy, with the sole exception of certain places along the Tjiliwong River; taking care to minimise exposure to the heat of the day and the chill of the night; continuing to dredge the Great River; urging physicians and surgeons to do their utmost when treating the patients, and above all, to consult each other.[168] In accordance with prevailing information, everything was done to check the air pollution, to insist that people keep their land and water clean, and to warn them against the dangers of extreme temperature changes.

The hospital trustees were naturally concerned about the high mortality rates and this concern dominated practically every meeting. By the same year, one member of the Batavian medical establishment had been included on the committee of trustees: the minutes of the meetings of the trustees not only mention the member of the Council of the Indies and its future Governor-General, Reijnier de Klerk, who acted as chairman, but also Adrianus Vogelzang (chief master of equipment), Major Claudicis Anthonij van Luepken, the building contractor Pruijmers, Colonel Jan Jurge Feber, and the Head of Surgery Jan de Put, the former superintendent of Tjipannas.

The increased losses of manpower, the inability to find adequate crews for the ships, the heavy strain on the physical ability to house the patients in the hospitals, all contributed to the fact that the costs of the Batavian medical organisation were too high and that disease seriously threatened essential trade. For instance, current epidemics and the consequent lack of manpower meant that no products were being transported between Batavia and the Preanger in 1757.[169] Drastic cost-saving measures were unavoidable. Batavia's hospitals were among the first to feel the effects of the (economic) downturn.

A missive sent by the Gentlemen XVII to the Council of the Indies in 1768, again, expressed their worries about and annoyance with the directors about the high mortality rates in Batavia. As a result, the council decided to appoint a commission of enquiry in order to shed light on the issue. Ten of the most prominent physicians and surgeons in Batavia were offered a seat on that commission: Jan de Put, Head of Surgery; Dr Kriel, City Physician; Dr Gerardus Maas, City Physician; Jan Adam Spenolt, Chief Surgeon of the Castle; Andries Johan Decker, Jan Dat, Gerrit Vollé and Caspar Ludeker, all of them full surgeons in Batavia; Dr Johannes Paulus Hofman and Hendrik Ernst Schreuder, both physicians in Batavia. Again, Reijnier de Klerk acted as chairman. The commission's report, with an introduction by Councillor De Klerk, was presented in October 1768. De Klerk had been especially charged with the supervision of hospitals during this period. The report referred mainly to the City Hospital because mortality rates in the Outer Hospital were not exceptionally high at that time. No agreement among the commission's members could be reached because of the animosity that existed amongst the commissioners. Head of Surgery, Jan de Put, nevertheless, summarised what the Council of the Indies wanted to know: (i) Are food and beverages of sufficient quality being served to the sick? (ii) Is the care offered patients of sufficiently high quality? (iii) Can anything that might be termed malpractice be discerned? (iv) What are the causes of the extremely high mortality rates? and (v) What can be done to prevent these unacceptably high levels of mortality?

Examining the first point, commission members believed that food and beverages were indeed of high enough quality, although some wished that more could be done towards individualising the patients' meals. The second question caused more disagreement among them. However, they admitted that a high degree of cleanliness was indeed usually observed in the care of patients but also that many serious complaints had been still brought forward. The general opinion was that the City Hospital, built for 600 patients, was much too small, since there were usually more than 1,000 patients accommodated there at any one time. Some members of the commission thought that the delivery of large numbers of new patients on the vessels might be the cause of the high fatality figures among convalescent patients. The third question was refuted completely and the fourth was generally considered to be too difficult to answer. All of the possible causes were discussed, but most of them were already present in earlier periods when mortality rates were lower. One surgeon thought that people could find the cause in the

Republic where unhealthy men were allowed to sail to Asia. It was generally felt that the Cape's hospital also had a negative influence on health. The members were convinced that the many diseases that broke out between the Cape of Good Hope and Batavia must have been because they had been incorrectly diagnosed as cured. The debates on the last question led to various demands and propositions such as, for instance, that an extension be added to the City Hospital so that the patients could be separated by diseases; the destruction of the mattresses and clothes of patients suffering from contagious diseases; the improvement of hygienic conditions on the vessels; the construction of a new hospital at the Cape of Good Hope; and more uniformity in the treatment of patients buttressed by the appointment of competent physicians to supervise that treatment. In an accompanying memorandum, J. Radermacher, a member of the Council of the Indies, stated that the outward-bound soldiers should first be allowed to acclimatise at the Cape of Good Hope where a new hospital was needed. He advised the Gentlemen XVII to exercise stricter control over enlistees and that people suffering from a disease should not be allowed to sail.[170] In the end, the Radermacher recommendations were never followed up by the Gentlemen XVII because they were considered too costly.

Finally, at the meeting of the Council of the Indies of 7 October, 1768, as a consequence of the reports, it was decided that both the City Hospital and the Outer Hospital should be expanded as soon as possible. Together they would then be able to house some 2,000 patients. The staff were again ordered to separate patients according to their diseases. Reverting to tried and tested methods, sprinkling vinegar, burning powder and saltpetre should be used to disinfect the air. A number of physicians were ordered to investigate the City Apothecary from which the City Hospital received its supply of medicines. Furthermore, the Gentlemen XVII were asked to place an extra surgeon's mate on each East Indiaman, which might help fill the need for extra surgeons. The Moorish Hospital's superintendent, Dekker, was put in charge of drawing up a report regarding life on board the ships in order to try to pinpoint how diseases could be avoided. Moreover, three physicians were hired to investigate the causes of mortality in Batavia.

These measures seemed to bear little fruit, however. The transfer of patients to the *Buitenhospitaal* caused an increase in mortality rates there and Batavian fatalities overall did not decrease after the inquiry of 1768. The physicians and surgeons' mission proved disappointing. In 1773, the hospital superintendents, all surgeon-majors, all full surgeons in town, and the City Surgeons were asked by the Council to formulate guidelines for the combatting of the endemic diseases. This also turned out to be a pretty futile exercise and nothing significant resulted from it. City Physician Kriel reported to the Council of the Indies that, in his opinion, the practitioners knew best how to treat their patients, and that any remarks he might make were merely of a minor nature.[171] The one measure the committee did accept was the re-instalment of the use of a hospital ship in the roadstead so that patients who were sick upon their arrival could be better accommodated.[172]

After 1777, the scales turned and Batavia briefly enjoyed somewhat healthier conditions. As a result of the declining number of patients, some medical positions could be and were indeed, abolished. The City Hospital let three practitioners go, leaving the superintendent to act as first practitioner, assisted by a second and a third practitioner and a dresser, and with some six surgeon's mates, six indigenous *derde meesters* and 50 slaves at his disposal. They had to make twice daily rounds of the patients. As compensation for the extra work, the superintendent was elevated to the rank of chief merchant so that he became the social equal of the Head of Surgery, with equal pay.[173] Further retrenching was to follow in 1779: as a result of the decision to transfer the patients on arrival to the hospital ship or the *Buitenhospitaal*, there were never more than 50 patients in the *Binnenhospitaal*. Therefore, all practitioners with the exception of the superintendent were dismissed.[174] The dresser was made second practitioner, assisted by three surgeon's mates and three European *derde meesters*, backed up by some servants and slaves.[175] In 1786, a new investigation into the diseases in Batavia was ordered as the mortality in the *Binnenhospitaal* grew again. However, the *Binnenhospitaal* lost its status as City Hospital: patients from the fleet were sent to the *Buitenhospitaal*, and Company servants in Batavia preferred the *Buitenhospitaal* too.

Concluding remarks

During its presence of nearly 200 years in Asia, the Company created a full-fledged health service, which was principally located in Batavia. What started as mere ship's surgery developed into an organisation that was comprised of various hospitals in Batavia and elsewhere in Asia (including Cape of Good Hope), with many qualified employees attending to numerous patients, a Dispensary, a City Physician, a City Surgeon, medical courses and lessons, and medical investigation committees, all created with the intention of curing sick Company employees and ensuring their fitness for future service.

This was a result that, indeed, could not have been foreseen at the beginning. The directors of the Company, the Gentlemen XVII, did not and could not provide the local Batavian authorities with a clear-cut blueprint for a successful health service; it was largely experimental. The health-care system in Asia developed in response to the needs of the time, and was dependent upon the views and ideas of local officials and proper financing. From the very outset the hospitals in Asia were considered centres of convalescence and healing, and not institutions where poor and infirm patients could be tucked away and kept under control.

There are solid grounds to argue that, in contrast to the situation at home, a long-term policy was pursued both by the Gentlemen XVII and by the Council of the Indies, namely to set up a permanent medical organisation to deal with the treatment of the ill and injured among their employees and, to some extent, the local people. To achieve this goal, the Gentlemen XVII dispatched the physician Dr Bontius to Asia in the early seventeenth century. He created the office of Head of Surgery and became the first to fill it successfully. He formulated and implemented a medical policy in close collaboration with the Council of the Indies, the main administrative body of the Dutch trading empire. From the days of Bontius, a Head of Surgery, to whom all ship's surgeons in Asia – on the ships and ashore – were accountable, was stationed there permanently.

The Council of the Indies assumed responsibility for the creation of a health service right from the start: in 1632 it had already appointed one of its members to deal with the medical problems of Company employees. This member was usually on the board of trustees of Batavia's hospitals . Consequently, the Council of the Indies was directly and perpetually involved in all of the current medical issues. The Company's medical organisation in Asia was deliberately centralised in Batavia unlike the decentralised, fragmented health-care system in the Dutch Republic. The Head of Surgery here was not just some advisor to the colonial authorities; he was actively involved in most of the medical decisions taken by the Council. The Council never took its most significant decisions without consulting the Head of Surgery. In the second half of the eighteenth century, the entire top of the Batavian medical establishment was fully involved in the decision-making process concerning health care.

This chapter argues that a long-term policy was pursued by the Gentlemen XVII, the Council of the Indies, and the Head of Surgery, which was designed to set up a permanent and properly functioning colonial medical service. And they did succeed in this! The foundations established by Bontius in the early seventeenth century did not change structurally during the Company's entire existence and even survived well into the nineteenth century. The same can be said about the physical infrastructure, namely the hospitals. They also survived. In the eighteenth century, the health-care system was repeatedly challenged by a number of health crises, both on the ships (largely caused by typhus) and in Batavia (where the chief culprit was malaria). Although other Asian settlements were stricken with serious diseases from time to time, these were never as serious and structural as those on board the vessels and those in Batavia. The Batavian policymakers tried to deal with these health crises to the best of their ability. They did so by establishing broad-based committees that examined the health problems and reported on their findings. They installed 'committees of inquiry' in 1750, in which the medical establishment's top brass were prominently represented. In that same period, a number of medical initiatives and innovations were introduced under the aegis of Governor-General Van Imhoff.

The maintenance of a health-care service required major infusions of financial assistance on the part of the Company directors. However, and herein lies the drawback of the Company's management, neither the directors back in the Republic nor the Council of the Indies were able or willing to vouchsafe the proper and sufficient level of funding necessary for a competent health organisation.[176] Few medical experts until 1750 were represented in the higher echelons of the Company's administration (with the exception of the Head of Surgery) and, if they were, they remained relatively low key. It was only after 1750 that Batavia's medical experts became fully involved in the medical administration of the city.

In short, the Company's health-care organisation originally fell within traditional paradigms. It was constrained – unavoidably – by a lack of modern medical knowledge, an inability, or rather unwillingness, to provide adequate funding which left the system unable to cope with the problems that arose. Leaving aside some of the less than successful decisions, in general the Company's health-care system was truly 'revolutionary' in the sense that it was set up to *cure*. It may not have created a totally modern *Krankenhuis* as we now know it, but it represented a new, transitional stage in which the old binary patient-healer relationship was replaced by a more modern triangular one, that of patient–health-care provider–physician (surgeon/healer). As often happens when a society is challenged by extreme conditions such as war, or, in this case, a sustained mass migration from Europe to Asia, social and institutional progress was achieved.

4. The geographic origin of the Company's surgeons

Who were the surgeons who sailed on the Company ships and worked in the Company settlements? To answer this question we will begin this chapter with another question: Where did they come from and why did they come? A knotty question, prudently evaded in the pertinent literature. This dodginess is understandable because this question is intimately tied to another question, namely that of the motives of the surgeons who sought employment with the Company. At first sight it does seem to be a rather foolish act of a youngster (or a somewhat older person for that matter), learned in surgery, to sail on an East Indiaman in search of distant shores, uncertain of whether he will ever see his home again. What moved him to exchange the certainty of the solid ground under his feet for the ever-moving deck of a ship? Why not just stay at home and make one's life there, for a less risky, and perhaps even better paid future? Was there no proper employment to be found in his own neighbourhood? Were these surgical men just simple adventurers or romantics? Was the 'lure' of the sea, the Siren's song of adventure, the common psychological parameter? Nicolaas de Graaff (1619-1688) may well have been one of these types who loved adventure. He made some 16 voyages as a ship's surgeon, of which five were for the Company. He professed that he had been seized by an uncontrollable urge to see the world and unusual things, with the added pleasure of interesting wounds and operations.[1] A very different point of view is expressed by Gijsbert Heeck (1619-1669), a master surgeon in the village of Bunschoten (near the city of Amersfoort), who decided to seek the Company's employ (again) to escape his feelings of sadness after the death of his wife.[2] Should the researcher then simply try to discover the common denominator in these psychological factors, which include self-sufficiency, the urge for self-development, courage, mere inquisitiveness or curiosity, the wish to prove oneself, the hope to strike it rich, the feeling of bereavement and loneliness, or a sense of filial duty to a widowed mother, to name but a few?

Perhaps some felt compelled by family tradition, like their colleagues in Württemberg, as it appears from a study by the medical historian M. Lindemann? There, the percentage of surgeons' sons who became surgeons themselves was more than 50 per cent![3] Or, if the father was a (ship's) surgeon, would the son(s) follow in his footsteps? Or, if a brother hired on with the Company, would his male siblings also follow suit? Nicolaas de Graaff' father had been in the employ of the Company and this may very well have motivated the son which may often have been the case in families.[4] At least four family members from the Vuijstingh family from Alphen aan den Rijn (near Leiden) served as ship's surgeons. Another possibility presents itself at this point. It is quite feasible that it became a contagious 'epidemic' among villagers and city dwellers: friends who heard from (the parents of) friends that they had embraced an interesting or adventurous calling as a ship's surgeon with the Company, became inspired by these tales to sign up themselves. The upshot of this contagion would be that a bunch of villagers or city dwellers would sometimes leave their hometowns to join the Company and sail to distant harbours at a short space of time.

Or were they just plain quacks or opportunists, seeking a fortune at the expense of Company personnel? This was, in fact, the image that the ship's surgeon acquired in the seventeenth century, and became even more poignantly so in the eighteenth century, echoes of which have been faithfully reported down through the centuries, and the ship's surgeon of the early modern period is usually still depicted as such in contemporary novels. This was also the opinion held by their contemporaries, as we have already seen. The seventeenth-century Company captain (*schipper*) and author Willem IJsbrantsz Bontekoe (1587-1657) tells us about ship's surgeons who 'after they had roamed the high seas and, like executioners, had tormented and ill-treated their miserable crews, such bunglers consider their education as complete and dare to establish themselves as qualified masters in the home-country'.[5] The French traveller J.B. Tavernier (1605-1689) informs us that the surgeons of the Company were young, callow boys, having not yet outgrown the barber's shop, who had few skills save shaving and dressing superficial wounds.[6] These opinions may well have been due to the lower standards set for the sea examination, which led to petty jealousies when ship's surgeons became successful in their lives. Eighteenth-century contemporaries advise us that, concerning the second half of the century, qualified surgeons were certainly hard to find.[7] But then, this particular complaint was not limited solely to ship's surgeons. It was equally relevant for recruited sailors and soldiers who were often paupers, children, and the enfeebled aged, as ship's surgeon L. de Sille on board the East Indiaman the *Amsterdam* wrote to his friends on 4 January 1780.[8] Most historians have noted that many down and out men sought refuge in the Company, including some who had gone bankrupt and even some criminals who managed to escape justice in the Republic on one of the Company vessels.[9]

For some of the ship's surgeons, the prospect of earning 'quick' money seems to have been the most compelling motive, an attitude which earned them the reputation as ruthless opportunists driven by not quite the honourable motive. Johan Andreas Muller, a German ship's surgeon in the employ of the Company, wrote to his parents in May 1748 while his ship *Westhoven* was anchored in the roadstead of Hellevoetssluis awaiting departure, and listed all the things he intended to make a profit on in the East:

Dear Parents, I am letting you know that I have here on the ship more than 2,200 Dutch guilders' worth of products like French and Rhinish wine, beer and gin, and pipes and textiles. I hope and pray that God may safeguard me from misfortune and that He may give me health; if so, I do not doubt that I will make a nice profit on these products so that I can come back and live in my native country and then I will earn my bread on land, if God grants that I shall live.[10]

There must have been many more like him who were lured by the prospects of private business dealings in the fabled treasures of the East, and whose ultimate goal was to return and live quietly in their home country. However, the immediate bread-and-butter motive has its irresistible appeal: the scarcity of a population to practise upon, too many surgeons in one area, or an economic depression in their region might compel some to leave their native villages and cities to seek employment elsewhere. In which case they could have been part and parcel of the so-called North Sea Migration System, which developed in the seventeenth and eighteenth centuries in northwestern Europe and consisted of a migration of labourers from the poor inland areas (well into Germany) to the North Sea coast.[11]

Whatever their origins or motives, the ship's surgeons constituted a special professional group. They were craftsmen, to whom the broadening of their expertise was important. This had been one of Nicolaas de Graaff's motives for seeking service as a ship's surgeon. German surgical journeymen, for instance, were compelled to travel around for several years in order to gain professional experience. Research in Münster has shown that many craftsmen made their way from Münster to the East Indies to gain experience.[12] Although this kind of journeying was not obligatory in the Republic, apprentice surgeons often switched masters over the course of several years in the same city. Did the Company's ship's surgeons belong to that tradition of these wandering craftsmen, who chose this option to broaden their expertise and horizons, like the German *Wanderburschen*, or their English and French counterparts, the Travelling Brothers and the *Compagnons*?[13]

Although the answer to the 'why' will, as a matter of course, remain hazy in the whirlpool of human motives, the answer to the question of their geographical origin may, sometimes, give an indication of the 'why', as an analysis of the 'where from' question at least holds the promise of a factual basis for the supposition that one or another factor may predominate among the many options outlined above, whether traditional, psychological, social, demographic, or economic.[14] Hereafter, we observe the results of tracing the geographical origins of the eighteenth-century Company surgeons, based on a sample of circa 3,000 of these surgeons during that period. The methodology used can be found in appendix 1. The Republic is, for the sake of this chapter, divided into seven areas: North (the provinces Friesland, Groningen, and the area Drenthe), East (the provinces

Overijssel and Guelders or *Gelderland*), Central (the province of Utrecht) and South (Limburg, Brabant: the *Generaliteitslanden*), North Holland (more or less today's *Noord-Holland*, including the city of Amsterdam), South Holland (today's *Zuid-Holland*), and Zeeland. Using the general historical practice, we will distinguish within North Holland between a *Noorderkwartier* (that part of the province of Holland bordering the River IJ on the south and on the north by the former West Frisian sea dyke) and *West-Friesland* (the area north of the *Noorderkwartier* and together with the *Noorderkwartier* called North Holland). The *Noorderkwartier* basically comprised the quadrangle formed by the towns of Haarlem, Amsterdam, Hoorn (excluding the towns themselves) and Alkmaar (including the town). *West-Friesland* is that area to the north of the *Noorderkwartier*, including the Wadden Islands. Chronologically, the eighteenth century has been divided into four periods: I (1700-1725), II (1726-1750), III (1751-1775), and IV (1776-1795). Results will be presented mostly for the demarcated Dutch areas; some specific attention will be paid to the Company's individual chambers; and because so many German surgeons were on the payroll, they will also be included in the analysis. A brief survey of the economic situation of the Dutch Republic and of contemporary labour streams precedes the results in order to provide the necessary background.

The economy of the Dutch Republic

The Dutch Republic had experienced a period of economic growth which stretched from circa 1460 to 1660, and it was linked to a dramatic growth in population.[15] In the eighteenth century, the Dutch Republic was gradually overshadowed by the expanding power of England at sea and France on land. The decline of Dutch trade was to a certain extent due to their competition.[16] During the second half of the century, most neighbouring states (had) developed aggressive mercantile strategies, from which the products of the Republic were excluded. The intra-European transport of most bulk products, such as corn, wood, wine, tar, and hemp, which until 1740 had been dominated by the Dutch, was progressively taken over by others, which inflicted further economic damage. At the same time, there was an unmistakable reduction in Dutch fishing and industry.[17] The Dutch economic system, which was so dependent on (the production and processing of products for) export, began to disintegrate.

For instance, according to Jonathan Israel, Amsterdam's processing industries were devastated, the number of tobacco-curing factories in the city, for example, shrank from circa 30 in 1720, to eight in 1751, a decline that was not compensated by the growth of Rotterdam's tobacco industry after 1750. The number of cotton presses in Amsterdam slumped from 80 in 1700, to 12 in 1796. The silk industry also experienced a decline.[18] In Leiden, the production of fine cloth and camlets was destroyed in the 1720s and 1730s. Haarlem's fine linen and bleaching industries disintegrated in the 1730s and 1740s. Salt-refining at Enkhuizen, Dordrecht, and Zierikzee collapsed. Bulk transport (Baltic grains and timber) shrank dramatically as Dutch herring, salt, and wine exports all dwindled, so that Hoorn's bulk-transport fleet inexorably shrank and that of Enkhuizen was all but ruined. Zeeland's herring industry had already collapsed some time earlier. The oldest industrialised area of the Netherlands, which had grown up along the banks of the River Zaan in the Noorderkwartier, had some 600 industrial windmills in simultaneous operation at the peak of its prosperity at the beginning of the eighteenth century, mostly used in the sawing of wood, grinding of oil seeds, manufacturing paper, fulling cloth, and husking rice.[19] A considerable number of these windmills fell into disuse and were demolished in circa 1750.[20] The Zaan region of the Noorderkwartier had been the most important centre in Western Europe for shipbuilding, the manufacture of canvas, and the whaling industry. In some villages there, like Graft, practically all of the seafarers worked in the whaling industry.[21] By the 1750s, whale oil, sail canvas, rope making, and shipbuilding, were all in steep decline.

The historian Johan de Vries, author of a still important monograph on the economic decline of the Dutch Republic in the eighteenth century, points out, however, that the textile industry in Twente as well as the peat-digging activities in Vollenhoven (both in the province of Overijssel) continued to thrive. He also drew attention to a persevering, sometimes rising economy in the provinces surrounding Holland.[22] In contrast, Israel concentrates on the collapse of Holland's inland economy after 1750. The Twente linen-weaving industry in Overijssel declined sharply in the 1750s and 1760s. The agrarian historian B.H. Slicher van Bath observed a rapid growth in the population in Overijssel after 1675, despite the rather meagre numbers of jobs available there. After 1750, the economy of Overijssel underwent a severe crisis; the textile industry and population growth declined.[23] Furthermore, in North Brabant, the textile industry in Helmond and surroundings rapidly declined as well. Harlingen, the main industrial town in Friesland, began also its steep decline after 1750.[24] Rural poverty in the inland provinces showed steady increases, especially in Overijssel, Gelderland, Drenthe, and States (or north) Brabant.[25]

In the end, Europe's long-distance trade network was transformed from one largely conducted via the Netherlands, with the Dutch as the all-important buyer-seller and shipper, to one of multiple routes and fierce competition. Although Dutch trade and shipping were able to maintain a level of activity they had reached by the end of the seventeenth century, they could no longer match the dramatic expansion of their French and especially English competitors during the eighteenth century. The eighteenth century concluded with the Fourth Anglo-Dutch War (1780-1784) and the conflict with revolutionary France, both more or less dealing deathblows to the glories of the Republic.

The population of the Dutch Republic

The economic historians Jan de Vries and Ad van der Woude have summarised various characteristics of the Republic's demography. Long before the Republic came into existence, a long-sustained demographic growth was already present, extending from 1460 to about 1660 (which pretty much doubled the Republic's population from one to almost two million). This was followed by a failure to participate in the general European revival of population growth in the second half of the eighteenth century. Furthermore, there were large regional differences in demographic behaviour over relatively short distances; a high level of urbanisation; a large volume of interregional and international migration; and a household structure of an apparently modern type.[26]

Immigration had been a significant factor in the population growth; Protestants and Jews had fled from religious persecution in the southern areas, bringing their business acumen, artisanal skills, and intellectual talents. They were joined by people from war-torn areas, and finally, people came in great numbers simply because of the attractiveness of the Dutch economy, which was accompanied by labour shortages. Demographic and economic development were intimately linked. The process of land reclamation in North Holland had led to an increase of no less than 40 per cent of the total area under cultivation with the Wormer, Schermer, Purmer, and Beemster lakes having been drained in the seventeenth century. Here, as elsewhere in Holland, there had been a tremendous rise in population between 1514 and 1622: the areas of West Friesland and the Noorderkwartier had seen a population rise of 150 per cent. The whole region formed part of the most densely populated rural area of the province of Holland. North-Holland became the cradle and major recruitment area for seamen and fishermen.[27] The towns lying along the Zuider Zee, and particularly the West Frisian towns of Hoorn and Enkhuizen, developed considerable trade and shipping industries of their own.

After the Peace of Westphalia (1648), immigration dwindled, only to increase again with the temporary influx of Huguenots from France (after the Revocation of the Edict of Nantes by Louis XIV in 1685). Meanwhile, the 'economic migration' from 'Germany' continued well into the nineteenth century. Despite these influxes, the overall effect was one of stabilisation: population decline in northern Holland and in the regions around the Zuider Zee was compensated by increases in the eastern and southern provinces.[28] In particular, the booming industries in the Noorderkwartier and West Friesland, where the towns of Hoorn, Enkhuizen, and Zaandam had profited from fishing, whaling, shipbuilding and agriculture as a result of the cultivation of reclaimed land, declined, as did the demand for (skilled) labour. The depression caused a population decline of some 40 to 50 per cent between 1650 and 1750.[29] Despite this, the historian Paul van Royen did not yet note any decline in the quantity or quality of seafarers in northern Holland in the period 1700-1710.[30] Indeed, the population decrease was not evenly divided throughout the area; some villages like Graft in the Noorderkwartier were affected much later by this trend. Graft's population was still 1,487 in 1747 and only began to show a decline in the second half of the eighteenth century, when by the end of the century, the population had decreased to 1,113.[31]

Increasing complaints by the Company and the Admiralties were heard that seafarers were nowhere to be found and that the mariners who did apply did not have the 'sea legs', in other words, did not have the seafaring qualities that they had been used to in previous decades, or worse, they represented the 'scum of the earth', scrounged together by the crimps who lured them in. This image became a popular stereotype. Although Van der Woude, the leading historian of the economic history of the Noorderkwartier area, noted a considerable improvement after 1760, there was no returning to the former prosperity.[32] Again, in Graft, the sailors' insurance policies (*zeevarende buidels*) show that it was only after 1768 that seafarers' insurance policy numbers declined drastically. In 1781, there were no applicants at all, and in 1793, it happened again.[33] There is ample evidence that the eighteenth century was a period of contraction and depression, though not simultaneously and conditions were not equally grave in all areas of Holland.

The sometimes spectacular decline in population was somewhat balanced by growth in other regions of the Republic. South Holland showed a period of substantial population growth between 1514-1622, and again after 1622, though not as spectacular as the earlier increases. The population of Rotterdam increased by over 172 percent between 1622 and 1795, albeit most of this occurred between 1622 and 1690; growth stagnated in the first half of the eighteenth century, to resume at a slow pace in the second half.[34] The Republic's eastern provinces underwent a natural increase in population, rather than one due to economic circumstances. In Overijssel, for example, the population increased from 97,253 in 1675, to 132,124 in 1764 and to 134,104 inhabitants in 1795.[35]

Labour migration streams

Mobility was the norm in pre-industrial Europe as so many had to travel to find work.[36] As L. Page Moch phrased it in her book *Moving Europeans*, 'the poor were the bulk of migrants on the roads of Europe, for their livelihoods were least secure'. This was because the children of landless peasants could not all be supported by their families and so they set out on their own to secure a future for themselves, resulting in large numbers of young men and young women migrating along the roads and seaways.[37] For northwestern Europe, the 1650-1750 period was a period of economic stagnation, in which the urbanised and industrialised Republic, along with a few other regions, formed an exception. Europe in that time was still mainly a rural world. The vast majority lived in villages or very small towns. Only one in nine lived in a city with a population of 5,000 or more.[38] Men and women married late, which meant that a large number of single people could move easily from one household to another. Networks of acquaintances and kin generated migration streams, as information about livelihoods was shared by families and friends,[39] leading to, for instance, an estimated 15,000 German workers who crossed the Zuider Zee to Amsterdam every year for seasonal work in Holland by 1700, to 25,000 by 1730, and probably 30,000 around 1790.[40]

In her study, Page Moch (re-)classifies certain migration patterns within pre-industrial Western Europe, namely local migration (in which people moved within their own home, land or labour market); circular migration (people moved back and forth as with seasonal migration); chain migration (in which social arrangements were made with people already at a destination, who helped newcomers find jobs and housing); and career migration (in which the needs and location of an employer rather than village contacts or family needs determined the timing and destination of migrants).[41] As will be shown, the ship's surgeon may fit in all of these patterns, except for the first, and as such these categories are not very useful for the professional group of surgical craftsmen. This having been said, the various migration patterns do somewhat add, refine, and overlap earlier migration pattern categories. It was customary to single out family migration, which was usually permanent. In pre-modern Europe, it was almost invariably due to religious persecution. In the sixteenth century, people in this category were largely immigrants from the Southern Netherlands, and in the seventeenth century it was the French Huguenots who emigrated to the Republic in 1685. The religious persecution-induced migration of Jews from Poland, Germany, and Central Europe acquired impetus after 1726, and was also usually permanent.[42]

Another category is that of seasonal migration, which characterises the early-modern period. This was the result of a symbiosis between areas with a labour surplus and mono-cropping regions with a strong seasonal labour demand. The seasonal labourers came mainly from East Frisia, Lower Saxony and Westphalia in Germany and they worked as seasonal labourers in Groningen and as peat cutters on the Drenthe moors. These labourers formed part of the North Sea Migration System and their arrival in the Republic was purely motivated by economics: they came in search of work. This *Hollandgängerei* began in the early seventeenth century when Germans from Westphalia began travelling to the Republic seeking seasonal work, where wages, at that time, were relatively high compared to wages in Westphalia. This group of seasonal workers included foreign labourers working in the alkaline lead-carbonate mills on the Zaan and in Amsterdam, in the linen bleacheries in Haarlem, and there were many foreign labourers in the 'mud' mills of Amsterdam and the Zaan. Grass mowing (*hannekemaaiers*) and reaping grain, harvesting industrial crops such as flax and madder, land reclamation, dredging and cutting peat, industrial jobs such as construction, brick-making and bleaching, logging on the major rivers, and peddling and hawking, were all seasonal jobs. The labourers, usually German, came to Amsterdam via three routes: via the Rhine on barges to Cologne, then to Nijmegen and on to Amsterdam; via the Elbe to Hamburg, by ship along the coast of Friesland, from Hasselt by boat via the Zuider Zee to Amsterdam; or through Lower Saxony to Groningen and Leeuwarden, and from Leeuwarden, traversing the Zuider Zee to Amsterdam.[43]

Seasonal and non-seasonal labour migration are both, as per the definition in J. Lucassen's thesis, *Naar de kusten van de Noordzee*, defined as workers employed too far from their homes that they are unable to return at night. These workers quickly made the transition from migrant labour to permanent migration, as most of them were young and single.[44] They include groups like the *Wanderburschen*, the English Travelling Brothers, the French *Compagnons*, as well as mercenary soldiers, long-distance sailors, domestic servants (maids), as well as itinerant traders, pedlars, and jugglers. An inevitable component of this category was also a mixed bag of vagrants, beggars, the wealthy, the professionals, and university students, who had the means to travel far and wide.[45] This was especially true of aspiring craftsmen whose families could afford an apprenticeship.[46] Clearly, a seafarer working for the Company was a non-seasonal migrant labourer according to the definition because Company fleets embarked for Asia around Easter, in September, and at Christmas (*Paasvloot*, *Kermisvloot*, and *Kerstvloot*) and were usually not expected back within two years.

As part of his thesis, Lucassen defined 'pull areas', which attracted labourers, and 'push areas' which people departed in search of work. An example of the first is the coastline of the North Sea roughly stretching from Calais to Bremen; an example of the second one is Westphalia, the northwest reaches of Brabant, the Liège and Hainaut/Picardy region, and parts of the Eifel and the Hunsrück. Together, they comprise the North Sea System. The 'pull area' had a number of distinct characteristics. The configuration of the means of production conspired to promote the emergence of mono-cropping, and was also affected by an insufficiency of available local labour to satisfy demand during peak seasons. Therefore, the work offered sufficiently attractive remuneration for labourers from elsewhere to leave their homes regularly each season. Such *foci* of attraction were counterbalanced by *foci* of expulsion, where the economic climate was not as sunny, usually in the hinterland.[47]

Basic wages were already fairly high in the Republic in the seventeenth century, certainly compared to Germany and Scandinavia, and these financial advantages attracted many to work in the Republic, even if only seasonally. The eighteenth-century Dutch recession induced a restructuring of the labour market, which became essential because of reduced employment opportunities. This caused a new increase of (redundant) non-seasonal migrant labourers who could be swept up as crews for the Company's ships. At the beginning of the nineteenth century, the labour attractive area was pretty much still the coast between Calais and Bremen. At that moment, the Dutch expulsion regions included the Veluwe, Overijssel, the Drenthe-Frisian peat moors to the Münster-Osnabrück-Minden-Lüneburg border, although most of the labourers from these areas migrated to Denmark and Mecklenburg.[48]

Maritime recruitment

Jan Lucassen divided the most important seagoing nations into four groups according to their recruitment policies: those with mixed systems of free and forced labour, as in France, Portugal, Spain, Venice and other Mediterranean countries, which prevailed until the abolition of the galleys; nations that recruited mainly national free labour, as in Scandinavia, Germany, and Great Britain, although press gangs were used in emergencies, and to a certain extent in France and Spain after the galley period. National recruitment of forced labour, occurred in Russia in the eighteenth and early nineteenth centuries, and national and international recruitment of free labour was the source of labour in the Dutch Republic.[49]

Recruitment of personnel is – of course – defined by the need for it. In Spain and in France, the demand surpassed 30,000. It was extremely exceptional if the annual demand for sailors in any Western European country prior to 1700 exceeded a total of 50,000. However, at the end of the seventeenth century, more than 50,000 men were indeed needed to man English and Dutch Republic ships (table T4.1).

Table T4.1: Estimate of sailors on Dutch vessels [50]

Year	1680	1725	1770
Total	55000	60000	60000

These seafarers should have been relatively easy to find in countries like France, with a population of circa twenty million, or England, with its circa ten million, or Spain (somewhat less than ten million). If one assumes that the male working population in these countries constituted one-quarter of the total population, this would mean that sailors represented one-half a per cent of the total workforce in France, circa two per cent in Spain and in England, but nearly ten per cent in the Republic, with its population of circa two million.[51] The governments of England, France, and Spain had their own methods to ensure that enough men were recruited to work their ships. The Company of Surgeons in London, for instance, had a nation-wide mandate to use press-gang methods to ensure that a sufficient number of surgeons joined the Royal Navy. The disadvantage was that it might press journeymen, or men who had only a limited licence, for instance, a practitioner in midwifery, or an optometrist, a cataract specialist, a dentist, a venereal 'specialist', a bone setter, and those who performed minor surgeries for hernias, wryneck, kidney stones, or a harelip. The London Company had the authority to send any of them to the ships to deal with war casualties or those incurred on the ships of privateers.[52] In contrast, the Dutch recruited free labour, which was quite another thing altogether.

The Company was the largest private employer in the Republic. On the more than 4,700 voyages made by the Company from the Republic to Asia between 1602 and 1795, nearly one million people departed from Dutch shores headed to the East. During the same period, somewhat more than one-third of them returned to the Netherlands. Some caution is due here as these figures are somewhat deceptive because they include men who went back and forth to the East several times.[53] In the eighteenth century, the emphasis of this labour migration lies on the outward-bound voyages. As bureaucracy intensified, consolidation of territories spread, and mortality ran high in Asia as well as on board, the Company needed ever-increasing numbers of seafarers and soldiers in the eighteenth century (graph G4.1).[54]

Graph G4.1: Total number of persons on board the Dutch East Indiamen (1602-1795)[55]

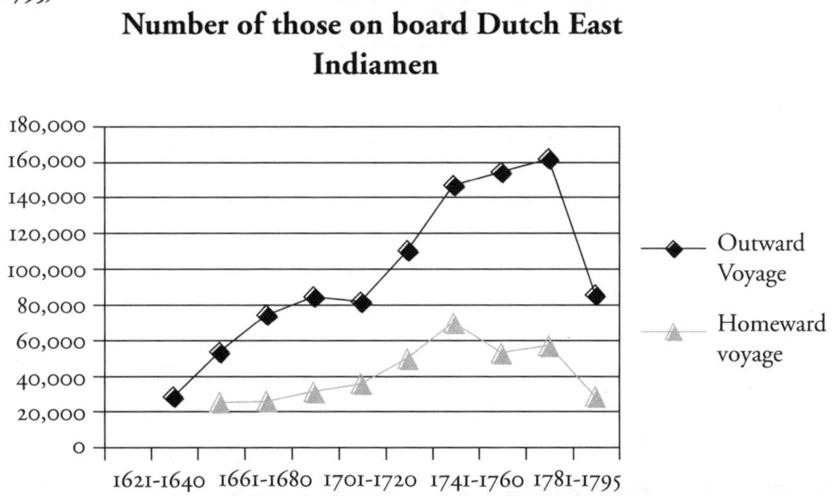

Of course, this could only be met if there was appropriate population growth within the nation, but this had come to a standstill since 1650. The Dutch Republic's population remained stable at circa 1,900,000 for nearly a century.[56] This had dire consequences on recruitment activities. A labour force had to be found elsewhere, in the interior and abroad, and the crews were often comprised of many Germans or Scandinavians during the course of the eighteenth century, as is demonstrated in table T4.2. It should also be noted, that no 'headhunters' were actively recruiting crews for the Company in these countries. These 'foreigners' arrived in the Republic's ports of their own accord in the wake of migration streams.

The Company was in much the same situation as the Dutch Admiralties. It was barely able to recruit sufficient and able manpower locally or nationally. Boxer expressed it as follows: 'One of the most striking differences between the *Gouden Eeuw* (seventeenth century) and the *Pruikentijd* (eighteenth century) was the real apparent decline of the Dutch Republic as a maritime power – a decline which was reflected in an increasing shortage of the native born seamen, *varend volk*.'[57]

Table T4.2: Geographic origins of Company sailors and craftsmen in percentages [58]

	1700	*1710*	*1720*	*1730*	*1740*	*1750*	*1760*	*1770*	*1780*	*1790*
Dutch Republic	77	76	73	62	59	50	56	47	54	48
North Holland	49	47	45	41	44	44	37	41	46	40
South Holland	26	30	28	32	30	27	28	25	23	24
Zeeland	12	9	9	10	10	9	12	12	5	12
Friesland	4	4	6	5	4	5	5	5	6	7
Utrecht	3	2	3	3	3	4	4	4	4	3
Other Provinces	6	8	9	9	9	11	14	13	16	14
Abroad	23	24	27	38	41	50	44	53	46	52
Scandinavia	27	26	21	29	21	29	15	23	21	16
German Coast	38	38	38	38	32	32	28	22	26	23
Rest Germany	11	13	13	12	20	14	21	23	23	27
Belgium, France, Luxembourg	11	10	13	9	11	7	13	12	8	8
Other countries	13	13	15	12	16	18	23	20	22	26

Various factors other than those specified above also helped determine the discrepancy between the Company's high demand for labour and the low supply. The increasing mortality rates on the ships and in Asia during the eighteenth century naturally raised the demand for manpower there. One major problem was that the Dutch autochthonous population was relatively small and a lack of flexibility and mobility prevailed within the various categories of seafarers: Dutch coasters and fishing crafts recruited virtually all their crew locally,[59] and seamen often proved loyal to their trade, ships, and captains, so much so that coastal seafarers stuck to their coastal sea trade or sea fishing activities, while merchant-fleet crews remained tied to the merchant fleet, and no whalers ever entered the employ of the Company.[60] The sailors of Graft usually sailed under the same whaling *commandeur* for years.[61] Another exacerbating factor was that working for the Company or the Admiralty was considered unsavoury, at least in the seventeenth century. In fact, West Frisians from the countryside were averse to going to Asia, to working for the Admiralty, or enlisting on an armed privateer's ship.[62] The West Frisian seaman was usually only driven by his penury to take service on one of the Company's risky voyages. Especially as there was more to be earned by signing on with mercantile, whaling, or herring companies than by being employed by the Company or Admiralty, although service at the Company did offer the possibility of the private trade in luxury goods such as spices from Asia.[63] Surgeon Nicolaas de Graaff, however, does not seem to display any of these characteristics. He sailed whenever his fancy took him, on a whaler, with the Admiralties or the merchant fleet, or to the East Indies. But then, perhaps a lack of flexibility was not applicable to ship's surgeons after all, or at least not in the seventeenth century?

The recruitment of sailors and soldiers by the Company had never been a sinecure. Graph G4.1, for instance shows that each year a greater number were needed to work the ships and/or in the settlements at the Cape of Good Hope or in Asia. The captains (*schippers*) of the ships were directly engaged by the 'managers' of the local chambers. The enlistment of sailors, soldiers, and petty officers was, however, a different matter altogether, and was usually done via mediation. There was no advertising policy at the chambers of the Company and no propaganda, except that prior to sailing, official Company drummers would rouse the town's men and implore them to enlist. It seems likely that the ship's surgeons were recruited by word of mouth, and this kind of recruitment 'procedure' was autonomous on the part of the Company. Migration information was shared by kin, friends, and acquaintances who often chose the same destination and helped each other find work.

These networks explain why the migrants concentrated on particular destinations and occupations. For instance, surgery had a good reputation in the Republic and for many a surgical journeyman or master surgeon in search of knowledge and experience, this must have been an adequate enough reason to visit the cities of Holland. The information passed on about a particular location created migration streams between a home area and a destination. Surgical migration streams were thus generated by webs of relationships.[64] When he was 12 years old, the Swiss-born David Henry Gallandat (1732-1782), for instance, travelled to the Dutch province of Zeeland to stay with his uncle on his mother's side,

Dr J.H. de Bruas. De Bruas was a city physician of Flushing (Vlissingen) and David was introduced to the profession by his uncle. He acquired nautical surgical experience in the merchant fleet, for which he was examined and certified as a first surgeon in 1751. Subsequently, he made three journeys to Guinea and the West Indies. In 1757, David travelled to Paris where the *Académie Royale de Chirurgie* elevated the surgical profession to academic status, to broaden his medical knowledge. On his subsequent return to Flushing in 1759, he opened a surgeon's shop there. The Flushing authorities acknowledged his great surgical expertise by offering him the function of City Surgeon and City Obstetrician in 1766. In 1772, he was promoted to the position of the provincial 'cutter of the stone' (*lands-steensnijder*). He crowned his surgical career by defending his doctorate degree on *De Sectione Caesara* at the University of Harderwijk in 1775, where Boerhaave had also presented his doctorate thesis.[65] In short, David's family used its relations to ensure his future. And so did the family of ship's surgeon Charles Ghislain Wilmet who was born in Gembloux (Austrian Netherlands). He lodged with a colleague in Rotterdam, master surgeon Van Putten, in 1779, from whose house he visited the authorities of the Chamber of Rotterdam in order to apply for surgical employment with the Company. Wilmet apparently used his surgical network, which determined his travelling to the Rotterdam Chamber of the Company.

Sailors and soldiers were often enlisted by the so-called *volkshouders* or crimps, and the (health-care) problems resulting from that type of recruitment were shown in chapter 2. Ship's surgeons, it is safe to say were generally not crimped. There is only the occasional indication of this practice regarding ship's surgeons in the financial records of the ships (*scheepssoldijboeken*), but no structural hard data. Besides, the reputation of these crimps was not unknown among the surgeons. One German surgeon wrote, upon arriving in Amsterdam in 1715, that those who wanted to sail would do better to find a good captain, a good, fast-sailing, sturdy vessel, and to avoid the crimps.[66] The results of an ongoing study of the recruitment practices of the sea officers at the Chamber of Hoorn, to which we will return in the next chapter, show that surgeons often requested specific surgical functions on specific vessels, which certainly does not support the crimp theories, as crimps would not have been particularly bothered about these details.[67] Over and above this, many of these prospective ship's surgeons were rejected by this chamber.

Eventually, a substantial number of foreigners were found among the crews of the long-distance vessels. On average, during the period of the Company's existence, 40 per cent of the sailors were foreign, as were 60 per cent of the soldiers on board. The number of foreigners in the service of the Company changed over time. In the first half of the seventeenth century, it rose to circa 50 per cent; then, a decline set in, also in absolute numbers. The recruitment of foreigners began to rise again after 1700 and surpassed that of Dutchmen after 1730. In circa 1770, 80 per cent of the soldiers on board and 50 per cent of the sailors were foreign.[68] Of the craftsmen on board between 1720 and 1750, 40 to 55 per cent were Dutch, and of the (60 to 45 per cent) foreigners 20 to 30 per cent were German.[69] By comparison, during the period 1700-1710, 20 to 25 per cent of the men in the Dutch merchant fleet, operating between Archangel and Portugal were foreign; 30 to 40 per cent of the crew on the Europe–West Africa–Caribbean route were foreign. Meanwhile, in the eighteenth century over 50 per cent of the warships crews were foreign; and 75 per cent of whaling fleet crews were foreigners.[70] Fortunately, the Republic could claim some kind of hinterland from which to recruit in the German states, the Southern Netherlands and even beyond that.[71]

Germans comprised the largest group among the Company's foreign seafarers. At the Chambers of Enkhuizen and Hoorn, half of this contingent of Germans serving on Company ships at the beginning of the eighteenth century came from the regions bordering the North Sea and the Baltic Sea. The foreign captains of the Dutch East Indiamen were nearly all German or Scandinavian and/or came from the North Sea or Baltic Sea areas. They were commonly from places like Bremen, Schleswig, Drammen, or Stockholm.[72] As the century progressed increasing numbers of these foreigners came from the inland areas of Germany.[73] The German surgeon Johan Andreas Muller was born in Magdenburg, in the region of Saxony-Anhalt, rather a long way from the Republic's coast. Muller had clearly wanted to make his fortune in Asia, to which end he took along products to Asia in copious quantities. His plans came, as we have seen, to nothing, leaving his mother not only bereft of her son but also attempting in vain to recover his initial investment of at least 2,200 Dutch guilders.[74] Muller was not the only Company employee who tried to profit from his employment. So willing were many of these employees that they did not even care what job they had on board, as a result of which the relationship between their standard of education – rank during tenureship with the Company – and function after Company tenureship were often quite different. Jurgen Andersen, for instance, after having received excellent schooling in Germany, sailed to Asia as a sergeant. After his employment with the Company, he became a public servant for the Duke of Schleswig-Holstein, and published his Company experiences. Johan von der Behr, enlisted as a soldier, later became a notary in Leipzig.[75] Many an educated German would enlist as a soldier on the Company payroll.

In the seventeenth and eighteenth centuries, many foreigners thought that it was almost impossible to work for the Company in any other capacity than as a soldier. This impression was to a certain extent true. The Company's policy was to ensure that the ship's officers and high-ranking administrative servants were mostly Dutch citizens to better ensure their loyalty to the Company.[76] As the function of ship's surgeon did not *a priori* mean managing a ship and/or a settlement, it might be supposed that this consideration was, perhaps, less important in hiring surgeons. However, it appears that these German surgeons were often employed in a lesser function than their educations warranted. Christoph Frik (1659, Ulm, Germany – after 1717, Batavia?) was trained as a surgeon by master surgeon Bartholomaeus Heking, the City Surgeon in Ulm.[77] After his formal training, he made several journeys through Austria, Switzerland, Bohemia, Saxony, and Silesia. However, for his first voyage for the Company, he was employed only as a surgeon's mate from 1681 to 1685.[78] Johan Jacob Merklein (1620, Windsheim, Germany – 1700), a physician's son and educated as a surgeon was hired as a surgeon's mate, and not as a full surgeon in 1644.[79] As there were usually more prospective surgeons than vacancies, the Germans played it safe and usually applied for several surgical functions on several outward-bound vessels. Philip Pieter Musculus, another German, was so eager that he applied for the functions of full surgeon, surgeon's mate and third surgeon on two vessels in 1731.[80] There must have been numerous German surgeons like Musculus, many of whom were rejected, and who then, quite plausibly, may even have found employment as Company soldiers, waiting for an opportunity to return to their former profession. They remained anonymous because they never published their experiences, but often returned to their home country, married and practised as a surgeon in their native villages, or they simply died too soon.

Of the sample of 3,000 surgeons, no less than 715 non-Dutch ship's surgeons entered the service of the Company in this capacity during the eighteenth century, one-quarter of the total sample. They became a significant group, especially after 1725, and they comprised nearly half of all of the Company surgeons by the end of the century (table T4.3). One may well wonder whether these non-Dutch surgeons were part of a particular labour migration stream as delineated by Lucassen.[81]

Table T4.3: Non-Dutch Company surgeons within the sample (excluding those of unknown origin)

Period	*Non-Dutch surgeons*	*Total Company surgeons*
1700-1725	86 (10%)	853
1726-1750	198 (23.5%)	843
1751-1775	210 (29%)	733
1776-1795	221 (40%)	559

The changes in the distribution patterns of all national and foreign employees of the Company are summarised in table T4.2. This table sets out the growing proportion of foreigners in the course of the eighteenth century in response to the demand/supply discrepancy. The question 'is a similar change in the ratio

Dutchmen/foreigners also to be observed among the category of Company ship's surgeons' is answered in table T4.4, which clearly demonstrates that the decline in Dutch participation as Company surgeons sets in after 1720. A recovery is seen after 1750, but after 1760 the decline sets in again, and now rather sharply. The percentage of non-Dutch surgeons in the employ of the Company is significantly smaller if compared to table T4.2, although it follows the same trend.

Table T4.4: Geographic origins of Company's surgeons in the eighteenth century [82]

	1700	*1710*	*1720*	*1730*	*1740*	*1750*	*1760*	*1770*	*1780*	*1790**
Republic	87%	97%	93%	85%	71%	53%	100%	61%	67%	55%
Non-Dutch	13%	3%	7%	14%	29%	43%	0%	35%	33%	41%

* 4 percent of unknown origin.

Besides filling medical or surgical vacancies at the Cape and in Asia, the basic need for ship's surgeons of the chambers, assuming that the average ratio between ships and surgeons should be at least 1:3 (three surgeons per one outward-bound ship) was, for most of the eighteenth century, adequately fulfilled for all of the chambers, although the Zeeland Chamber appears to have had some problems in the second period; Rotterdam in the first two periods; and Delft in the first and fourth periods (table T4.5). Despite complaints heard during the century about the lack of surgeons at the Company, the Amsterdam Chamber grew in significance as surgical recruiter. The Batavian cry for more surgeons was answered by an intensified recruitment in the latter period, when occasionally six to seven surgeons were employed on an outward-bound vessel.

Table T4.5: Ratio between ships and surgeons supplied to the ships per chamber

Chambers: *Period*	*Amsterdam* *Ratio*	*Zeeland* *Ratio*	*Hoorn* *Ratio*	*Enkhuizen* *Ratio*	*Rotterdam* *Ratio*	*Delft* *Ratio*
1700-1725	1:2.9	1:2.9	1:2.9	1:3.2	1:2.9	1:2.9
1726-1750	1:3.0	1:2.5	1:2.9	1:3.0	1:2.9	1:3.0
1751-1775	1:3.1	1:3.2	1:3.0	1:3.0	1:3.0	1:3.0
1776-1795	1:4.0	1:3.6	1:4.0	1:3.2	1:3.7	1:3.0

If a particular chamber experienced recruitment problems, did this show up in the chamber's pattern of recruitment areas?

Dutch recruitment

Around 1700, nearly 90 per cent of the Company's ship's surgeons recruited were Dutch. The majority came from the Dutch maritime provinces Holland (60 per cent), Zeeland (17.5 per cent) and Gelderland and Overijssel (12 per cent). Only 8 per cent of the ship's surgeons were non-Dutch, and four-fifths of this group were German. By the end of the Company's existence, the recruitment patterns had shifted quite radically. Dutch surgical participation on the Company's labour market had declined from 89 per cent to 52 per cent; this decline was the most dramatic for the eastern region and northern Holland, and extremely striking for Zeeland, only somewhat balanced by the recovery of Dutch participation in South Holland and the southern region (table T4.6).

Table T4.6: Geographical origins of Company's surgeons around 1699/1700 and 1789/1790

	Period	*998/999*	*998/999*
Total		64	100
Dutch		57 (89%)	52 (52%)
of which:	North (Friesland, Drenthe, Groningen)	3 (5%)	4 (8%)
	East (Gelderland, Overijssel)	7 (12%)	3 (6%)
	Central (Utrecht)	2 (3.5%)	2 (4%)
	South (northern Brabant and Limburg)	1 (2%)	5 (10%)
	North Holland	20 (35%)	14 (27%)
	South Holland	14 (25%)	22 (42%)
	Zeeland	10 (17.5%)	2 (4%)
Unknown origin		2	5
Non-Dutch		5 (8%)	43 (43%)
of which:	Germany	4 (80%)	24 (80%)

Of the sampled ship's surgeons in the service of the Company during the entire eighteenth century, 72 per cent were Dutch and 24 per cent were non-Dutch, the remaining 4 per cent were of unknown origin.[83] As is demonstrated in table T4.7, Dutch surgical recruitment was largely concentrated in Holland. The coastal province of Zeeland was much less significant as a supplier of surgeons than North and South Holland, and ranks almost lower than the East region. The 'Holland' recruitment regions declined in significance after 1725; Zeeland declined spectacularly after 1775. In view of the small numbers of surgeons from the North, South, and Central regions, we may conclude that these areas were in fact negligible as recruitment areas.

Table T4.7: Recruitment of Dutch surgeons per area (in absolute numbers and percentages) within the sample

Period	*North*	*East*	*Central*	*South*	*North-Holland*	*South-Holland*	*Zeeland*	*Total Dutch surgeons*
1700-1725	28 (4%)	69 (9%)	20 (3%)	9 (1%)	312 (41%)	231 (31%)	88 (12%)	757
1726-50	32 (5%)	88 (15%)	18 (3%)	20 (3%)	200 (33%)	167 (28%)	79 (13%)	604
1751-75	11 (2%)	58 (12%)	18 (4%)	12 (2%)	182 (36%)	153 (30%)	74 (15%)	508
1776-96	18 (6%)	27 (9%)	9 (3%)	24 (8%)	113 (37%)	100 (33%)	17 (6%)	308

Northern area

The northern area, consisting of the provinces Friesland, Groningen, and Drenthe (the last being an 'area' which had come directly under the States-General's jurisdiction in 1594) was mainly agricultural. Just 3 per cent (89 ship's surgeons) of the total number of Dutch ship's surgeons in this sample came from this region to try their luck with the Company. Of these, 63 per cent went to the Amsterdam Chamber. The surgical trek from this area to Amsterdam confirms the trend recognised in Hart's study about labour migration from Friesland and Groningen to Amsterdam, which became a well-trodden path during the first half of the eighteenth century, followed by a sharp decline during the second half.[84] In Friesland, the surgeons came mostly from the larger cities (Leeuwarden, Harlingen, and Dokkum). According to Israel, the Frisian economy underwent a severe depression (i.e., Harlingen) after 1750, which coincides with the decline in the numbers of Frisian surgeons in the employ of the Company.

The Groningen surgeons left in groups: one party left in the 1720s, another one (another 25 per cent) in the 1730s, yet another (25 per cent) in the 1770s, the remaining 25 per cent in between; most of them stated they had come from the provincial capital, Groningen. Hart's study also shows that the city of Groningen yielded the most migrants who left this province for Amsterdam in search of work in general,[85] although it is unclear if all of these migrants actually came from the city of Groningen as no birth registers were checked; they may well have originated from the surrounding countryside (*Ommelanden*). Amongst the Frisian and Groningen ship's surgeons-to-be, no family relationships, which could have served as a motive for seeking employment, were detected. In all probability, these professionals influenced one another with their migration stories and experiences, as they left in groups, and they all came from an urban environment.

Of the 15 surgeons from the Drenthe area (in our sample), four appear to have been related, and came from the city of Meppel: Hermanus and Josephus Bolle were brothers, and so were Jan and Lambertus Donk. The family connection must have played a role in their reasons for wanting to seek employment with the Company. Meppel was the only significant city in Drenthe in terms of trade and industry and it was the only city in the area with a Latin School, the essential preparation for any academic pursuits.[86] Furthermore, Meppel was the place to find physicians, pharmacists, and surgeons.[87] Also in Drenthe, the *trek* took place in the first half of the century, with Israel noting an increase in rural poverty after 1750.

To recap, surgical recruitment from this northern area was primarily an urban one. The surgeons came mainly from the cities of Groningen, Harlingen, Leeuwarden, and Meppel (appendix 2, Map A2.1). This recruitment took place mostly in the first half of the century, and was mainly associated with the Amsterdam Chamber.

Eastern area

The eastern region was out of tune with the rest of the Dutch Republic as it continued to experience peacetime population growth between 1650 and 1750, as the result of the introduction of labour-intensive crops (tobacco), the spread of rural industrial employment (paper and linen), and employment in the peat bogs. The decline, however, began in 1750, in contrast to the rest of the Republic.[88] Some 242 ship's surgeons departed from the eastern agricultural provinces Gelderland and Overijssel (within the sample taken here) during the eighteenth century, with totals being more or less evenly divided between the two provinces. Of these, more than half were employed by the Company Chamber of Amsterdam, although after 1750 the Chambers of Enkhuizen and Hoorn became more attractive as prospective employers. There was a steady flow of surgical migrants from Overijssel to the coastal areas along the North Sea during the century, but the emphasis on migration to the chambers of the Company occurred mainly during the period before 1760 (80 surgeons). Of the Overijssel surgeons, one-fifth came from the Twente area, especially Oldenzaal. Family ties among the surgeons were strong among those from Overijssel as one-fifth of them were related, with the Bello family of Zwolle being typical with no less than five family members joining the Company. Besides Oldenzaal, the cities of Kampen, Zwolle, and Deventer also supplied surgeons for the Company. The historian and archivist S. Hart claimed that general labour migration from Overijssel (to Amsterdam) showed a steady plateau during the first half of the century, which was followed by a decline after 1750. Slicher van Bath, Israel, De Vries, and Van der Woude all noted a sharp economic decline in this area in the 1750s and 1760s.

The same applies to the surgical migration from Gelderland to the Company chambers, although the peak of surgical migration to the Company occurred in the second quarter of the century. A sharp decline of (surgical) migration to Amsterdam occurred after 1760. Half of the Gelderland surgeons came from the Achterhoek region, especially the cities of Doesburg, Bredevoort, and Zutphen. Other Gelderland towns that figured prominently were Arnhem, Elburg, Nijmegen, and Winterswijk (appendix 2, Map A2.2). In all probability, family ties were a motive for joining the Company as 9 per cent of the Gelderland surgeons were related to each other, for instance, Johannes Jaspers and Lucas Johannes Jaspers from Bredevoort; Hendrik and Jan Haagelbos from Doetinchem; the Elburg brothers Gerrit and Hendrik Kuilenburg; the Groenlo brothers Jan and Pieter Crabbenburg; and even a grandson from Nijmegen followed his grandfather's footsteps: Hermanus and Pieter Heijligers.

The migration of surgeons from the eastern area to the various Company chambers was, like its northern counterpart, an urban recruitment effort; concentrated on the regions of Twente and the Achterhoek; and the bulk of it mainly took place during the first half of the eighteenth century. For instance, during the period 1700-1750, the cities of Arnhem, Bredevoort, Dalfsen, Doesburg, Deventer, Elburg, Hasselt, Groenlo, Kampen, Oldenzaal, Nijmegen, Zutphen and Zwolle each supplied more than four surgeons. In the period 1750-1776, there were only four cities left in this area with any significant contributions of surgeons, namely Arnhem (4), Doesburg (4), Kampen (9), and Zwolle (9). In the last period, only Nijmegen managed to supply four surgeons, as recruitment of this area became more diffuse and less significant.

The south and central areas

Although the surgeons from the province of Utrecht were mostly attracted to the Chamber of Amsterdam, those from the South (Brabant and Limburg) applied mainly to the Rotterdam and Zeeland Chambers, probably because of their geographical proximity. These two regions managed to supply 128 ship's surgeons (according to the sample). Family tradition did not appear to play a role in Brabant, and most of Brabant's surgeons (70 per cent) were recruited after 1740 (with two peak decades being 1740-1750 and 1780-1790, in which migration information must have been a significant factor). Here as well, the recruitment was mainly an urban and regional phenomenon as the surgeons came predominantly from cities such as Breda, 's Hertogenbosch (or Den Bosch, Bois-le-Duc), and Bergen op Zoom, although this area became an expulsion area as its economic decline began in 1747, when the transit route for products (once centered on the capital 's Hertogenbosch) disappeared as a result of the shift towards Liège.[89] At the same time, both Limburg and Brabant enjoyed population growth between 1750 and 1795, corresponding to the development of industry and commerce in the Austrian Netherlands (Belgium).[90] Limburg underwent successful urbanisation as exemplified by the city of Maastricht in the eighteenth century, which was possibly attributable to the stimuli this city received from the metallurgical and textiles industries from the nearby Liège region.[91] Only 18 surgeons came from Limburg and most of them were born in Limburg's capital of Maastricht (appendix 2, Map A2.2 and Map A2.3).

Geographically, the province of Utrecht is the central province of the Republic. A slight emphasis in the surgical migration from Utrecht can be seen during the second half of the eighteenth century. The major part of the Utrecht surgical labour migration to the Company took place between 1770 and 1780. Of the 65 surgeons in the sample, 42 came from the capital city Utrecht, and six from Amersfoort. From this province, the ship's surgeons-to-be left in batches: twenty-five of them left before 1730, then a decline in surgical migration set in, only to flare up again in a one-decade peak in 1770-1780, when ten surgeons left the province.

North Holland

Most of the surgeons recruited were born in North Holland, not surprisingly as this area was also the cradle of many a Dutch sailor. In this area alone, we find three Company chambers, those of Amsterdam, Enkhuizen, and Hoorn. North Holland delivered some 807 of the sampled sea surgeons (27 per cent of the total number of ship's surgeons sampled; 37 per cent of the total number of Dutch sampled ship's surgeons). The Noorderkwartier region did not offer much to the Company in the way of a surgical recruitment area (appendix 2, Map A2.4). This is understandable, as this region had few urban areas. It delivered only 31 surgeons sampled (1 per cent of the total number of surgeons) to the Company, and most of them went to the Chamber of Hoorn (18 surgeons) and that of Amsterdam (ten surgeons). Overall, the recruitment accent lay on the second half of the century. Most *Noorderkwartier* surgeons were natives of Alkmaar (17).

West Friesland includes the cities (and Chambers) of Hoorn and Enkhuizen. Enkhuizen had a population of circa 20,000 inhabitants in 1640. Its economy was based on the fishing fleet (herring), the merchant fleet (salt, grain, tar, and wood), the Company, salt-works and sugar refineries, and the whaling fleet. The seafaring and fishing industries of Hoorn and Enkhuizen all dwindled during the century, and, in 1795, the population of Enkhuizen had fallen to 6,803.[92] Hoorn also functioned as an administrative centre (for instance, the Admiralty of the

Noorderkwartier had its headquarters there) which cushioned it to some extent from the economic and population decline. In circa 1650, it had approximately 15,000 inhabitants; in 1810, this total had declined by one-third to circa 10,000.[93] From this area of West Friesland, 329 surgeons (15 per cent of the total number in the sample) departed on Company ships, especially during the first four decades of the eighteenth century (236 surgeons). This contrasts sharply with the observations of the archivist and historian P. Boon on the seventeenth-century population of West Friesland which, he argues, was quite unwilling to work for the Company and they preferred careers with the whaling or merchant fleets. It is only after 1740 that a drastic decline set in among the surgeons. Although the decade 1740-1750 still produced some 27 surgeons for the Company, this fell to 17 in the next decade. The places vacated were mainly taken by German surgeons. Each period, more or less, saw a halving of its West Frisian surgeons. Most of the surgeons sought employment in Enkhuizen (197), and Hoorn (131). After 1750, a mere 40 surgeons from Enkhuizen and a mere 27 surgeons from Hoorn entered Company service, and the recruitment also became more diffuse.

Because North Holland was such a significant recruitment area, it may be enlightening to list the major recruitment cities (table T4.8). In this table only those cities are mentioned from which more than three surgeons took employment with the Company during any one period. As has undoubtedly been established, the role of the recruitment of surgeons tended to concentrate more and more on Amsterdam during the course of the eighteenth century. That of Enkhuizen fell sharply in the second and the fourth periods, whereas Hoorn's surgeons were almost spectacularly absent during the third period. The ratio of ships to surgeons was rather strained during those periods (table T4.5). Smaller cities such as Alkmaar, Haarlem, and Medemblik lost their significance. The attraction of Amsterdam as a surgical recruitment area just continued to increase while that of Enkhuizen and Hoorn was all but destroyed. To some extent, this must be related to the standing of surgical education which was increasingly gravitating towards Amsterdam. Clearly, the prosperity of North Holland declined significantly during the second half of the century.

South Holland

South Holland (*Zuid-Holland*) also supplied the respectable number of 651 sea surgeons sampled (22 per cent of the total number of surgeons within the sample; 30 per cent of the total number of Dutch ship's surgeons), which should be placed in the context of the two Company Chambers of Delft and Rotterdam in this area (appendix 2, Map A2.5). The emphasis on ship's surgeons employed from this province fell in the first half of the eighteenth century; after 1750 a gradual decline set in. The cities of Delft and Rotterdam provided the largest number of

Table T4.8: Surgical recruitment in North Holland (in absolute numbers and in percentages of the total per period, according to the sample)

Cities/Period	*1700-1725*	*1726-1750*	*1751-1775*	*1776-1796*
Alkmaar	8 (3%)	3 (2%)	4 (2%)	2 (2%)
Amsterdam	120 (39%)	81 (41%)	120 (66%)	80 (71%)
Enkhuizen	100 (32%)	47 (24%)	34 (19%)	7 (6%)
Haarlem	6 (2%)	6 (3%)	4 (2%)	4 (4%)
Hoorn	59 (19%)	49 (25%)	11 (6%)	13 (12%)
Medemblik	4 (1%)	3 (2%)	1 (1%)	0
Total number of surgeons northern Holland	312	200	182	113

surgeons from South Holland. This region was even more densely urbanised than North Holland, although some cities such as Delft and Leiden were in decline. The population of Dordrecht, however, stablilised during the period 1633-1795, as did those of Schoonhoven and Den Briel. Rotterdam grew during this period, as did The Hague and Schiedam.[94] South Holland was characterised by regional differences in population growth and economic prosperity, which is reflected in the surgical recruitment which was, as elsewhere, largely urban. Family motives certainly played a role as in some thirty instances more than one member of a specific family was employed by the Company in a surgical function. The supply of surgical recruitment from Alphen-aan-den-Rijn during the period of 1751-1775, for instance, was entirely made up of members of the Vuijsting family. Two Jans, one Frederick, and one Salomon from this one family set sail for Asia.

The principal places the surgeons came from are listed in table T4.9. As in table T4.8, only those places that supplied more than three Company surgeons during one period are listed. The gradual economic growth of Rotterdam is demonstrated by surgical participation that increased from 28 per cent to 44 per cent during the last period. As in the case of Amsterdam, the trek from the surrounding countryside to Rotterdam diminished, which was counterbalanced by the growing significance of the city of Rotterdam itself. The decline in prosperity and the concomitant drop in the population of Leiden is demonstrated by the surgical participation of this city, which fell from 25 per cent to 11 per cent. The Hague, on the other hand, the seat of the Dutch Republic's government, was not insignificant and grew from 8 per cent to 12 per cent.

Table T4.9: Surgical recruitment in South Holland (in absolute numbers and in percentages of the total per period according to the sample)

Cities/Period	*1700-1725*	*1726-1750*	*1751-1775*	*1776-1796*
Alphen aan den Rijn	1	1	4 (3%)	0
Delfshaven	10 (4%)	4 (2%)	2 (1%)	1 (1%)
Delft	57 (25%)	42 (25%)	27 (18%)	11 (11%)
Den Briel	6 (3%)	8 (5%)	2 (1%)	2 (2%)
The Hague	19 (8%)	15 (9%)	11 (7%)	12 (12%)
Dordrecht	13 (6%)	6 (4%)	4 (3%)	3 (3%)
Gorinchem	0	0	4 (3%)	0
Leiden	12 (5%)	3 (2%)	13 (9%)	7 (7%)
Maassluis	4 (2%)	0	0	1 (1%)
Rijswijk	4 (2%)	2 (1%)	0	0
Rotterdam	65 (28%)	53 (32%)	62 (41%)	44 (44%)
Schiedam	3 (1%)	5 (3%)	4 (3%)	3 (3%)
Vlaardingen	4 (2%)	1	0	0
Total number of surgeons from South Holland	231	167	153	100

Zeeland

The coastal province of Zeeland is where the Zeeland Admiralty's offices were located, as well as two companies trading in the West Indies (*Middelburgsche Commercie Compagnie* and the *West-Indische Compagnie*), and a Company chamber (second only to the Amsterdam Chamber). Zeeland supplied a mere 232 ship's surgeons to its Company chamber, two-thirds of whom were born in Middelburg (within the sample) and 64 per cent were employed before 1750 (appendix 2, Map A2.6). Economically speaking, this province had endured a prolonged demographic and economic decline, although it is difficult to find figures to substantiate this decline more precisely. There can be no doubt that the basic trend was that Zeeland ports were declining in significance and being forced to relinquish their power to those in Amsterdam and Rotterdam, which also exerted a similar effect on Hoorn and Enkhuizen in North Holland. All of them shrank to nearly half of their peak populations and by the late eighteenth century were considered mere backwaters.[95]

The Chamber of Zeeland itself employed some 400 ship's surgeons (within the sample), of whom half were from Zeeland itself. As was seen in table T4.5, surgical recruitment tension occurred in the second quarter of the century. The number of surgeons employed by the Chamber Zeeland gradually declined during the century, with a sharp decline after 1775. Most Zeeland surgeons came from the city of Middelburg (167 of the 232 sampled Zeeland surgeons, 68 per cent). This, however, cannot be verified because the archives with the relevant baptism records no longer exist. The Chamber of Zeeland employed most of its ship's surgeons between 1700 and 1770, with a peak during the period 1720-1730, when 40 surgeons set sail, after which a gradual decline set in, which assumed dramatic proportions after 1770 (table T4.10). The recruitment areas were primarily those of the provinces of Zeeland and South Holland during the first decades. One could argue that in the fourth period, the Fourth Anglo-Dutch war (1780-1784) must have played a significant role. The insecure seas on which the Company's ships could be over-powered by the English made the employment conditions somewhat hair-raising. In 1781, no Company ships left the harbours as it was deemed too dangerous. It was also a time during which the Dutch men-of-war were short of manpower (and among them, ship's surgeons), and a highly competitive situation between the Admiralties and the Company emerged.[96] Cogently, this was also valid for the other chambers, which had not suffered the same

Table T4.10: Geographical origins of recruited surgeons of the Zeeland Chamber (according to the sample)

	Period	*1700-1725*	*1726-1750*	*1751-1775*	*1776-1795*
Total		122	109	95	66
Dutch		112 (92%)	91 (83.5%)	81 (85%)	24 (36%)
	North	1 (0%)	2 (2%)	1 (1%)	0
	East	5 (4%)	4 (4%)	3 (4%)	0
	Central	3 (2,5%)	2 (2%)	1 (1%)	0
	South	2 (2%)	5 (5 %)	3 (3%)	2 (3%)
	North-Holland	6 (5%)	0	0	6 (20%)
	South-Holland	15 (13%)	4 (4%)	8 (10%)	3 (10%)
	Zeeland	80 (71%)	74 (81%)	65 (80%)	13 (43%)
(Of which	*Middelburg*	*52 (65$)*	*54 (73$)*	*50 (63$)*	*11 (85$))*
Non-Dutch		9 (1%)	14 (13%)	13 (14%)	36 (55%)
(of which	*Germany*	*5 (56$)*	*6 (43$)*	*8 (62$)*	*27 (75$))*
Origin	Unknown	1	4	1	6

drastic declines. Thus, this war cannot be considered the sole cause of the decline of surgical participation from Zeeland on the Company fleets; the change had set in well in advance of the outbreak of hostilities, although the war must have amplified its effects.

In fact, participation of surgeons born in the province of Zeeland declined after 1765, and only stabilised after the outbreak of the Fourth Anglo-Dutch war (table T4.11). No adequate explanation, such as employment by another maritime employer, decline of apprentices solicitations at the surgical guilds, or the attraction of Amsterdam at the expense of Zeeland, has been found for this sharp decline in the numbers of Zeeland's ship's surgeons.

Table T4.11: Surgeons from Zeeland in absolute numbers (according to the sample)

Period	*Number*	*Period*	*Number*
1751-1755	20	1771-1775	9
1756-1760	19	1776-1780	5
1761-1765	17	1781-1785	4
1766-1770	10	1786-1790	4

In short, we have seen that the main influx of Dutch surgeons was recruited in the province of Holland (North and South Holland), although the eastern area and the province of Zeeland did provide a substantial number of surgeons (especially in the earlier period). The other areas were negligible in this context (graph G4.2). The recruitment was an urban one and strongly linked to the demographic and economic growth of the specific area or city. Surgeons seeking employment from areas experiencing an economic decline simply stopped showing up at the Company chambers. The adventure had either become too expensive, or their families had become impoverished so that it was no longer possible for them to get a surgical education (appendix 2, Map A2.7a-d).

The surgeons came from cities and the larger villages where a surgical education was available. During the course of the eighteenth century, this recruitment, as we already mentioned, began to become increasingly centred in Amsterdam, at the expense of the Chambers of Hoorn and Enkhuizen, which definitely began encountering recruitment problems after 1725. In Zeeland, this decline in Dutch surgical recruitment became dramatic after 1760, although the chamber did manage to find enough surgeons for its vessels. It might perhaps add to our insights if we were to take a closer look at the recruitment of the other chambers.

Graph G4.2: Surgical recruitment per area (based on Table T4.7).

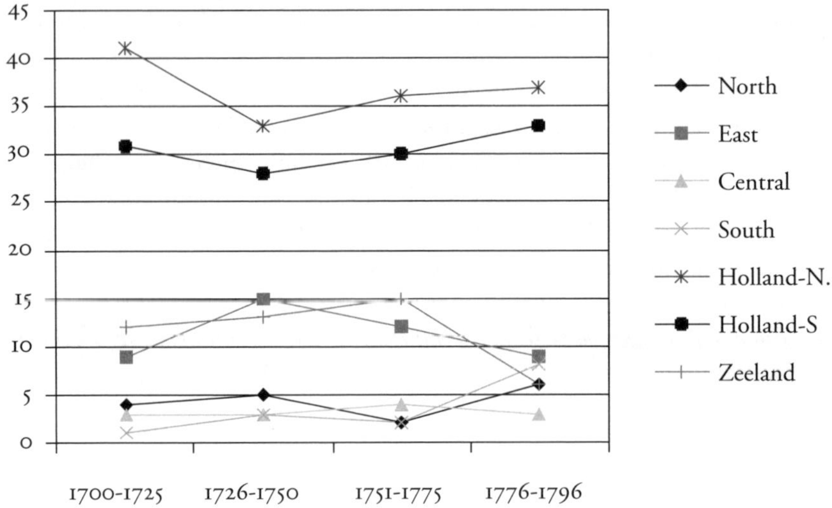

Amsterdam Chamber

Most ship's surgeons in search of a job were attracted by the Chamber of Amsterdam, which meant that this chamber experienced *de facto* no severe problems regarding the ratio of ships to surgeons. Surgeons from Amsterdam figured prominently in the first and third quarters of the eighteenth century (T4.8). The participation of those born in Amsterdam was halved in the second quarter and again in the last quarter century. This decrease was partly compensated for by an increase of surgeons from the north (Groningen, Friesland, and Drenthe), and, during the first and second periods, by surgeons from the eastern region (particularly Gelderland). From the South Holland area, even though it had two chambers of its own (Delft and Rotterdam), no less than 49 sea surgeons joined the Amsterdam Chamber, mostly from the cities of Leiden and The Hague.

Table T4.12 below shows that Holland and the eastern region were distinguished by their relatively high supply of ship's surgeons to the Amsterdam Chamber, although the eastern-region surgeons'participation declined after the second period. The surgeons from the northern provinces entered the Amsterdam Chamber on only a small scale, as the Amsterdam-born surgeons made up practically all of North-Holland's recruits (circa 90 per cent). German participation doubled, in absolute terms, during the second period, and German surgeons constituted approximately 90 per cent of all foreign surgeons. Non-Dutch participation began to hover at approximately one-third after 1725. Although the number of Dutch ship's surgeons from this chamber dwindled steadily during the eighteenth century – especially during the period 1725-1750 and after 1775 – the first decline was offset by a sharp increase in foreign, mainly German, surgeons, who showed an increase of 200 percent in the second quarter of the century. The relative and absolute decline of Dutch participation in ship's surgery was at least compensated for by German participation during this period. The third period was marked by increased participation of surgeons born in Amsterdam, while the number of foreign surgeons (again, German in particular) began to decline. The Scandinavian countries were represented by the odd three Swedish surgeons; obviously, Scandinavian surgeons were not attracted to the Company Chamber of Amsterdam, which contrasts strongly with the general inclination of the Scandinavians because they usually represented about one-fifth of the entire crews (table T4.18).

Table T4.12: Geographical origins of recruited surgeons of the Amsterdam Chamber

	Period	*1700-1725*	*1726-1750*	*1751-1775*	*1776-1795*
Total		284	280	250	163
Dutch		223 (79%)	164 (58%)	164 (66%)	95 (58%)
	North	16 (7%)	21 (13%)	9 (6%)	8 (8%)
	East	45 (20%)	48 (28%)	28 (17%)	12 (13%)
	Central	10 (4.5%)	10 (6%)	8 (3%)	5 (3%)
	South	5 (2%)	5 (3%)	3 (2%)	3 (2%)
	North Holland	121 (54%):	68 (42%)	100 (61%)	58 (61%):
(Of which	*Amsterdam:*	*106 (88%)*	*62 (91%)*	*94 (94%)*	*52 (90%))*
	South Holland	28 (12%)	7 (4%)	15 (9%)	9 (8%)
	Zeeland	0 (0%)	2 (1%)	1 (1%)	0 (0)%)
Non-Dutch		55 (18.5%)	99 (35%)	78 (31%)	58 (35%)
(of which	*Germany:*	*48 (91%)*	*88 (89%)*	*71 (91%)*	*52 (90%))*
Origin	Unknown	6	17	8	10

The Chambers of Hoorn and Enkhuizen

As table T4.13 shows, the decline in Dutch surgeons on the Company payroll plainly begins after 1725, when a drop of some 20 per cent was experienced by the Chambers of Hoorn and Enkhuizen. After 1750, these chambers lost their Dutch contingent of surgeons in aggregates of 10 per cent in each subsequent period. This loss was most particularly felt by the Hoorn Chamber which was already functioning under the recommended ratio of vessels to surgeons (table T4.5), which was only partly counterbalanced by surgical participation from the eastern region. Surgeons from South Holland also came to help these chambers after 1750. The north, central, and south regions were not significant as recruitment areas of Hoorn and Enkhuizen. Gradually, non-Dutch surgeons came to comprise a significant portion of employees at the Hoorn and Enkhuizen Chambers. By the early years of the eighteenth century, Germans already occupied some 85 percent of the foreign-filled positions. Overall, the picture confirms West Friesland decline both in terms of population and the economy.

T4.13: Geographical origins of recruited surgeons of the Hoorn and Enkhuizen Chambers

	Period	*1700-1725*	*1726-1750*	*1751-1775*	*1776-1795*
Total		216	233	197	168
Dutch		200 (93%)	171 (74%)	121 (61%)	81 (48%)
Of which:	North	8 (4%)	8 (4%)	0 (0%)	9 (11%)
	East	9 (4%)	24 (14%)	20 (17%)	9 (11%)
	Central	0 (0%)	2 (2%)	6 (5%)	3 (4%)
	South	0 (0%)	1 (0,5)	1 (1%)	3 (4%)
	North-Holland	181 (90%)	127 (63%)	76 (63%)	45 (55%)
(Of which	*Enkhuizen:*	*101 (56%)*	*46 (36%)*	*33 (43%)*	*7 (16%))*
	Hoorn	*59 (33%)*	*49 (39%)*	*11 (15%)*	*13 (29%))*
	South-Holland	2 (1%)	9 (5%)	16 (13%)	9 (11%)
	Zeeland	0 (0%)	0 (0%)	2 (2%)	2 (1%)
Non-Dutch		13 (6%)	52 (22%)	72 (37%)	73 (41%)
Of which:	Germany	10 (85%)	41 (82%)	66 (92%)	57 (83%)
Origin	Unknown	2	9	4	15

The Chambers of Delft and Rotterdam

After the first period, the Chambers of Delft and Rotterdam experienced a drop in Dutch surgical participation. In contrast to Hoorn and Enkhuizen, this decline more or less stabilised after 1725, and Delft and Rotterdam maintained a large contingent of regional surgeons, which was mainly attributable to the fact that the area was highly urbanised, and experienced growth in both population and in terms of prosperity. The eastern provinces of Gelderland and Overijssel played a less significant part in the supply of surgeons for these chambers than in the Amsterdam Chamber and in those of Hoorn and Enkhuizen. The north, central and Zeeland regions were also fairly irrelevant as recruitment areas for Delft and Rotterdam. However, the southern provinces of Brabant and Limburg became noteworthy after 1775. The non-Dutch contingent rose during the course of the eighteenth century, but never assumed the large numbers found at the Chambers of Hoorn and Enkhuizen.

Table T4.14: Geographical origins of recruted surgeons of the Delft and Rotterdam Chambers

	Period	*1700-1725*	*1726-1750*	*1751-1775*	*1776-1795*
Total		223	218	185	161
Dutch		213 (95%)	174 (79%)	138 (74.5%)	105 (78%)
Of which:	North	2 (1%)	0 (0%)	0 (0%)	1 (0%)
	East	10 (5%)	13 (7.5%)	8 (6%)	6 (6%)
	Central	7 (3%)	2 (1%)	4 (3%)	1 (1%)
	South	2 (1%)	8 (5%)	5 (5%)	12 (12%)
	North-Holland	3 (1%)	4 (2%)	8 (6%)	5 (5%)
	South-Holland	189 (87%)	147 (84.5%)	113 (82%)	80 (75%)
(Of which	*Delft*	*54 (29%)*	*42 (29%)*	*27 (24%)*	*11 (14%)*
	Rotterdam	*65 (34%)*	*53 (36%)*	*62 (55%)*	*44 (55%))*
	Zeeland	0 (0%)	0 (0%)	0 (0%)	0 (0%)
Non-Dutch		9 (4%)	34 (15%)	47 (22.5%)	54 (33%)
Of which:	Germany	4 (50%)	32 (99.9%)	35 (75%)	38 (72%)
Origin	Unknown	1	10	0	2

German recruitment

Some attention should obviously be paid to the Company's recruitment areas in Germany, since Germans constituted by far the greatest number of non-Dutch surgeons. Since Germany did not exist in the seventeenth and eighteenth centuries as we know it today, we mean the various states of the Holy Roman Empire. It should be emphasised that no baptismal registers have been checked and that the statements of place of origin have been taken here at face value. Moreover, no specific research has been done regarding the economic, social, and demographic history of Germany, which will be sketched in rather general terms, when necessary. It would not serve the purposes of this book to provide an in-depth study of the socio-economic circumstances in which the German surgeon found himself. Therefore, the remarks and conclusions presented here about German recruitment are only tentative.

In 1500, Germany occupied a leading position in Western Europe, both economically and culturally, but by 1600 it showed evidence of backwardness and provincialism.[97] The German universities attracted fewer and fewer students as these students came to prefer other centres of cultural and intellectual life in, for instance, Leiden or Paris. The Hanseatic League, officially dissolved in 1669, had become a mere shadow of its former self long before that date. Parts of Germany were devastated and disintegrated by the Thirty Years' War (1618-1648), the subsequent economic stagnation and the slow demographic recovery, which led to a lack of employment opportunities that convinced many people that they had to be 'on the move'. The over 300 German states were virtually sovereign powers after the Peace of Westphalia in 1648, leaving essentially no centralized government to pull the region's economy together.

As much as one-third of Germany's population perished during the war and poverty was the rule throughout, although not evenly divided across the Empire.[98] Some regions or cities, such as Brandenburg, Magdeburg (besieged ten times), Hesse, Franconia, Bavaria, Swabia, and Alsace, suffered more than others. The areas that lost between one-half to two-thirds of their populations included Pomerania, Mecklenburg, Thuringia, Trier, the Palatinate, and Württemberg. Some areas, such as Westphalia, Lower Saxony, and Schleswig Holstein, felt the effects less.[99] The Palatinate War (1688-1697) and the War of the Austrian Succession (1740-1748) also wrought havoc. These successive wars and crises were not conducive to economic recovery in Germany. There was a lag in development that was not only an outcome of war, but also from the regional differences in mentality. The traditional-feudal, inward-looking areas of the east (such as Brandenburg, Prussia, Bavaria, and Saxony) displayed a tendency to turn away from the Atlantic world trade orientation.[100] It was only after the Seven Years' War (1756-1763) that social and economic life in general found some stability.

As in other European states, there were various groups of medical practitioners in Germany, such as the physicians, the surgeons (*Wundarzte*), the military surgeons (*Feldscher*), the barber surgeons, the bathmasters (*Bader*), the midwives, and the specialists or quacks who were not part of a guild. The surgeons in Germany, however, were incorporated into a guild. The requirements for becoming a surgeon were intimately linked to the *numerus clausus* and other guild restrictions. The guilds were politically fairly powerful, and had obtained so many privileges that they could sometimes act more or less independently of the city authorities. Until the medical reforms were launched in Germany with the Imperial Trade

Edict of 1731, the surgical guilds or the cities had more or less freely distributed the right to practise as a surgeon to the highest bidders until the Prussian king Frederick William I (1688-1740) began enforcing the new reforms.[101] The 1731 Edict forbade the guilds to proscribe economic practices considered advantageous to their own self-interests and eliminated obstacles to the attainment of future masterships; in short all of the guilds, not just the surgeons' guild, had to forfeit much of their autonomy and power to the state. This reform was rapidly enforced in Austria and Prussia and gradually spread throughout Germany. However, the old distinction between 'medical surgery', as represented by the university graduates with no practical experience; and 'practical surgery', as represented by the uneducated barbers and feldshers, who practised surgery with little insight into their art, prevailed. It was only towards 1775 that the distinction began to disappear and practical surgery was introduced as an academic discipline at some universities.[102]

Germany contributed the largest number of non-Dutch ship's surgeons to the Company during the eighteenth century. In the sample, some 597 German ship's surgeons entered the Company's service, comprising one-fifth of the total number of ship's surgeons and four-fifths (83 per cent) of the total number of non-Dutch surgeons. How much can we learn about the origins and motives of the German surgeon who sought employment with the Company?

Non-Dutch participation rose dramatically in the second quarter of the century (from eight to 20 per cent), after which the growth stabilised to five per cent in each period.

Table T4.15: German surgical participation in absolute numbers, in relation to non-Dutch surgeons (in percentages) and in relation to the total number of surgeons (in percentages).

	1700-1725	*1726-1750*	*1751-1775*	*1776-1795*
Germany	69 (80%) (8%)	170 (85%) (20%)	180 (86%) (25%)	178 (80%) (31%)
Non-Dutch	86	198	210	221
Total	853	843	733	559

Conventional wisdom would have it that many of these surgeons would have come from the ports of northern Germany and from the Baltic ports, such as Danzig, Lübeck, Königsberg, and Stettin, which had also been the case with many of the captains and soldiers employed by the chambers of the Company. In fact, these surgeons came mainly from Lower Saxony, Saxony, and Westphalia, although after 1750, the relative participation of Germans from these areas – while remaining high – declined. Saxony-Anhalt began to figure prominently after 1725.

It was these four regions of Germany that were the main recruitment areas for the Company. Compared to these four, the other major regions in Germany did not contribute significant numbers of recruited surgeons (table T4.16).

Table T4.16: Regional German surgical participation in absolute numbers and in relation to the total German participation in percentages

	1700-1725	*1726-1750*	*1751-1775*	*1776-1795*
Lower Saxony	24 (35%)	42 (25%)	43 (24%)	32 (18%)
Westphalia	13 (19%)	42 (25%)	32 (18%)	33 (19%)
Baden-Württemberg	1 (1%)	4 (2%)	14 (8%)	8 (4%)
Bavaria	2 (3%)	2 (1%)	2 (1%)	11 (6%)
Brandenburg	3 (4%)	11 (6%)	6 (3%)	9 (5%)
Hesse	2 (3%)	4 (2%)	9 (5%)	15 (8%)
Mecklenburg-Vorpommern	2 (3%)	4 (2%)	4 (2%)	2 (1%)
East Prussia	3 (4%)	0 (0%)	1 (1%)	3 (2%)
Pommerania	0 (0%)	1 (1%)	3 (2%)	2 (1%)
Prussia	0 (0%)	1 (1%)	1 (1%)	1 (1%)
Rhineland-Palatinate	0 (0%)	3 (2%)	3 (2%)	6 (3%)
Saarland	0 (0%)	0 (0%)	1 (1%)	0 (0%)
Saxony	6 (9%)	8 (5%)	15 (8%)	9 (5%)
Saxony-Anhalt	4 (6%)	24 (14%)	21 (12%)	21 (12%)
Silesia	0 (0%)	2 (1%)	1 (1%)	4 (2%)
Schleswig-Holstein	4 (6%)	11 (6%)	9 (5%)	2 (1%)
Thuringia	2 (3%)	5 (3%)	7 (4%)	9 (5%)

Westphalia and Lower Saxony were densely populated areas and they had not suffered as much as other German areas during the Thirty Years' War. Furthermore, the Counter Reformation never reached these areas, and thus, they generally remained Protestant. It must be kept in mind that the Company was more attractive to Protestant job-seekers than to Catholics, which meant that most German employees of the Company came from the Protestant German countries (north and central).[103] Moreover, the regions of Westphalia and Lower Saxony, as we have seen, produced the three traditional migration routes to the Republic. Also of importance was the fact that, unlike Mecklenburg-Vorpommern, Pommerania, and

Prussia, where landowners controlled the economy and ruled their estates with absolute authority, these areas had no history of feudal structures. In the feudal regions, the peasants were still serfs, and entirely dependent on the nobles who could even buy and sell them with or without their property. The few surgeons recruited from Mecklenburg came from the coastal cities.

The maps A2.8a-d give some insight into differences within the German recruitmen regions (appendix 2, Map A2.8a-d). There are three main recruitment zones. One lay along the coast of Lower Saxony and Schleswig Holstein, and the coastal areas of Mecklenburg and Vorpommern, getting thinner as it went eastwards. The second is a broad strip from Enschede, Lingen, Meppen, Bentheim via Osnabrück, Hannover, Brunswick, Wolfenbüttel, which penetrates the regions of Saxony-Anhalt and Saxony. In Saxony-Anhalt, the places the surgeons came from lay particularly in the south, north of the Harz Mountains. In Saxony itself, the recruitment was diverse. Together, Lower Saxony (appendix 2, Map A2.9), Saxony (appendix 2, Map A2.10) and Saxony-Anhalt (appendix 2, Map A2.11) delivered more than 40 per cent of the Company's surgeons during the eighteenth century. Westphalia had two belts: one in the north bordering on Lower Saxony (which belonged to the migration route of Lower Saxony), and the other followed the migration route to the Republic via the Rhine and the Ruhr (appendix 2, Map A2.12).

The other regions (appendix 2, Maps A2.13-A2.19) show no specific and clear-cut patterns, except Baden-Württemberg (appendix 2, Map A2.20) where surgeons came mainly from north of the Black Forest. As for Hesse, the recruitment was focused mainly around the cities of Frankfurt and Hanau; while for Brandenburg it centered on Berlin and Potsdam. Bavaria and Thuringia were insignificant contributors. The maps show the changing patterns in recruitment areas during the eighteenth century. In the first period, German recruitment was sparse and diffuse but already showed the broad belt which cut Germany into two. The second period shows extensive recruitment in Westphalia, along Hamburg, Saxony, Thuringia and around Berlin. The third and fourth periods are marked by centres of recruitment in the north of Baden-Württemberg (around Kirchheim) and in Bavaria (around Neuremberg). Lower Saxony was always represented among the German surgeons, and the emergence of the independent city of Hamburg takes place in the second period.

Lower Saxony

Lower Saxony bordered the Dutch Republic and was a traditional recruitment area for migrant workers for the Republic (appendix 2, Map A2.9). As such, it might have been almost natural for surgeons in this area to follow the great migration stream towards the North Sea to fulfil their *Wanderschaft* obligations. During the first period, surgeons from the East Frisian ports figured prominently;

Embden and Esens produced more than one-third (table T4.17). The importance of this area declined at the same time as this area was assigned to Prussia at the Convention of Emden in 1744. Until that time, East Frisia had been governed by the States-General of the Dutch Republic. Probably an even more significant factor was the founding of the Royal Prussian-Asian Company (1751-1756), as a result of which, East Frisian ship's surgeons now sailed from Emden.

Surgeons from Hamburg left for the Republic especially in the second and third periods of the eighteenth century. Hamburg had been part of the Hanseatic League and, while the League itself began to weaken, Hamburg continued to thrive. In fact, Hamburg was the only Hanseatic town that showed rapid progress in the seventeenth and eighteenth centuries.[104] Hamburg gradually emerged as the most significant commercial port for half of Europe, especially in the eighteenth century, a growth which was also accompanied by a population explosion. There was a set back at the end of the Seven Years' War, when Hamburg experienced an economic depression that persisted into the 1780's.[105] At the same time, the number of Hamburg surgeons on the Company pay roll declined.

The Quakenbrück and Brunswick areas were also significant suppliers of ship's surgeons in Lower Saxony during the third and fourth periods, which coincides, at least for Brunswick, with a period of flourishing trade and culture after 1750, when the cultivation of an array of crops had created a diversified and well-developed agricultural economy, that even exported grain. This was also a period in which mining and refining grew into major industries and the population of Brunswick increased markedly after 1750.[106] In 1753, the Guelph rulers moved their residence from Wolfenbüttel to Brunswick, which gave this city an extra economic boost. In sum, Brunswick's economy improved during the eighteenth century, with increasing speed after 1750. At the same time, medical reforms established an ethical code for practitioners and elaborated the medical bureaucracy, which intensified medical and surgical criteria for physicians, surgeons, apothecaries, barber surgeons, as well as midwives. The *Collegium Medicum* to which the practitioners were responsible was founded in Brunswick in 1747, and thereafter, they had to be examined before they were allowed to establish a practice. Surgeons had to follow surgical-anatomical courses at the *Collegium*.[107] The table T4.17 below shows details of the distribution of surgeons recruited from Lower Saxony. At the beginning of the eighteenth century, surgeons came mostly from Lower Saxony's coastal towns, while in the second half they came more from the interior areas.

Table T4.17: Sampled ship's surgeons from Lower Saxony in absolute numbers and percentages (only those cities are mentioned that produced more than one Company surgeon during a specific period.)

Lower Saxony	*1700-1725 (24)*	*1726-1750 (42)*	*1751-1775 (43)*	*1776-1795 (32)*
Braunschweig	0	0	3 (7%)	5 (16%)
Embden	6 (25%)	8 (19%)	4 (9%)	3 (9%)
Esens	3 (13%)	0	0	0
Göttingen	0	0	0	3 (9%)
Hamburg	2 (8%)	8 (19%)	9 (21%)	2 (6%)
Hannover	1	1	1	2 (6%)
Hildesheim	0	0	2 (5%)	1
Lingen	0	0	4 (9%)	2 (6%)
Meppen	0	0	0	3 (9%)
Norden	0	2 (5%)	2 (5%)	0
Oldenburg	0	0	2 (5%)	0
Osnabrück	0	3 (7%)	0	3 (9%)
Quakenbrück	0	6 (14%)	4 (9%)	5 (16%)
Wittmund	2 (8%)	0	0	0
Wolfenbüttel	0	0	2 (5%)	0

Recruitment from other areas

The Austrian Netherlands (Belgium)

It would be natural to assume that the non-Dutch surgeons came from northern and western Germany as well as from other neighbouring countries such as the Austrian Netherlands (nowadays Belgium). However, the significance of the Austrian Netherlands as a surgical recruitment area for the Company was small: the participation percentage varied between 1 and 2 per cent during the entire eighteenth century. It could be that religious motives (the Catholic Austrian Netherlands versus the Protestant Company) exerted a negative influence, or they were influenced by economic reasons. After the Scheldt was blocked by the Dutch during the Dutch Revolt at the end of the sixteenth century, the economy of that area declined. Many traders and craftsmen migrated north. It was only after 1750 that new industries began to develop in the northeastern part of present-day Belgium, the area around

Liège. The recruitment of Belgian surgeons for the Company's vessels, low as it may have been, dates particularly after 1750. These surgeons went mainly to the Rotterdam and Zeeland Chambers. Ship's surgeon Charles Ghislain Wilmet, for instance, was employed by the Rotterdam Chamber for all his Company voyages.

Switzerland and Scandinavia

The Calvinistic and German-speaking part of the Swiss Cantons, which has no maritime tradition at all, supplied more ship's surgeons to the Company (19 surgeons in the sample) in the eighteenth century than Lutheran Scandinavia (nowadays Norway and Sweden) with its nine surgeons in the sample. Because of the skills and initiatives of Protestant refugees from Italy, the Swiss towns had already developed important export industries such as silk and wool by the eighteenth century.[108] This may have generated trading networks from which the Swiss surgeons profited. The Swiss ship's surgeons hired by the Company began to arrive in the Republic from 1730, as did the aforementioned David H. Gallandat. They came mostly from Zürich, and they all but disappeared from the Company's bookkeeping – except one – after 1774. During that time, a medical-surgical trading network must have been established. The favourable reputation of Dutch surgery (eventually surpassed by Paris in the second half of the eighteenth century) may well have been a strong motive for these surgeons to come to the Republic.

The Scandinavian ship's surgeons could, of course, more easily find employment in their own East India company for their maritime surgical experience. The wages of the Swedish Company's crews were higher than in the navies and the rest of the shipping world, which must have been an incentive for Scandinavian surgeons to join the Swedish Comapny.[109] Moreover, Danish surgery flourished in eighteenth century Copenhagen, which had its *Theatrum Anatomico-Chirurgi-*

Table T4.18: Surgical participation from Belgium, Scandinavia, Switzerland, and France in absolute numbers (within the sample)

	1700-1725	*1726-1750*	*1751-1775*	*1776-1795*
Total non-Dutch surgeons	86	198	210	221
Denmark	0	3	2	2
Norway	1	1	0	0
Sweden	2	3	0	2
Switzerland	0	5	13	1
France	4	6	3	11
Belgium	5	2	8	11

cum and elevated the status of the surgeons, thus creating more attractive career opportunities than sailing aboard an East Indiaman.

France

France (24 surgeons in the sample) was also more significant than the Scandinavian countries as a supplier of ship's surgeons. During the first three-quarters of the eighteenth century, the French ship's surgeons appear from almost every region in France, although the second quarter was dominated by surgeons originating from the Languedoc. The Languedoc was at the time a 'push' recruitment area; cogently, large parts of the Languedoc were (and still are) Protestant. Guillaume Teisseire, fom Castres, was a surgeon from this area who for unknown reasons travelled to the Republic in early 1730. After having been examined on his surgical skills, he was employed by the Chamber of Enkhuizen, for which he departed as third surgeon on the *Vis* in 1732. After his arrival in Batavia in 1733, he continued to work there, first at Batavia Castle where he was promoted to surgeon's mate in 1741. On 19 February, 1744, he left the service of the Company and became a free citizen of Batavia (*vrijburger*), practising as a surgeon among the population of Batavia until his death on 31 December, 1760. His daughter married another Frenchman and Company surgeon in Batavia, François Aurous (also from the Languedoc), and their son became one of the most successful inhabitants of Batavia. After 1775, French surgeons mainly hailed from Strasbourg, which had experienced an economic boom in the eighteenth century, as a communication centre between Germany and France.[110]

As the numbers of Company surgeons originating from the Austrian Netherlands, Scandinavia, France, and Switzerland were so small, it is impossible to draw any conclusions or construct any structural patterns about them. Only for France do the data hint that in the first half of the century surgeons from the Languedoc favoured the Republic, and after 1775 it was the Strasbourg surgeons who felt attracted to join the Company.

Discussion and conclusion

According to the sample, the recruitment of Dutch surgeons was primarily a regional one, namely from Holland and Zeeland, mainly from the larger cities and their direct surroundings. Pertinently, this recruitment showed a two-phased decline in the course of the eighteenth century. The decline set in after 1725 and came to a conclusion after 1775 (tables T4.19 and T4.20).

Table T4.19: Geographical recruitment of surgeons in the eighteenth century

Period	*Coastal Areas: North-Holland, South-Holland, Zeeland*	*Other Dutch Areas*	*Non-Dutch*
1700-1725	74%	17%	9%
1726-1750	53%	19%	28%
1751-1775	56%	14%	30%
1775-1795	41%	13%	46%

The recruitment from the more inland Dutch areas, especially Gelderland and Overijssel (eastern area), which in part counterbalanced the decline in coastal recruitment, declined as well, although not as sharply as along the coast. South Holland, or more specifically, the city of Rotterdam, made a slow comeback as the supplier of surgeons after 1750, while during that same period, Zeeland slipped away into oblivion. The zest for ship's surgery in the northern (Groningen, Friesland, and Drenthe) and southern (Brabant and Limburg) areas had never been high and remained insignificant. Germany emerged as the main surgical recruitment area after 1725, in which the surgeons from the regions of Lower Saxony, Westphalia and, later, Saxony-Anhalt particularly figured highly. Scandinavia, the Baltic shores, the Austrian Netherlands, France and Switzerland, although not absent, were not that important as recruitment areas.

Table T4.20: Dutch and non-Dutch surgeons per Chamber (excludes surgeons of unknown origin)

Period	*Amsterdam Dutch/ Non Dutch*	*Hoorn/Enkhuizen Dutch/ Non-Dutch*	*Delft/Rotterdam Dutch/ Non-Dutch*	*Zeeland Dutch/ Non-Dutch*
1700-1725	78%/18.5%	93%/6%	95%/4%	92%/1%
1726-1750	58%/35%	74%/22%	79%/15%	83.5%/13%
1751-1775	66%/31%	61%/37%	74.5%/22.5%	85%/14%
1776-1796	58%/35%	49%/41%	78%/22%	36%/55%

Coming up with a simple list of the countries from which surgeons came does not give us enough information about the changes over the period of time in question. One should also ask why they came from a particular area in such abundance. There were several motives mentioned at the beginning of this chapter for surgeons wanting to join the Company, such as traditional, psychological, social, demographic, or economic reasons, when they faced questions about the future of their careers. The sample shows a number of instances of typical family recruitment in which fathers and sons, and other members of the same family opted for a career with the same employer, the Company. Those surgeons who left their cities in groups might have been influenced by information about the work, which was shared by kin and friends. The sample shows that, particularly in the north and central areas, groups of villagers or citizens left their homes in a short period of time. These surgeons may have influenced each other to seek employment with the Company. It is impossible for the modern researcher to pinpoint one specific motive as the decisive factor regarding the question 'Why did they join'? It is very plausible that, given the personal identity of each surgeon, one or the other motive, or a combination of them, might have determined his decision. However, it is impossible not to see that for many surgeons a significant motive was the pursuit of an interesting and important professional experience, plus the possibility of amassing an attractive fortune in the East.

One pattern that we see emerge during the research was that surgeons only took employment with the Company when their home areas were experiencing periods of prosperity, usually accompanied by population growth. This is in sharp contrast to the generally accepted theory that the Company's crews came mostly from poor inland areas desperately seeking some kind of employment. This theory may hold (although it is still unproven) for the Company soldiers and sailors however.

The ship's surgeons originating from the north (Groningen, Friesland and Drenthe) chose not to join at the West Frisian Chambers of Hoorn and Enkhuizen, which is curious since it was convenient and close by. But Friesland was more oriented toward Amsterdam when it came to shipping. Thus, most of the surgeons from the north went to Amsterdam, which was, apparently more attractive to most including those from the north. In West Friesland and the Noorderkwartier, an economic decline combined with depopulation which reigned since the early eighteenth century made the Chambers of Hoorn and Enkhuizen perhaps less attractive than Amsterdam. Two-thirds of the ship's surgeons from the northern area had already left *before* 1750, when the north was still relatively prosperous; when the economic decline occurred in Friesland *after* 1750, few surgeons came from Friesland to seek employment with the Company. This may in part be due to the fact that the economic deterioration of the north caused a disinclination to enlist. The general economic deterioration in North Holland resulted in a drop in surgeons at the Chambers of Hoorn and Enkhuizen after 1725. It certainly substantiates the notion that there could well be a positive correlation between the prosperous economic climate of the area of origin of the surgeon and his willingness to hire on with the Company. It also appears that there was a positive relationship between the economic climate of the areas where the chambers were located and the surgeons' eagerness to seek employment there.

The fabric industries of Twente in Overijssel declined sharply during the 1750s and 1760s; again, of the 23 ship's surgeons in the sample who were from Twente, most of them (17) joined the Company *before* 1750. The same is true of the entire eastern area of Gelderland and Overijssel: two-thirds of the ship's surgeons from this area left their native soil in the first half of the eighteenth century. Israel records increased rural poverty in the inland provinces especially in Overijssel, Gelderland and Drenthe *after* the 1750s. Rotterdam, after it had experienced a depression in the first half of the eighteenth century, came back in the second half; as a result, an increasing number of local and regional surgeons were willing to take service at the Rotterdam Chamber. Delft was already slipping away into economic oblivion during the seventeenth century, and thus it was difficult to recruit any significant number of ship's surgeons there. There are similar explanations for the sharp fall of Dutch surgical recruitment in Zeeland in the last period. When we turn to the German surgeons, at least those originating from Brunswick and Hamburg were caught up in the same process; we see that a serious depression in Hamburg after the Seven Years' War dilapidated the supply of Hamburg's surgeons joining the Company.

It is therefore argued that, in the case of the recruitment of the ship's surgeons for the Company, the more their native areas experienced an economic decline, the less inclined they were to join the Company. It could also be argued that, *vice versa*, the more an area experienced a period of growth and prosperity (for example Rotterdam and Hamburg), the more ship's surgeons from that area sought employment with the Company's. It is clear that the Company's recruitment of ship's surgeons was diametrically opposed to the generally accepted idea of the recruitment of the sailors and soldiers: they, apparently, were recruited from areas undergoing economic slumps, which forced inhabitants to migrate and hire on with the Company. In the case of Dutch and German ship's surgeons, the sample points to the reverse: the influx of surgeons dried up as soon as their native areas deteriorated economically.

It might be fitting to conclude that the Company did not attract the surgical 'scum of the earth' in bad times. This is made all the more plausible because most of them came from fairly well-to-do families. Many of them had already been educated by a master surgeon, which would have required some financial means. They probably went into Company service with the knowledge that, upon their return, they could easily set up their own practices in the Republic or in Germany. They could afford a 'foreign adventure' and a novel educational experience, such as a voyage as a ship's surgeon, knowing there was no danger of being made redundant upon their return home. If the prospects of a future career were promising, the ship's surgeon certainly belonged to the wandering craftsmen of the early modern period. The moment that his home province or city began to deteriorate (economically or otherwise), he decided to stay home to secure employment there; he could then ill afford the luxury of a foreign experience. As enough other surgeons, for example from outside the Republic, offered their services to the Company, Dutch surgeons were less needed by then.

5. The career of the Company surgeons

The Company offered its surgeons an environment in which a career could be pursued. Some 10,000 surgeons grasped this opportunity during the seventeenth and eighteenth centuries. In responding to this challenge, these men made a contribution to the physical welfare of their colleagues in the Company on board its ships and in its hospitals in Asia and the Cape of Good Hope, and also, to some extent, to that of the slaves and the local inhabitants of the 'colonial' settlements. If not ahead, they were at least abreast of their times, often fascinated by their unfamiliar surroundings. The Company ship's surgeons were interested in the scientific nature of the world around them and in the tropical diseases suffered by its inhabitants. A prime example of such a man is the Duch ship's surgeon Wouter Schouten, born in 1649, who wrote a description of Madura foot in his *Aanmerkelijke Voyagie, gedaan door Wouter Schouten naar Oost-Indien* ('Remarkable Voyage made by Wouter Schouten to the East Indies', 1676).[1] Company surgeon Caspar Schambergen was invited to Edo in 1649 to instruct the Japanese in surgical matters. The Swedish ship's surgeon Carl Peter Thunberg (1743-1828) used his time on Deshima in Japan (in the employ of the Company) to collect hundreds of plants, and his botanical drawings were published as *Flora Japonica* in 1794. Thunberg had studied medicine at Uppsala University and had graduated in 1770 before he travelled to Leiden, Amsterdam and Paris to study their botanical gardens. Although he was a physician he accepted a position as ship's surgeon to the Company in order to collect (Japanese) plants for the Dutch botanical gardens. Profiting from the Dutch presence on Deshima, the Japanese scholars (*Rangakusha* or 'Hollandologists') threw themselves into the study of Western medicine, astronomy, mathematics, botany, physics, chemistry, pharmacy, geography and the military arts – all studied in Dutch.

Of course, many surgeons died before they had a chance to leave their mark on the scientific world in general or on the Company medical organisation in particular. Those who did not, often remained unacknowledged, and it was precisely these anonymous men who, in the centuries that followed, acquired the reputation of being nothing more than illiterate barber's mates, capable of not much more than the shaving of beards, or of being opportunistic charlatans or quacks, who had no idea of how to treat a sick man.[2] One may well wonder if this was a truly faithful picture of the (Company) ship's surgeon, and if not, how did he acquire such an unmerited reputation.

Precious little is known about the surgeons' (working) lives in general. In nineteenth- and twentieth-century historiography, specific diseases from which the Company's personnel suffered as well as some deserving Company surgeons have been highlighted and brought to the attention of a wider audience.[3] The anonymous body of Company ship's surgeons, however, has not been so fortunate, even though it was this body that shaped the medical organisation in Batavia and elsewhere, and which raised, in all likelihood, medical care and medical science to a more advanced level, whereas in Europe, the organisation of medical services only began making considerable progress in human survival rates after circa 1850.[4] We should therefore take a closer look at the careers of these men and, in order to define them more clearly as a professional group, a number of aspects of their careers should be examined.

Career is here defined as the development of a ship's surgeon's professional status within a certain period of time measured by formal parameters such as pay and rank, or, phrased rather differently, a profile of the positions a ship's surgeon occupied during a certain time span while exercising his profession. The purpose of this chapter is to provide the answers to the following questions: What kind of schooling did the surgeon receive before signing a contract with the Company? What sort of career could he pursue in the context of the Company? Could and did he amass a fortune during his service? What was the time span in which he could make a career? Was he, indeed, nothing more than a junior barber unqualified for the task he was called upon to perform? The factors that should be included in these considerations are his social origins, the age at which he entered Company service, his level of education at the time of his first contract or first voyage, and the number of voyages he made and the number of changes in rank he experienced reflecting his responsibilities. For the methodology used in this research, please refer to appendix 1.

Social origins

A surgical career usually began with a proper education. The training involved in becoming a master surgeon was deemed a decent education in the Republic, one which fit into the broad range of professions considered suitably by the middle class in the Dutch Republic. Within Dutch society, distinctions were made based on a man's ability to pay taxes. For instance, according to the 'tax authorities' in Haarlem at the end of the seventeenth century, 20 per cent of the population of Haarlem lived more or less on hand-outs from charitable institutions; 7 per cent were 'people of substance' as they possessed capital of more than 1,000 Dutch guilders, while the rest (circa 70 per cent) belonged to Haarlem's middle class, which was also characterised by finely drawn distinctions: there was a top layer of circa 10 per cent which included religious leaders, physicians, brewers, coopers, and some silversmiths. They were considered *brede burgerij* or upper bourgeoisie. The rest were assigned to the *smalle burgerij* or petty bourgeoisie and consisted of petty merchants, surgeons, smiths, schoolmasters, carpenters, and midwives.[5]

In villages like Graft in the Noorderkwartier, the master surgeon was invariably counted among the elite of the village, if an elite may be defined as those belonging to the local magistrature. They were taxed accordingly, which meant that the surgeons of Graft were considered of high status.[6] In large cities like Amsterdam and Rotterdam, however, not all surgeons were this prominent as a social class. While it is true that some did belong to the cream of urban life, most of them were the sons of respectable families of the petty bourgeoisie or *smalle burgerij*. During the second half of the eighteenth century, the master surgeons of Amsterdam shed the barbering aspects of their work in order to concentrate more on the surgical side of their profession.[7] This elevated their social status accordingly. By this time, surgeons had come to look down on this purely practical side of their profession, which was usually learnt empirically and did not require any 'bookish' knowledge. In Middelburg, the capital of Zeeland, this trend only developed in the early nineteenth century.[8]

The Dutch Company surgeons tended to come mainly from respectable upper- to lower-middle-class families, although the number of surgeon's fathers in the sample of whom the profession is known is small.[9] Those who we know about were often surgeons themselves. Professions related to the church, such as sexton, organist or minister, came second. Occupations from the lower middle class (*smalle burgerij*) up to the higher middle class (*brede burgerij*) are also mentioned among their fathers' professions: hatters, innkeepers, schoolmasters, mastmakers, merchants, manufacturers, master mariners, notaries, and magistrates. Six of the 132 ships surgeons who were natives of Hoorn had been born into magistrates' families in their native city.[10] In Württemberg, Germany, during the period 1742 to 1792, the percentage of surgeons' sons who became surgeons, was more than 50. Artisans, a few pastors, and an equally small handful of apothecaries were also stated as professions. In Württemberg, few sons of prosperous parents seemed to have chosen surgery as a profession.[11]

An interesting comparison is that the Company captains (*schippers*) seem to have been an equally motley crowd as far as their social origins are concerned.[12] In the English Navy, the social status and professional ability of surgeons also varied widely: in general, their pretensions to gentility, if any, were based on rather insecure claims.[13] In 1787, they were still ranked equal to that of warrant officers. It was only because the English Admiralty wished to attract more surgeons into the Navy (just at a time when the physicians and surgeons demanded a rank more or less equal to that of army officers), the surgeons of the English Navy were finally accorded officer status in 1805.[14] The Company's senior (first) ship's surgeons on board had always been ranked as equal to or as being part of the officers group: they messed together with the (other) officers, whilst the surgeon's mates ate with the petty officers such as the steward, the cooper and the quartermasters. In the first half of the eighteenth century, the first surgeon on board got his own private cabin. From the earliest days of the Company they were considered to be as respectable as the master surgeons ashore in the Republic.

The Company: A refuge for drop-outs?

In most cities in the Republic, passing a master's examination (*huisproef*) and receiving a diploma were obligatory before a master surgeon could settle in a city. This was regulated by the local surgeon's guild and the municipal authorities. The countryside – lacking such governmental centralisation and infrastructure – was more liberal in this respect: a practitioner was more or less able to settle as a surgeon there without having to pass the master's examination, although this varied from one area to another. As a consequence, the countryside could and sometimes did form an outlet for those who had not rounded off their surgical educations in the cities or for those who were purely empirically trained (such as those trained in the army, in the fleet, or in the countryside). There is a tendency to think the same about the Company, which also employed those who had not completed their educations by taking the final examination of a surgeon's guild. Even then, a surgeon could have a successful career with the Company, as was the case with Jacobus Ellerie. Ellerie was born in the tiny village of Uithuizen in the province of Groningen, where his father Alexander, by whom he was trained, was the local surgeon. He began his surgical career as a surgeon's mate in 1749 and made eight voyages with the Company. Upon his retirement in 1770, he had received one of the highest monthly salaries the Company had ever paid to a ship's surgeon, namely 50 Dutch guilders for his last three voyages.[15] It must thereby not be forgotten that Jacobus Ellerie was examined by the Company on his surgical abilities before he was hired. He was promoted to first surgeon after some four years of working as a surgeon's mate. Again, this promotion was subject to his passing a Company examination.

When Simon Teijling, a country surgeon in the small village of Durgerdam just north of Amsterdam, retired in 1737, an announcement of the vacancy for a village surgeon of Durgerdam was placed in the *Amsterdam Zaterdagsche Courant* of 22 February, 1738. At least three of the ten candidates, namely Albertus Grubee of Amsterdam, Arnoldus Toreman of Harderwijk, and Siwert Ros of Edam had pursued or, in the case of Siwert Ros, would pursue a career in the service of the Company. Siwert Ros was rejected in Durgerdam and three years later, in 1740, he was employed by the Company as ship's surgeon's mate. Arnoldus Tooreman, born in Harderwijk in 1708, already had some experience as a ship's surgeon, as he had been employed as a surgeon's mate at the Hoorn Chamber from 1732 to 1736. He was also turned down for the Durgerdam position and he returned to the Company, where he joined the Enkhuizen Chamber as senior (first) ship's surgeon in 1740. The Durgerdam vacancy was offered to Albertus Grubee of Amsterdam. Grubee remains a bit of a mystery. Nothing about his previous career is known, except for the fact that he had made a three-year voyage for the Company as senior ship's surgeon from 1734 to 1737.[16] Therefore, he must have been a fairly experienced (ship's) surgeon. After accepting the position in Durgerdam, he bought himself a prestigious pew in the village church in October 1738, as was the wont of all prominent villagers. Perhaps the choice was not felicitous because, within the year, Grubee had disappeared from Durgerdam. No trace of him can be found in the Amsterdam archives, except that he filed for bankruptcy in 1742 as he could not pay his debts, which amounted to 20,000 Dutch guilders.[17] Unexpectedly enough, it is in the VOC archives that he turns up again. For one reason or another, he left the Republic in 1739, again as a senior surgeon for the Company, for a short voyage to the Cape, from which he returned in July 1740. He then bought a surgical shop in Amsterdam, which went bankrupt in 1742. He joined up again with the Company after his bankruptcy, and he died in 1745 while still in the Company's employ.[18] In order to evade his debts or to make a new fortune, this defaulter had sought refuge in the Company's ever needy surgical service. In that sense, the Company indeed could not be said to have attracted the high and mighty of society, although Grubee can only be accused of financial mismanagement and not of having lacked surgical experience.

Another group that needed an outlet was the army surgeons. Army surgeons were usually discharged as soon as a war ended, for instance, after the Peace of Utrecht in 1713. It seems that many of them then sought careers as country surgeons[19] and there is good reason to suppose that they also sought out maritime services, although, in the sample used for this chapter, no actual proof has been found of former army surgeons in the service of the Company.

Education

As we saw in chapter 1, in order to become a fully qualified master surgeon ashore in the cities of the Republic (having passed the tripartite master's examination), an aspiring surgeon began as a pupil or apprentice (*leerknecht*), rising via journeyman (*knecht*) to the position of master. The quality of the education of the pupils depended upon the master in whose house the pupil lodged. The pupil assisted with the shaving, the cleaning of instruments, minor operations, and the treating of wounds. Furthermore, at least in most Dutch cities, there was a kind of standardised programme of instruction for the surgeons-to-be. Textbooks were agreed upon among the surgical guilds, and there was usually a set curriculum that included practical training at the master's shop, at the *Hortus Medicus*, and in the hospitals. Anatomy was learned by dissecting cadavers in the hospitals or in the anatomy theatres.

At the end of this learning period, the master provided the pupil with a *leerbrief* (literally 'teaching letter'), a certificate which testified to the apprentice's performance during the first half of his training. The *leerbrief* also served as a certificate of good behaviour. Shown to the local guild, it was a prerequisite to becoming a journeyman, and gaining experience as such. It would enable him to attend the lectures given by the *praelector* of the city, and to take the master's examination (*huisproef*) or surgeon's sea examination (*zeeproef*) after a couple of years of practical training with another master surgeon. Once he had taken possession of this *leerbrief*, the journeyman could change masters. The German journeyman, for instance, often went on a *Wanderschaft*, gathering experience in his craft and in life by travelling from one master surgeon to another; travels which could take him as far as the Dutch coast and beyond. With this certificate, the *knecht* could also join the army as a *veldscheer*, seek work as a country surgeon, or perhaps try to find employment as a ship's surgeon with the Admiralty, the merchant fleet, the West India Company or the (East India) Company. The period served as a ship's surgeon was accepted as the equivalent of the obligatory practical training years before one could take the masters' examination.

Research by H. Ketting for his masters' thesis in 1988 revealed that the number of journeymen listed at the Amsterdam surgeons' guild who eventually passed its master's examinations declined during the eighteenth century. This was primarily because *knechten* (apprentices) left the guild to earn their livelihood elsewhere, for example, as a surgeon's mate with the Company or somewhere in the countryside. Those who did complete their training often took 11 to 12 years (from pupil to master).[20]

Indeed, it certainly occurred that pupils, to gain experience, signed a contract with the Company after which they completed their training in the Republic. This was the case of Matthijs van Brugge, born in Schiedam in 1725. He sailed for the Company as surgeon's mate in 1746, returned in 1747 and obtained his *leerbrief* in 1748, eventually passing his master's in 1754.[21] Hendrik van Ette, of Amsterdam, entered the surgeon's guild as pupil in 1754. To broaden his experience and knowledge he made two voyages with the Company, one as a surgeon's mate in 1766, and another one as first surgeon in 1768. Returning in 1770, he passed his master's examination (*huisproef*) the same year.[22] This is typical of a number of other ship's surgeons as well. The records of the surgeons' guild archives of Amsterdam show that most surgeons who passed their surgeon's sea examination (*zeeproef*) were nearly always qualified for the function of surgeon's mate (*ondermeester* or second ship's surgeon), but rarely for that of a first surgeon. This does not conform to the text of the Enkhuizen regulation of 1636 (which is thought to have been in force in all chambers) which stipulated that those who successfully passed the surgeon's sea examination could obtain the rank of first surgeon on board.[23] Apparently, the Amsterdam Chamber was inundated by such an abundance of aspiring ship's surgeons that the Chamber could easily afford to hire applicants at a rank lower than what they were qualified for.

This abundance also seems to have been the case in the Chamber of Hoorn: research in the archives in Hoorn by the amateur historian H. de Vos shows that during the years 1725 to 1765 the Hoorn Chamber received 733 applications for surgical vacancies on the ships. The authorities of this chamber turned down 492 (67 per cent) of these surgical candidates and were apparently not so desperate for ship's surgeons that it employed every willing candidate.[24] According to De Vos, the candidates for ship's surgeon applied for a particular vacancy on a certain ship, or for several vacancies on certain ships, and not for the position of ship's surgeon on any ship of that particular Chamber. The candidates expressly mention the ship(s) they want to be employed on. This practice does not confirm the generally accepted idea of a structural and deepening lack of surgeons willing to serve on Company vessels. Although the enthusiasm of Dutch surgeons to join the Hoorn Chamber declined (in the period 1726-1750, 80 per cent of the ship's surgeons were Dutch, in the period 1751-1775, this percentage fell to 59), overall, German surgeons filled the gap left by the Dutch. Furthermore, these candidates were not 'choosy' about the positions they applied for: they applied for the positions of surgeon's mate and senior surgeon, or for third surgeon and surgeon's mate, at the same time. For instance, Johan Allorath of Stockholm applied for the positions of both senior (first) ship's surgeon and surgeon's mate on the *Vrouwe Petronella*. Andreas Hendrik Angelocnator, from Magdenburg, applied for the vacancies of surgeon's mate on the *Baanman* and on the *Geertruid* and for the position of third surgeon on the *Baanman*, the *Buis*, and the *Geertruid*, all in 1727. Jan Meteren Daum, of Frankfurt, applied for the positions of surgeon's mate on the *Langewijk* and as first ship's surgeon on the *Land van Beloften*, both in 1734.[25] The ship's surgeons were, of course, a special professional group on board, and as such, perhaps not comparable to the sailors because surgeons were educated and wanted to broaden their expertise in whatever surgical position that was available.

Usually, the third surgeons (and surgeon's mates) were already in possession of the *leerbrief* before seeking employment with the Company, meaning that they had had at least three years of surgical schooling before they were employed by the Company as a mere third. The sample and research in the surgical guilds archives have shown that if a first surgeon was employed by the Company for the first time, he had had an average of nearly 13 years educational experience since his entry into the surgeon's guild as a pupil; a surgeon's mate had nine years of training; and a third surgeon had six years before being hired by the Company (table T5.1). Sometimes a surgeon, although fully qualified as a master surgeon was hired as a ship's surgeon's mate, a lot that befell Augustinus Eckhart of Amsterdam. He was born in 1742 and was apprenticed by his father at the age of 11. It took him another 11 years to pass his master's examination at the surgeon's guild of Amsterdam (1764). Despite his ample qualifications, he accepted a job as surgeon's mate for the Company in 1769. He died on the return voyage.[26]

Table T5.1: Level of education at first contract during the eighteenth century

Number of Surgeons (143)	Rank at first contract VOC	Amount of time between first entry surgeon's guild and first VOC contract
24	First Surgeon	13 years
49	Second Surgeon	9 years
70	Third Surgeon	6 years

The ship's surgeons in table T5.1 had all enjoyed a surgical training before they accepted a Company job as ship's surgeon. The time that elapsed between apprenticeship and the passing of one's surgeon's sea examination or a master's examination was quite long, which confirms Ketting's observations. Furthermore, the Company, and particularly the Amsterdam Chamber, could afford to offer fully qualified master surgeons (whose schooling was broader and longer than that of a surgeon who had passed a surgeon's sea examination) a position that was not commensurate with their education and these offers were accepted, which raises the question of why? It certainly does not agree with the general complaints by contemporaries whose jeremiads averred that qualified ship's surgeons were difficult if not well-nigh impossible to find, nor does it agree with prevailing historiographical ideas about the profession of ship's surgeons and their social status.

It appears that these men were very willing to work as a ship's surgeon, although this did not necessarily mean they were clamoring to be hired by the Company. For instance, among the names of the men who passed their surgeon's sea examination (*Zee-examen*) in the city of Hoorn, there are many who do not appear on the Company's pay rolls, such as Jan Bruel who passed his *Zee-examen* on 20 September, 1776; Jan Hendrik Blok on 2 April, 1778, as well as Pieter Dekker on 16 March, 1780; and Christiaan de Wolf on 10 July, 1787.[27] They preferred to sign on with another maritime employer. As in Zeeland, there were certainly other (maritime) employers, which many a Dutch ship's surgeon may have preferred after 1775, vide the drop in the numbers of Dutch surgeons employed by the Company in the last period of the eighteenth century (discussed in chapter 4).

This eagerness by ship's surgeons could be explained by their possible motives. As we saw in the previous chapter, it is very probable that those surgeons who applied to the Company did indeed want to broaden their professional horizons, and that they were more or less indifferent to what position they ended up in as long as it was surgical. The professional experience on board the Company vessels or at the Company settlements in Asia and South Africa was always more comprehensive and diverse than what they could ever acquire in their native countries in Europe, where the master surgeon was limited to the practice of surgery, and the surgeon's mate was limited to assisting the master, and the pupil was limited to the cleaning of the shop and the washing of beards. It has already been shown that a third surgeon or surgeon's mate on board stood a fair chance of learning of matters far beyond the limited scope of his peers and masters ashore in the Republic, if he could withstand the physical dangers inherent in being a seafarer with the Company.

Another possible explanation for the enthusiasm may have been the possible lack of employment opportunities in Europe, which forced the local surgical guilds or municipal authorities to apply stricter protective measures to limit the entry of non-local surgeons, as we saw in Flushing. Unfortunately, this particular aspect remains outside the scope of this research, and is, for now, an unanswered question. Other plausible explanations may be that the status of a ship's surgeon was not as low as has generally been supposed, which is quite a plausible hypothesis indeed as there were even some seventeenth- and eighteenth-century physicians who sailed to Asia as ship's surgeons – among them Carl Peter Thunberg who was interested in tropical plants. Engelbert Kaempfer (1651-1716) was also a German physician and botanist in the employ of the Company as a surgeon. Thunberg and Kaempfer clearly had scientific motives, which must have been a priority in their employment. Another motive may have been the remunerations of a ship's surgeon, which were well beyond the expectations of the (master) surgeons ashore in Europe.

An adequate reward may have led to a satisfactory supply of ship's surgeons. Surely, these aspiring ship's surgeons must have had some idea about the (financial) rewards signing on with the Company could offer them?

Average age

The ages of surgical pupils upon accepting their apprenticeships show no great deviation if these ages are divided between the ranks of first, second, and third surgeons. This is to be expected: in general, apprentice surgeons commenced their training around their fourteenth year. The ages of first, second, and third surgeons do differ somewhat at the outset of their Company careers, which can also be expected because those who were engaged as first surgeons at the time of their first Company voyages, having been in training longer, were older. Moreover, some of these men could have also had some maritime surgical experience elsewhere, for instance, with the *Westindische Compagnie* or one of the Admiralties. This background enabled them to obtain better positions. Research regarding seafarers from the Zeeland and/or employed by the Chamber Zeeland of the Company (1500-1800) by P. Poortvliet, a retired naval officer turned maritime historian, has shown that these seafarers had no difficulty switching from one employer to another.[28] They felt no particular loyalty to the Admiralty, the WIC, the Company or the *Middelburgsche Commercie Compagnie*, the last one being a local company trading in the West Indies, which loyalty to maritime employer is presumed among the seventeenth-century seafarers of northern Holland (as discussed in chapter 4). Bartholomeus Nebbens, from Veere; Jan de Winter, from Middelburg; Johannes van der Riet, from Bergen op Zoom; Pieter Evertsen, from Middelburg; Elias van Zeilighem, from Veere; Cornelis Lammers, from Middelburg; Petrus Callenfels, from Serooskerke; and even the German, Hendrick Nicht, from Wandersleben in Germany (but employed as ship's surgeon in Zeeland) had all worked for the Admiralty of Zeeland once or twice, or the WIC or the MCC before hiring on as a ship's surgeon with the Company.[29] Others switched to another seafaring fleet after their first voyages with the Company, changing employers as easily as changing hats. Since no such research has been done on the seafarers in the other provinces, no conclusions can be drawn about the seafarers in general. Nonetheless, the data from the province of Zeeland may serve as an indication. In all likelihood, the often presumed loyalty to a particular naval employer was not as strong as previously supposed. It certainly does not apply to the professional group of ship's surgeons employed by the Chamber of Zeeland.

The average age for first surgeons when they first became apprentices was 14. In general, there was a span of fifteen years between their becoming an apprentice and their first voyage with the Company. The surgeon's mates averaged 15 years when they became a surgeon's pupil. The third surgeons were in general around 13 years of age when their names were registered at the surgeon's guilds. By the time the third surgeons sought employment as a Company ship's surgeon they were usually 20 years old (table T5.2). Therefore, it should be possible to conclude that Company ship's surgeons were fairly well educated by the standards of those times and their rank, as well as being fairly experienced. Consequently, the idea that they were merely illiterate, uneducated young barbers, although there were exceptions, should be consigned to the realms of mythology.

Table T5.2: Span of time between apprenticeship and first VOC contract (of sampled surgeons)

Group F1 (F1=72 surgeons)	*Average age at start apprenticeship ('E1')*	*Average age at first contract ('A')*	*Average time between A and E1*
First surgeons (16)	14 years	29 years	15 years
Surgeon's mates (24)	15 years	23 years	8 years
Third surgeons (32)	13 years	20 years	7 years

Do their ages at the time of their first voyages change over time during the eighteenth century, influenced by circumstances such as shortages of surgeons so that younger (less educated and/or less experienced) surgeons were being hired or promoted? This question was investigated among the 776 ship's surgeons sample with birthdates that were retrieved. Only the ages of the first surgeons and surgeons' mates differ slightly from time to time, but these variations are fairly insignificant. The average ages of third surgeons at their first Company departure were more or less the same, being around 22 and 21 years old (table T5.3). Thus, it is an obvious conclusion that the age of being employed as first, second, or third ship's surgeon upon signing on for the first time remained the same throughout the entire century. The often postulated shortage of surgeons which would presumably have resulted in the employment of younger, less experienced, or less schooled surgeons thus did not exist, especially if the recruitment practices of the Amsterdam Chamber (employing surgeons in lower ranks than what they were actually qualified for) and those of the Hoorn Chamber, which actually rejected more than half of its applicant surgeons are taken into consideration.

Table T5.3: Average age per period of sampled surgeons (Group A)

Period	A	Average age on first VOC contract as:		
		(nr.) First	Second	Third
1700-1725	232	(33) 31	(117) 23	(82) 21
1726-1750	179	(25) 29	(54) 24	(100) 21
1751-1775	198	(23) 30	(76) 22	(99) 21
1776-1795	167	(40) 29	(71) 23	(56) 21
		(121) 30	(318) 23	(337) 21

The average age of a full first ship's surgeon commencing his career with the Company in a *lesser* rank on an earlier voyage, was 29 years, although it dropped slightly during the century from 30 to 28 (table T5.4). Here the supposed lack of qualified ship's surgeons also did not lead to the promotion of lesser qualified surgeons to the position of a senior ship's surgeon prematurely. Table T5.4 lists the average ages of Company's surgeons who, having climbed the promotional ladder, reached the rank of first surgeon during the eighteenth century.

Table T5.4: Average age first ship's surgeon top of career (Group A)

Period	*Average age VOC first ship's surgeons having started at the Company in a* lower *rank*
1700-1725	30 years (62 surgeons)
1726-1750	29 years (45 surgeons)
1751-1775	28 years (43 surgeons)
1776-1795	28 years (16 surgeons)

A brief comparison with other professional seafaring groups or with surgeons working with another East India Company might be interesting, but alas there is a lack of sufficient data. The Swedish East India Company's senior ship's surgeon was circa 32, although it is unclear if this average age was for first voyages as such.[30] On the English West African fleet, the majority of ships' surgeons were in their late 20s or early 30s, although also here it is uncertain at what age they began their nautical careers.[31] Unfortunately, there are no data for the English East India Company's surgeons, as far as I know. We do have some data pertaining to the officers of the Dutch Admiralties and the *schippers* (captains) of the Company. More than half of the Admiralties officers were over 30[32] and, considering a sample of some 300 eighteenth-century Company captains, it was established that the average age of a captain of a Dutch East Indiaman was around 34 to 35 years of age. But by then, this freshly appointed captain had had some ten years experience as a mate. [33] On average, a Company captain was the veteran of some two to three outward-bound voyages (some making only one voyage, others making three or four) after his ten-year apprenticeship as a mate. No *schipper* undertook seven voyages or more during the eighteenth century in that capacity, the reason for which was mostly caused by the high mortality rates.

In comparison, all ship's surgeons in the sample (S), that is senior surgeons, surgeon's mates and *derde meesters* (third surgeons) taken together, made some 5,000 outward-bound voyages on Company ships (as is shown in table T5.5). The resulting average of nearly two journeys per surgeon (1:1.7) does not seem to make much sense, because these journeys were not evenly distributed among them: nearly two-thirds made only one voyage for the Company; others made ten voyages or more. The intra-Asiatic journeys are not taken into account as they are deemed to belong to the tenure the surgeon signed on with the Company for each departure.

Table T5.5: Number of sampled surgeons and their departures per Chamber

Group S	*Amsterdam*	*Zeeland*	*Rotterdam*	*Delft*	*Hoorn*	*Enkhuizen*	*total*
Surgeons	977	410	440	347	396	418	2988
Outward Voyages	1794	874	624	593	543	623	5051

For the Company's senior surgeons (*oppermeesters*), the average number of contracts was less than that of the *schippers*: 1.6 voyages per first ship's surgeon, which is consistent with the whole population (S) as can be seen in tables T5.5 and T5.6. However, like the Company captains, these senior surgeons had made several voyages in a lesser capacity, averaging three earlier voyages as third surgeon and surgeon's mate.

Table T5.6: Eighteenth-century VOC-captains and first ship's surgeons

		Average number of voyages (out-ward bound) in such capacity
Number of captains	300	2.5
Number of first ship's surgeons	1115	1.6

Although the age of the senior surgeons at the moment they were promoted first surgeon was lower than that of a captain when the latter topped off his maritime career (mate-captain), for one reason or another, a senior surgeon was not able to or chose not to make more than one or two voyages in that capacity. The difference can be partly explained by the fact that a captain was never stationed at a trading settlement in Asia during his working life for the Company, which could and did happen to the ship's surgeon. While the captain always sailed his ship, the ship's surgeon treated patients, either on board or ashore at one of the settlements. As a result, the surgeon made fewer voyages, being settlement-based as often as on board, and the voyages he did make (departure from the Republic – settlement – repatriating to the Republic) were generally of a longer duration. Another factor affecting the discrepancy could have been the increased mortality risk. Because of his frequent contact with his patients, the surgeon ran a higher risk of contracting a fatal disease, which could lead to an earlier death. The captain as a rule did not come into daily contact with his crew: he had his own cabin, his own food, and his own segregated work area on the vessel away from the crew during working hours. Lastly, a ship's surgeon was, of course, able to retire sooner from the Company's service in order to start a practice ashore in Europe, which he might have wanted to pursue after only one or two voyages. A captain always needed the sea and a vessel to exercise his profession.

Positions and rewards

In 1682, ship's surgeon Lodewijk de Fuijter humbly requested Governor-General Speelman and the Council of the Indies for permission to repatriate to the Republic as 'his fantasies about the financial gains a surgeon could earn in Asia had burst like a bubble'.[34] Apparently, for him, and for many others, the Company's sea routes had turned out to be a *cul-de-sac*.

As a result of the disastrous mortality rates on board and in Asia during certain periods of the Company's existence (notably in 1690-1695, 1730-1750 and 1770-1775), the Gentlemen XVII had deliberated about how to ensure good surgical/medical services for their sailors and soldiers and how to counter the heavy death tolls. The increase in salaries to attract more and better surgeons was never really considered a solution, as companies (then or now) are often wont to think. For instance, in the wake of the heavy mortality rates suffered in the years 1690 to 1695, the Gentlemen XVII in 1695 issued regulations, which formalised the duties of a Company ship's surgeon. These regulations would not undergo any basic changes during the entire eighteenth century. It took nearly three-quarters of a century, in 1760, that the Gentlemen XVII tried financial rewards to keep their experienced surgeons working for the Company by paying a first surgeon on his first voyage the usual monthly 36 Dutch guilders; while on his second contract he earned 40 Dutch guilders; on his third voyage, 45 Dutch guilders; and on his fourth a monthly 50 Dutch guilders.[35]

Even before 1760, though no official decision has been found in the Company's archives, the surgeons' payrolls note that from 1745 on a premium was paid at the conclusion of the voyage. Thus, when Arnoldus Grubee died on his return voyage in 1745, his daughter Anna Catharina received not only the wages her father had earned but also an additional 500 Dutch guilders, called the *douceur* for surgeons, although this sum was hardly enough to cover the debts incurred by her father's bankruptcy.[36] Surgeon's mates would receive 300 Dutch guilders, and third surgeons 150 Dutch guilders at the successful conclusion of the voyage. Sometimes, over and above that, an extra month's salary was included. Nor did the perks stop there. There were premiums for sailing around Scotland (*achterom*), which was done during the wars with England, to evade a confrontation with the English Navy in the narrow Channel, or in other situations when the Channel proved too risky.

In 1783 the Gentlemen XVII decided to use a new, and what they thought would be cheaper, incentive. The ship's surgeons would receive a bonus sum for every sailor they delivered to the Cape alive. A chief surgeon would receive three Dutch guilders for every living man on board at the Cape of Good Hope and a surgeon's mate 1.10 Dutch guilders. This soon proved too expensive (the mortality rates on board the outward-bound vessels had for some time been improving), and the Company then re-introduced the premium or *douceur* for surgeons: the senior ship's surgeon received 150 Dutch guilders and a surgeon's mate received 100 Dutch guilders if the voyage was reasonably 'healthy'.[37] In practice, however, the surgeons were paid the *douceurs* introduced in 1745.

Moreover, for an extended period of time a Company servant was guaranteed a fixed income with free board and lodging, if he survived. For the family back home, this meant some financial security for a number of years, because part of the income earned by the employee on the ships and/or in Asia could be paid out to them, or was saved up during the term of employment and was paid out either upon a premature death or upon his return home.[38] Customarily, a portion of each bachelor's wages was withheld and deposited in the Republic. Whenever a man married overseas, his salary could be paid out there in full.[39] This long-term security must certainly have been attractive for many a surgeon's mate: he was guaranteed work (experience needed for the masters' examination), food, lodgings, and pay.

The Company and the Admiralties of the Republic paid their seafarers less than their counterparts in the merchant or whaling fleets.[40] As compensation, Company seafarers were allowed to take private commodities along to sell in

Asia on the outward-bound journey, and such wares as cotton, tea and *atjar* (all in small quantities) on the return voyage to sell at home. If posted ashore in Asia or at the Cape, he was given extra pay in products such as wine and beer. To demonstrate the course of an ordinary surgical career with the Company, let us turn to Adriaan van Brakel.

Van Brakel, born in Delft in 1733, joined the Company as a third surgeon in 1751 with a monthly salary of 14 Dutch guilders.[41] He cashed in a two-months' pay advance from his employer, which was common practice; the ship's surgeons were even allowed to have a third months' advanced pay in order to buy surgical instruments (usually lancets). Moreover, Van Brakel was allowed an advance of 5.15 Dutch guilders (five guilders and fifteen pennies or *stuivers*) to pay for a surgical chest. The Company provided the medical chest. Consequently, before he set sail on 20 October, 1751, he was in debt to the tune of 33.15 Dutch guilders. Van Brakel did not make use of the common practice of reserving a yearly three months' pay to be handed over to parents or wife, having neither. Having arrived in Batavia after a voyage of seven months, he had earned (seven times 14 guilders minus his debt of 33.15 Dutch guilders) an amount of 61.50 Dutch guilders. Whilst in Batavia, he again took a three-months' pay advance (perhaps to invest in buying some local products). Then he returned to the Republic on the same ship, which landed on 5 July, 1753. He received an amount of 404.50 Dutch guilders (comprised of 21.5 months' wages, as well as the *douceur* of 150 Dutch guilders minus the sums borrowed). Three months later, he set sail again as a surgeon's mate.

Table T5.7: The earnings of Adriaan van Brakel [42]

Voyage data	*Ship*	*Function*	*Monthly pay*	*What he received at the conclusion of his voyage in rounded figures (minus advances)*
1751-1753	Erfprins	third surgeon	NLG 14.00	NLG 405
1753-1755	Erfprins	third surgeon	NLG 14.00	NLG 406
1756-1762	De Hoop	Surgeon's mate	NLG 24.00	NLG 1,932
1762-1764	Overschie	Surgeon's mate	NLG 26.00	NLG 692
1764-1766	Bleiswijk	first surgeon	NLG 36.00	NLG 1,139
1767-1774†	Bleiswijk	first surgeon	NLG 40.00	NLG 4,558
			Total	NLG 9,131

The 9,131 Dutch guilders that Van Brakel received over some 25 years (400 Dutch guilders a year) is in fact less than the actual sum he earned. Deducted were his debts for buying instruments, surgical chests, and for the loans he took whilst in Batavia in order to buy native products. Cogently, Van Brakel did not have any living costs, such as board and lodgings, during his contract.

Van Brakel was never posted to one of the settlements for any period of time. A senior ship's surgeon on the Company's fleet rarely earned more than a monthly 45 Dutch guilders, an annual sum of 540 Dutch guilders, so he should have considered himself well paid. To earn more, he would have needed to have been posted in an important settlement, such as Batavia, the Cape of Good Hope, or Ceylon. And to really succeed, once posted at a settlement, he should have switched to the civilian service of the Company and acquired the rank of 'merchant', the highest rank at all the Company settlements in Asia in terms of social status and financial rewards. This step was usually not feasible for a Company surgeon but it did not mean a surgeon could not advance his career in the Company hierarchy. Willem Timmers of Schiedam, for instance, made his first voyage for the Company as surgeon's mate at the age of 25 for the Chamber of Delft in 1701.[43] He returned in 1703, and again departed – this time as first surgeon – in 1704. Having made various intra-Asiatic voyages, he settled in Batavia in 1710, where he remained for the rest of his life. In 1719, he became the superintendent (*eerste chirurgijn*) of the *Binnenhospitaal.* Ten years later, he was the best paid surgeon in the sample (S) of ship's surgeons with a monthly salary of 90 Dutch guilders (1,080 Dutch guilders annually).[44] In Galle in Ceylon, a senior surgeon could earn up to 70 Dutch guilders per month (840 Dutch guilders annually). As was already lamented by surgeon Lodewijk de Fuijter, the official Company stipend was not really what attracted the surgeons. The greatest lure was the opportunities offered to earn extra money, such as the premiums, the *douceurs*, and the private trading. This is made abundantly clear in a closer look at the incomes of the master surgeons practising in the city of Amsterdam (table T5.8).

The Amsterdam master surgeons improved their financial position in the course of the second half of the eighteenth century. More than half of them earned more than one thousand guilders annually while a senior ship's surgeon at the Company with, say, 45 Dutch guilders a month, would earn a mere 540 Dutch guilders yearly. This is to some extent counterbalanced by the fact that a ship's surgeon did not have to invest in a surgical 'shop', or pay for food or lodgings. Together with the premiums and the (illegal) trade opportunities, the Company's ship's surgeon could end up better off financially.

Table T5.8: Annual incomes of master surgeons in Amsterdam[45]

Yearly Income	*1741-1750*		*1776-1780*		*1781-1790*		*1791-1800*	
in Dutch Guilders	*no.*	%	*no.*	%	*no.*	%	*no.*	%
0 - <1,000	14	49	8	33	13	35	20	36
1,000 - < 2,000	10	35	9	38	6	16	18	33
2,000 - < 6,000	3	10	5	21	7	19	11	20
6,000 - < 12,000	1	3	-	-	4	11	5	9
12,000 and more	1	3	2	8	7	19	1	2

A comparison of the ship's surgeons' stipends with the wages of labourers working in the Republic reinforces the idea that the Company's wages were not *a priori* tempting, and that there must have been other incentives that made the Company attractive to (prospective) employees. The German agricultural workers or *Hollandgänger* worked some nine months in the Republic before returning home with their savings, which amounted to some 100 guilders; those who worked only two months in the Republic took home no more than 30 guilders.[46] The daily wages during the eighteenth century in the Republic averaged around one guilder in the countryside in the western provinces of the Republic; in the southern and eastern provinces they were somewhat less, fluctuating between half a guilder and one guilder. The annual income of an unschooled labourer averaged circa 240 Dutch guilders, whilst that of a third ship's surgeon on the Company vessels was circa 168 Dutch guilders. After 1680, the average income in the Republic was circa 383 Dutch guilders; while most people earned less than 600 Dutch guilders annually.[47] A ship's surgeon would only receive that official annual salary when he reached the top ranks of his profession with the Company. Clearly, the official Company salary could not have been the chief motive to the aspiring Company surgeon.

Company personnel were not averse to trading in contraband, smuggling, the so-called *morshandel* (spillage trade). This *morshandel* offered money-making opportunities on the private trading of (Asian) goods above the limit set by the Company, although this was officially forbidden. Should he so wish, an employee could also earn extra by handling money transactions, which meant the manipulation of bills of exchange which, with the Company's permission, could be cashed at home in the Republic for higher sums than they were bought for in the Asian Company settlements.[48] Many a ship's surgeon attempted to augment his income in this way. Although the private trading activities of the Company's surgeons have not been researched, the personal documents of these ship's surgeons such as wills, powers of attorney and letters leave the strong impression that many of them did take part in such transactions, and if not for themselves, then on the behalf of others, which will be discussed in more detail in chapter 6.

Officers (senior surgeons amongst them) employed on the Company ships were allowed to take commodities to trade along the way to Asia on behalf of Dutch merchants in the Republic. These included compasses, watches, razors ('shaving knives'), combs, snuffboxes, tobacco, and hats.[49] In 1745, senior surgeons demanded that they be allowed to take along larger quantities of goods on their outward-bound journeys, this being granted to them as an extra inducement as 'senior surgeons for the Company's vessels were hard to find'.[50] As noted earlier, there was, in general, no lack of surgeons for the outward-bound vessels. The crux lay in the East, as a result of the particular circumstances in the settlements, notably at the Cape and in Batavia, where the filling of vacancies was dependent on those who arrived from the Republic. It was there that a lack of surgical employees was often noticeable. Virulent diseases raging on the vessels strained the hospital's capacities at the Cape; there was not just a shortage of beds, but trained employees were sometimes hard to find. Surgical vacancies there were usually replaced by seafaring employees who were then taken from the vessels, which subsequently meant that the vessels were short of surgeons from the Cape bound for Batavia. The diseases that raged in Batavia produced similar problems. Then, during the period 1726-1750, for the first time it was felt that Dutch ship's surgeons were withdrawing from their participation in the Company's surgical labour-market, leading to a complaint by Company management that surgeons had become hard to find.

The increase in private trade for seafaring personnel was extra incentive to encourage (Dutch?) ship's surgeons to seek employment with the Company. There is plenty of evidence they did indeed make use of it. They stocked their chests with trade commodities in which they invested heavily, occasionally having to resort to borrowing to do so. Evidence exists in the financial administration of the Enkhuizen Chamber of repatriating surgeons being served with a writ of attachment by merchants in the Republic, to be repealed only after the surgeons paid their debts owed these merchants. In 1792, the widow of Merchant Van der Valk, for instance, thus distrained the wages of Senior Surgeon Jacobus Adolph Nies until his debt to her of 350 Dutch guilders was paid.[51] The Amsterdam merchant, Joseph Weesing served a writ on the wages of Wilhelm Hendrik Bekken in 1788, which was withdrawn when Bekken repaid his debt of 169 Dutch guilders.[52] The surgeon James Fredrik Christiaan Hendrik Nietsch, who repatriated with the *Resolutie* in 1784, found himself in the same predicament. He had to repay his debt to the Amsterdam merchant Dirk Boerrigter.[53] The surgeon Johannes Verwoert had borrowed substantially, a loan which he had to repay upon repatriation in 1782: his wages were distrained by J.F. Schepen; by Hendrik Hugo de Barnij (175 Dutch guilders); by Messrs Hendrik de Put, B. van Deijl and J.St.L. Maurenbrecher; and by the Amsterdam merchant Paulus Hansen (600 Dutch guilders).[54] When he repatriated after five years in 1714, the ship's surgeon Abraham Rosendaal was reminded by some Dutch merchants that he not only had to repay his debt but also the interest and costs of one-half percent, which had been agreed upon in a notarial deed.[55]

Social networks and private trading

These surgeons left the shores of the Republic, their chests full of trade commodities, their bags stuffed with letters of introduction to friends of friends who would promote, sponsor, and vouch for them in Asia. Letters of introduction were very important to every Company employee, as the Company could offer a wealth of opprtunities with respect to financial rewards and social status at the settlements, and, if a person had the right social connections, the ambitious man could achieve much. It was well known at the time that the prospects were good for improving one's position, socially and financially in Asia. Because of the high turnover rate of Company employees in Asia, with three- to five-year contracts compounded by high mortality rates among Europeans, jobs and positions had to be filled quickly from the limited number of available Europeans employees in Asia. Thus positions frequently fell vacant and it certainly helped to have the right connections.[56] In the East, one could marry prudently, that is to say, wed advantageously!

In Batavia, under the Company's political and economic structure, promotions were largely controlled by patronage in which family relationships played a key role. The crucial links were those between a man and his in-laws, as sons born of European parents in Asia were sent back to the Republic for schooling, while their sisters remained with their parents in Asia.[57] Ambitious employees marrying in Asia, therefore, sought a bride with powerful connections. Daughters of influential parents and/or widows left comfortably off by influential husbands were firm favourites.

Superior social networks, therefore, were significant to the career man. When the ship's surgeon set out from the Republic on his way to Asia, he usually knew some 'friends' to approach upon his arrival there. These 'friends', whom the surgeon in question would never have met, were acquaintances of his parents, or of his uncles, or of his family's neighbours. In his luggage, he carried letters of introduction to these friends, as did the surgeon's mate Jan Pietersz. Gouwenaar, from Enkhuizen. Departing from the Republic in 1752, he took along letters addressed to Governor General Jacob Mossel (1704-1761) in Batavia.[58] The third surgeon (*derde meester*) Simon Walmeester (1733-1752), also from Enkhuizen, not only had letters for His Excellency, he also carried along six tongue sausages and three hams for His Excellency's equerry, Colonel W.H. van Ossenbergh.[59] It is not very likely that Gouwenaar and Walmeester were close friends of Mossel, but Mossel was born in Enkhuizen as were Gouwenaar and Walmeester, and this connection could have been advantageous to these surgeons in their careers if they had lived long enough. Unfortunately, they never had the chance to deliver these letters and delicacies personally to the top man in Asia. They both died in 1752, never having set foot in Batavia.

The influential friends were courted and the relationships were maintained by an extensive correspondence. This private correspondence and its significance to the authors thereof were of extreme importance to anybody's career. Family ties were also deemed necessary for social survival and served as a motivation to seek a career with the Company. As discussed in chapter 4, many brothers, sons, and cousins of ship's surgeons were found on the Company payrolls.

Arnoldus op den Ool started his career as a third surgeon with a monthly stipend of 14 guilders in 1747. He arrived in Batavia that same year, and subsequently made several intra-Asiatic voyages as a ship's surgeon. In 1751, he was posted to Batavia as a surgeon at the *Arm en Weeshuis* (the Poorhouse and Orphanage). He swiftly became the chief surgeon of that institution (in 1755), earning a monthly salary of 45 Dutch guilders in 1754 (540 Dutch guilders annually), which was raised to 50 Dutch guilders (annual VOC income 600 Dutch guilders) in 1762.[60] However, these fine incomes were nothing compared to his real transactions. His aspirations reached much further. In 1761, Op den Ool became warden (*buitenregent*) of the *Lazarus*house on the island of Purmerend. He worked in this capacity, in a close relationship with the other warden, Joseph van den Berge, whose wife, Petronella Blanket, had superior connections. Her guardian was François Rijkloff van Goens, descendant of one of the former Governors General. The family Van den Berge-Planket was fairly well off, and Arnoldus befriended them. Together they bought a small rigged ship (*Pantjalang*) in 1763, restored the ship, and together they bought three slaves to serve as crew; all this for the sum of 2,000 Dutch guilders. Their intention was made all too clear in the notarial deed they drew up with Notary Gousset in Batavia: the profits made from the trade by means of the *Pantjalang* were to be divided between Messrs Van den Berge and Op den Ool.[61]

Profits made from what, one may well wonder? A notarial deed drawn up two months earlier gives some indication. Apparently, Op den Ool had asked a colleague, Senior Surgeon Pieter van den Sprenkel, to supply him with some products from the Republic. Van den Sprenkel consequently left the Republic in 1758 with the commodities in his chests. He made several intra-Asiatic voyages, and having spent time at Cochin between 1760 and 1761, he was now posted to Surat (1762-1766). In the notarial deed of 27 July 1763, Op den Ool empowered the Company Merchant R. van Hedin, who was also posted to Surat, to take charge of these products which were in the custody of Van den Sprenkel.[62] Op den Ool requested that other colleagues supply him with products from the Republic, including chests of red wine, Delft pipes, chests of Dutch gin (*jenever*), 50 hams, 60 cow tongues, 50 boxes of butter, 400 bottles of spring water, 50 cheeses, dozens of knives, 600 pairs of shoes, some 100 mirrors, and some 50 drinking glasses.[63] The assumption of private trading is soon reached, if we do not accept the idea that some hundred mirrors served Op den Ool's vanity.

How did Surgeon Op den Ool pay for all this? The short and simple answer is: He borrowed. Sometimes relatively modest sums, like 500 Dutch guilders from the free Christian woman, Anna Michiels (a freed slave), and sometimes large sums, such as 7,500 Dutch guilders from the Company merchant, Jacobus Johannes Craan. As security, he pledged his 11 slaves.[64] As his business grew, his very 'partner in crime' died. Van den Berghe passed away in July 1764; three months later, Op den Ool married Van den Berghe's widow, Petronella Planket.

These practices were certainly not unique for Company surgeons. Those involved in the English West-African trade also devoted themselves to non-medical pursuits while on a voyage: one aspect of their careers is their extra employment as independent traders and factors.[65] It is highly probable that these practises sprang up wherever opportunities presented themselves.

Climbing the ladder via promotions

Surgeons who accumulated experience during a number of voyages were fairly certain of being promoted. Promotion from third to second and ultimately to the rank of chief or first surgeon depended primarily on the numbers of vacancies. Some surgeons reached the rank of *merchant*, a status symbol so many servants of the Company strived for. The way to succeed beyond the rank of senior surgeon and to reach the top commercial functions in the Company was to follow a career in the civilian service in Batavia. This could only be done successfully if one possessed the necessary social connections, the correct European descent (Dutch/European), and the only true (Protestant) religion.[66]

Cornelis Willebrinck, Stephanus ten Holder, and Johannes Winkelaar sailed as senior surgeons or surgeon's mates on their first Company contract. Cornelis Willebrinck, sailed another three times in the same capacity but on his fifth, in 1721, he went as a merchant.[67] Stephanus ten Holder reached the rank of assistant merchant in 1729 on his fourth voyage,[68] which Johannes Winkelaar achieved on his third in 1732.[69] After one voyage as a third surgeon (in 1772), Gillis van Laarbeek, from Middelburg, preferred a real nautical career: He switched to master gunner's mate (*constabelsmaat*) in 1775 and became a captain (*schipper*) over the course of 14 years.[70] Those in the sample who switched careers were mainly employed by the Chamber of Zeeland. In all, eight surgeons from the Company's Zeeland Chamber switched careers halfway through their working lives, meaning nearly three per cent of the sampled ship's surgeons of that Chamber. This is in effect a very small percentage, as a consequence of which we might conclude that the majority of (Zeeland's) ship's surgeons went to sea primarily to work purely as ship's surgeons, and had no inclination to climb the ranks beyond that, or did not live long enough to be able to pursue another profession. Again, the uniqueness of the ship's surgeons' profession must be stressed.

Those who entered Company service as a *derde meester* were the ones who had, of course, the best prospects for a career. They were young(er) and stood at the bottom of the promotional ladder. Accordingly, we must take a closer look at their careers. In this context this excludes the Company's ship's surgeons who signed just one contract for one voyage and who repatriated within five years never to work for the Company again, as well as those who also signed just one contract, did not repatriate but died within five years. The number of those who signed just one contract and repatriated fairly soon (within five years[71]) and did not sign a second contract with the Company is 390, or 12 per cent of S. It is highly likely that these surgeons went to sea with no intention other than to broaden their knowledge. They were satisfied with the one maritime adventure and afterwards carried on with their normal surgical career ashore.

Table T5.9: Sampled surgeons (N) repatriated within five years never to take service again

Period	*Number of surgeons (N) (percentage N of 'S per period')*	*Total of S per period*
1700-1725	132 (16%)	853
1726-1750	114 (14%)	843
1751-1775	76 (10%)	733
1776-1795	68 (12%)	559

The number of those who died within five years and consequently could not make a career at the Company is impressive: 1,059 ship's surgeons, being 35 per cent of S. Especially in the third period, no less than 10 per cent of the entire sample died within five years of their first departures. These surgeons will also not be taken into consideration here because they were obviously unable to pursue a career in the Company. This mortality rate increased by 10 per cent in the third period, i.e., after 1750.

Table T5.10: Surgeons who died within five years after first departure

Period	*Number of surgeons (N) (percentage of S)*	*Total of S per period (percentage N per period)*
1700-1725	226 (8%)	853 (27%)
1726-1750	268 (9%)	843 (32%)
1751-1775	304 (10%)	733 (42%)
1776-1795	261 (9%)	559 (47%)

This leaves us a group of 1,539 sampled ship's surgeons (Group E) who signed up for several voyages, who stayed abroad at the various settlements, or who made intra-Asian voyages as ship's surgeons, and/or who died after five years making just the one departure. This is the group that will be examined here in some detail. It should be borne in mind, that these men (Group E) constitute half of the original surgical workforce of the Company, as 50 per cent were unable to follow (as a result of mortality) or did opted to not pursue a career with the Company. I have chosen to take a special look at the second departures, because of the short life spans these surgeons had, with the result that there are relatively fewer third and even fewer fourth and fifth voyages.

In the first period, 17 per cent of third surgeons were promoted to senior surgeon (first or chief surgeon). This was a major promotion indeed, which occurred in the second period as well, with a relatively high portion of 15 per cent, after which these major promotions dwindled, slipping from 7 per cent to 3 per cent.[72] One-fifth of these men had been posted at a trading post such as Batavia, Surat, Cochin, Japan, Macassar, Colombo, and Semarang for several years, during which time they had been promoted to surgeon's mate; after 1750 this post was usually Batavia. The promotion could also take place on board. Albert Pijl of Enkhuizen was promoted to surgeon's mate on the *Geertruijd* within a year of his first Company contract.[73] Interestingly, these promoted surgeons had remained at home quite a long time before they signed a second contract as first surgeon in the first half of the eighteenth century. It is highly plausible that in those years, the ship's surgeon finished his education and graduated at his guild. This is substantiated by the facts that these promoted surgeons were predominantly Dutch, and their number became significantly less during the third and fourth periods, while at the same time, the periods spent at home also grew significantly shorter.

Table T5.11: Group E (1,539 surgeons) Promotion to First Surgeon

	1700-1725	*1726-1750*	*1751-1775*	*1776-1795*
Number of third surgeons first contract	129	175	159	31
Number of those promoted to first sea surgeon at second contract	22 (17% of 129)	23 (13% of 175)	11 (7% of 160)	1 (3% of 31)
Average time between first and second contract	7 years	8 years	7 years	6 years
Average time staying abroad	4 years	4 years	5 years	5 years
Average time between repatriation and second departure	3 years	4 years	2 years	1 year
Average number of voyages after being promoted to first ship's surgeon	2	2	1.5	1

Table T5.12 shows that the majority of third surgeons were promoted to surgeon's mate on their second voyage. They had, on average, just the one year at home between their first and second voyages, which may have just been long enough to take the surgeon's sea examination (*zeeproef*); or they were deemed experienced enough by the Company after one voyage as *derde meester*. The trend during the eighteenth century was to promote fewer thirds to seconds, except during the last period. However, that trend is not significant by any modern statistical standards.[74]

Table T5.13 provides us with the number of third surgeons who were not promoted to a higher position on their second voyage, which grows and peaks in the third quarter of the century, after which it drops off again to the level of the first quarter. It is peculiar that it was precisely during this period of heavy mortality rates on board (1770-1775) that so few third surgeons (30 per cent) were promoted.[75] This awaits further clarification. What undoubtedly does emerge is that the third period is the difficult one. This can only be explained by the fact that high mortality among the ship's surgeons of the Company struck in Asia after 1750,

Table T5.12: Group E (1,539 surgeons) Promotion to Surgeon's Mate

	1700-1725	*1726-1750*	*1751-1775*	*1776-1795*
Number of third surgeons first contract	129	175	159	31
Number of those promoted to second sea surgeon (surgeon's mate) at second contract	92 (71% of 129)	122 (70% of 175)	104 (65% of 160)	26 (84% of 31)
Average time between first and second contract	4 years	3 years	3 years	3 years
Average time staying abroad	3 years	3 years	3 years	3 years
Average time between repatriated and second departure	1 year	<1 year	<1 year	<1 year
Average number of voyages after being promoted to surgeon's mate	1	2	2	1

which presented major problems to the authorities who were left wondering how to fill the vacancies. Perhaps neither the physical nor the professional quality of the ship's surgeons was up to par during this period.

Table T5.13: Group E (1,539 surgeons) Not promoted

	1700-1725	*1726-1750*	*1751-1775*	*1776-1795*
Number of third surgeons first contract	129	175	159	31
Number of those again as third surgeons second contract	15 (12% of 129)	30 (17% of 175)	45 (28% of 160)	4 (13% of 31)
Average time between first and second contract	3.5 years	3 years	3 years	3 years
Average time staying abroad	3.5 year	2 years	2 years	2 years
Average time between repatriated and second departure	< 1 year	1 year	1 years	1 year
Average number of voyages from second voyage onwards	1	2	2	2

In conclusion, most of the third surgeons (*derde meesters*) were promoted to surgeon's mates on their second voyage. During the first half of the century equal numbers remained third surgeons or were promoted to first surgeon. This changed after 1750 with a substantial part of the thirds remaining so on their second voyages.

If we examine the promotions of surgeon's mates, table T5.14 demonstrates that roughly two-thirds of the surgeon's mates were promoted to senior surgeon with their second contract. This percentage remains the same, even though the time between first and second contracts diminished in the third period.

Table T5.14: Group E (1,539 surgeons) Surgeon's Mates promotions

	1700-1725	*1726-1750*	*1751-1775*	*1776-1795*
Number of surgeon's mates first contract	177	105	100	46
Number of those promoted to first sea surgeon at second contract	115 (65%)	67 (64%)	63 (63%)	29 (63%)
Average time between first and second contract	5 years	6 years	3 years	5 years
Average time duration abroad	4 years	3 years	2 years	3 years
Average time between repatriation and second departure	1.6 years	< 1 year	< 1 year	1 year
Average number of voyages after being promoted to first ship's surgeon	1.8	1.8	1.8	1.4

It follows that circa one-third were not promoted on their second voyages for the Company, which is shown in table T5.15.[76]

Table T5.15: Group E (1,539 surgeons) Surgeon's Mates not promoted

	1700-1725	*1726-1750*	*1751-1775*	*1776-1795*
Number of surgeon's mates first contract	177	105	100	46
Number of those staying surgeon's mates at second contract	62 (35%)	38 (36%)	37 (37%)	17 (37%)
Average time between first and second contract	4 years	3 years	3 years	3 years
Average time duration abroad	3.21 years	2.16 year	2 years	2.1 years
Average time between repatriated and second departure	< 1 year	1 year	0.6 year	half a year
Average number of voyages from second departure onwards	1.87	1.68	1.88	1.29

In short, according to the data listed in tables T5.11-T5.15, it seems that a promotion of a third surgeon to surgeon's mate was slightly more difficult during the period 1725-1775, whilst the promotion to first surgeon with the second contract became virtually impossible after 1750. This substantiates the idea that quality criteria became stricter over the course of the eighteenth century. There was no change in the Company's promotion policies regarding surgeon's mates during the century.

Soldiers and surgeons

At the Cape sailors and soldiers were occasionally taken into the service of the local hospital. After a period of what served virtually as an apprenticeship, this soldier/surgeon submitted himself to an examination by the senior surgeons of the hospital and was granted a certificate of fitness to practise.[77] The promotion to the rank of *onderchirurgijn* or *ondermeester* (surgeon's mate or second surgeon) was made by a board of examiners composed of senior surgeons at the Cape Hospital, and of senior surgeons from visiting vessels who were summoned to assist in the examination.[78] Burrows states that, at the Cape of Good Hope, it was common practice to promote a soldier to the rank of third surgeon, as the number of replacements for surgical staff by surgeons arriving from the Republic often proved insufficient. It is needless to point out that these occasions, born of necessity, on which soldiers (or sailors), and, as we will see, Asians and Eurasians, were admitted into the surgeon's craft, did little to enhance the status of the craft in the eyes of those in Europe who already looked down on the profession, and may well have contributed to the increased disdain.

At this point, it is important to recall that historian R. van Gelder pointed out that many educated foreigners were employed as soldiers by the Company.[79] And it may well have been that especially those educated, perhaps even surgically schooled, soldiers were recruited into the medical ranks at the hospitals at the Cape of Good Hope and in Asia. Johan Christoffel Heinse, from Magdenburg, sailed as a soldier to Batavia on a monthly salary of 9 Dutch guilders in 1744. Upon his arrival in Batavia, he was posted to the *Binnenhospitaal* as a third surgeon. He must have shown some talent or already had some surgical experience and must have passed some examinations because he was promoted from third to second, and from second to senior surgeon during his nine-year residence in Batavia, where he died in 1753. Again, this was never done without the permission of the medical authorities in Batavia (or of those at the Cape of Good Hope, for that matter). They were called 'soldiers at the surgery' or 'pupils at the surgery', and they ranked – in general – lower and were paid less than a third surgeon (*derde meester*). These pupils, but for the occasional exception such as Heinse, were trained over a period of at least five years at a hospital before they became third surgeons. During their training, these pupils acquired far more experience than a surgeon's pupil would have gained in the very limited practise of a master surgeon in Europe. They assisted the surgeons on their clinical rounds in the hospitals on a daily basis. Cogently, these pupils saw the entire scope of medicine, as opposed to the limited exposure that master surgeons in Europe had, who usually ran a barber's shop besides his surgical activities. Company Surgeons were, as we saw, not obliged to trim and shave beards.

Soldiers also became surgeon-pupils at the hospitals in Galle (Ceylon). In 1760, the hospital's surgical staff consisted of the first surgeon, Barend Frederik Runstorff, surgeon's mates, Johannes Engelbregt and Mijnder Huijberts, and the third surgeon, namely the 'soldier at the surgery', Jonas Theering.[80] This certainly occurred at all of the trading settlements, out of sheer necessity as not enough surgeons were available, although the extent to which this happened cannot be determined.[81]

The same process happened on board, although rarely; not more than a handful in the sample ever switched careers from sailor or soldier to surgeon. For instance, when surgeon's mate Jan Gouwenaar died on the 16 August, 1752, the council of officers of the *Orangezaal* decided to conditionally promoted Simon Walmeester from third surgeon to surgeon's mate, which would only become official after he passed an exam given by the authorities in Batavia. The first surgeon on the *Orangezaal* lacked a loblolly boy at the time, and so the council decided to promote the soldier Gabriel Hendrik Kemper to third surgeon (*derde meester*).[82] Still, everything depended on the ratification of these promotions by the authorities in Batavia. We have already seen that the prevailing idea among historians of the Company, that it became increasingly difficult for the Company to recruit sufficient manpower and that the Company, therefore, on the whole, could not afford to be selective,[83] did not apply to the surgeons, as there were safeguards to guarantee the quality of the ship's surgeons. Although the Company, particularly at the Cape and on board the vessels, did promote soldiers (or sailors) to the function of loblolly boys, these were invariably examined on the spot and again after they arrived in Batavia, or the Republic. A further promotion was also only valid after training at the hospital and a thorough examination. If anything, quality criteria became stricter over the course of the eighteenth century.

Life span and mortality

After 1658, seafarers, soldiers, and craftsmen were all contracted for five years, which excluded the outward-bound and homeward-bound voyages.[84] In short, they had to serve five years in Asia. This obligatory tenure, which also applied to the surgeons, was in effect a 'dead letter': According to the exigencies of the moment (such as sudden vacancies), the authorities at the Cape of Good Hope or those in Batavia (the Head of Surgery) decided where and how long a newly arrived ship's surgeon would stay in Asia. If, for example, a surgeon on his outward-bound journey might arrive at the Cape of Good Hope and, if the return fleet from Asia happened to be anchored there and was in dire need of surgeons, this surgeon found himself, whether he liked it or not, placed on the return fleet, resulting in his unexpected return to the Republic within a year. At least one-quarter of the sample of ship's surgeons was back in the Republic within three years of their departures.

The numbers of those who died while under contract to the Company within five years of the date of their first departure, is impressive – no less than 1,059 ship's surgeons of the sample S. It means that more than one-third of the ship's surgeons died within five years of their first departure. As is seen in table T5.16, the mortality rates of ship's surgeons was incredibly high and continued to rise during the century. A plausible answer to the question of why these rates were so high may be that, in addition to the alimentary and climatological risks of the voyage, the ship's surgeon ran the risks of his craft: daily and intensive contact with the ill. Patients suffering from contagious diseases were, if possible, kept apart from the rest of the crew, or placed in a hospital. The surgeon, who had to treat these patients, came into contact with malaria, typhus, and dysentery sufferers and the like several times daily, as a result of which it may be supposed that the life expectancy of the ship's surgeon was lower than that of other professional working for the Company. However plausible this may seem, this is not true. Indubitably, the surgeon's life span in the service of the Company was affected by the prevailing infectious diseases on board, but it seems that his life span in the service of the Company was, if anything, the same or even somewhat longer than that of his fellow seafarers, although it must be stressed that it is rather difficult to compare the surgeons' mortality rates with that of other professional groups of Company personnel, as there are no data available for such groups.

Mortality data on board were discussed in chapter 2. During the seventeenth century, the overall mortality rate on the outward-bound Dutch East Indiamen had been 6.7 per cent and in the eighteenth century 7.3 per cent. But during the years 1690-1695, 1730-1750, and 1770-1775 it rose to 20 per cent, 9 per cent (two decades!), and 23 per cent respectively. That of the ship's surgeons on the outward-bound vessels (within eight months of departure from the Republic) was 9 per cent for the years 1730-1750, and 18.7 per cent for the years 1770-1775. The high mortality rates on board the vessels sailing to Asia during those years were in all probability attributable to typhus. It has been suggested that the soldiers employed by the Company during the years 1690-1695 carried lice in their clothes, and that these lice were infected with typhus (Ricksettsia).[85] Dysentery may have played a role, and sometimes outbreaks of hostilities lengthened the voyages by forcing the vessels to take the back route (*achterom*); contrary winds could be responsible for ships floating for long periods in the doldrums or even as early in the roadstead, as the vessels were forced to lie windbound. Severe epidemics may have been incidentally catastrophic. It has also been suggested that the practice of overcrowding the vessels was a contributing factor, as well as the detoriating physical health of the crews.[86] No real proof has been found for this qualitative decline in Company personnel, which was often a cause for complaint by Company officials, particularly after 1750. All inferences are based on indirect evidence, like these complaints and the increasing difficulties encountered in recruitment and consequent measures to deal with the problem such as the engagement of native labour in Asia and the recruitment in Europe of ever more sailors and soldiers from a wider (German) hinterland.[87] Returning to the ship's surgeons, then, although indeed there were more surgeons recruited from a wider hinterland, there is no reason to suppose that these men were of an 'inferior physical and professional quality' as there is no shred of evidence to support this. The only plausible cause is their encounters with disease which proved, given the particular circumstances (such as the crowding on board and in the hospitals), all too often fatal.

Table T5.16: The mortality of Dutch and non-Dutch ship's surgeons during their VOC tenure [88]

Period	*Total surgeons*	*Dutch*	*non-Dutch*	*Mortality Dutch*	*Mortality non-Dutch*
1700-1725	852	756 (89%)	86 (10%)	429 (57%)	47 (55%)
1726-1750	844	605 (72%)	199 (24%)	400 (66%)	124 (62%)
1751-1775	733	510 (70%)	210 (29%)	349 (68%)	152 (72%)
1776-1795	559	328 (59%)	228 (41%)	205 (63%)	138 (61%)

After the first quarter of the eighteenth century, the participation of Dutch surgeons in the surgical workforce of the Company diminished dramatically (by 17 per cent) which was repeated after 1775 (by 11 per cent), as has been discussed in chapter 4. The relationship between mortality rates of the Dutch and non-Dutch ship's surgeons shows only marginal differences between 1725 and 1775. Therefore, it may be concluded that the health (or physical quality) of Dutch and non-Dutch ship's surgeons did not differ very much. However, it should be noted that mortality among Dutch ship's surgeons jumped up in the second period by 9 per cent while that of the non-Dutch increased by 7 per cent. During the third period, mortality rates among the non-Dutch increased by no less than 10 per cent, a rate not matched by that of the Dutch surgeons, which only increased by 2 per cent. After 1775, mortality among both groups declined. Changes in the professional quality of non-Dutch surgeons remain to be proven, as no hard data have been found to corroborate these ideas, although the fact that promotion became more difficult after 1750 could be interpreted as such.

In taking a closer look at the surgeons' life span we find that those who stayed at home after one voyage, lived longer than those who made relatively shorter but more voyages. Those who kept on working as ship's surgeons pure and simple, and who were not posted to any Asian settlement, came in second place. After 1750, their life expectancy dropped to circa 33 years, which emphasises a far greater risk of unhealthy conditions on board. Surgeons who settled somewhere in the East, soon died, and on average lived no longer than the age of 27. Although apparently sadly young, the average age of 27 years was still higher than the life expectancy of people in cities like Amsterdam and London. There, the average age of mortality was around 24. To this we must add the provisio that this was mainly attributable to the monstrously high infant mortality rates, which kept the average age down and is therefore not a proper comparison. For instance, in Hanover during the years 1778-1787, in general the life expectancy was around 31, but of those who survived the first four years of life, could look forward to reaching the age of at least 49, an age, a Company surgeon seldom reached.[89]

Table T5.17: Average age at demise of sampled surgeons (in years)

Group H: Average Age at death	*1700-1725*	*1726-1750*	*1751-1775*	*1776-1795*
Surgeons with a minimum of two departures, not posted to settlements	38	38	33	34
No second departure, but remaining behind in a settlement	27	27	27	27
No second departure but repatriating after three years	58	70	60	no data available

One might suppose that those ship's surgeons who did survive their maiden Company voyages, and subsequently acquired some immunity, would have had better prospects. However, this supposition does not prove true, as is shown in the tables T5.18. - T5.20.

Table T5.18: Surgeons' mortality on further voyages (Group I)

Period	*Number of surgeons second voyage*	*Number of those dead within 8 months*	*Number of those dead within 1.5 years*	*Number of those dead within 3 years*
1700-1725	377	8 (2%)	35 (9.3%)	73 (19%)
1726-1750	328	19 (6%)	35 (10.7%)	57 (17%)
1751-1775	304	33 (16%)	59 (19%)	82 (27%)
1776-1795	103	5 (1%)	24 (23%)	29 (28%)
Surgeon's mortality on third voyage				
1700-1725	191	9 (5%)	15 (8%)	44 (23%)
1726-1750	160	19 (12%)	32 (20%)	40 (25%)
1751-1775	154	15 (10%)	27 (17.5%)	36 (23%)
1776-1795	27	4 (15%)	9 (37.5%)	7 (26%)

We can thus conclude that the high mortality rates were not the result of the first voyage when a tyro most certainly encountered strange diseases both on board and again in Asia, for which no immunity had been built up. This immunity could only be reached via a prolonged stay in Asia, particularly after 1750. A Darwinistic 'survival of the fittest' does not play a role here, as death rates remained high. In general, those surgeons who made only one voyage and who did not repatriate to the Republic could look forward to an average life span after the date of sailing from the ports of the Republic of 4.7 years in the first period; to 5.2 years in the second period; to 3.38 years in the third period; and to 2.8 years in the last period, as is shown in table T5.19. The ones who lived prosperously and peacefully in the East for 30 years or more are included in these figures!

Table T5.19: Average life span (Group I: one voyage, no repatriation)

Period	*Number of surgeons*	*Average life span after first departure and no repatriation*
1700-1725	275	4.7 years
1726-1750	337	5.2 years
1751-1775	314	3.4 years
1776-1795	285	2.8 years

It could be argued that these figures are only valid for those who indeed died while under contract to the Company and that there must have been many a surgeon who, after a couple of Company voyages, returned to the Republic, opened a shop and lived until the end of his days. Modern statistics enable us to calculate the average chance of living in which the total group of S has been valued, such as those who died early (let us not forget that one-third of the surgeons died within five years of their first departure), as well as those who made several uneventful voyages and returned to the Republic and thus leave in the sample, as they are never heard of again. That calculation is found in graph G5.1 and table T5.20, which present us with a 50 per cent chance that someone would survive his first voyage. As is demonstrated in both table and graph, the trend declined from circa ten years in the first period to three years in the last period.[90]

Table T5.20: Survival rates after first departure (Group S)

Period	*Median*	*Confidence Interval*
1700-1725	10.52 year	9.49-11.56 years
1726-1750	8.07 year	7.03-9.10 years
1751-1775	6.27 year	5.31-7.23 years
1776-1796	3.00 year	2.42-3.57 years

Graph G5.1: Survival rates after first departure (Group S)

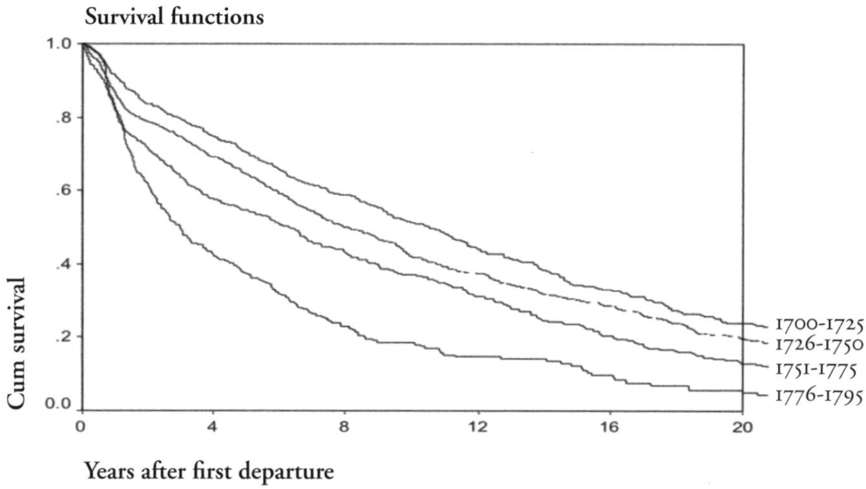

In view of these figures, it seems quite unbelievable that European surgeons were still willing to take service with the Company at all. It is difficult to escape the idea that prospective employees in the Republic must have had an impression, however vague, of these health risks. Perhaps Dutch ship's surgeons did indeed know, as their eagerness to enlist with the Company declined drastically after 1725, and even decidely after 1775.

Malaria

As we have seen in chapter 3, Van der Brug determined that malaria was the main killer in Batavia after 1733 where, after the construction of fishponds, the mosquito, the vector of the malignant form of malaria, multiplied and attacked the drifting population of Batavia. The data pertaining to the ship's surgeons, however, do not correspond with Van der Brug's findings. It is only after 1750 that their life expectancy notably diminished. With that in mind, I have researched the mortality under the ship's surgeons arriving in Batavia in certain intervals of time: within eight and ten months after departure from the Republic (more or less the duration of the voyage to Batavia); after one and a half years; after two years; and after three years (table T5.21). In this sample, the mortality rates of the ship's surgeons dying within eight months after first departure was seven per cent during the entire eighteenth century, which is more or less consistence with the entire Company's mortality rate on the outward-bound vessels during this century. During the years 1725-1775, the mortality rate of the ship's surgeons more than doubled from three to eight per cent and to thirteen per cent in the third quarter of the century within eight months of first departure on the outward-bound ships. These surgeons must have fallen victim to the diseases rife on board.

Table T5.21: Ship's surgeons' mortality compared to N and to the increase of N-mortality over time (Group G)

Period	*A (8 months)*	*B (10 months)*	*C (12 months)*	*D (18 months)*	*E (2 years)*	*F (3 years)*
1700-1725 N=267	9 3%	13 (+4) 5% (2%)	17 (+4) 6% (2%)	36 (+18) 14% (7%)	55 (+19) 21% (8%)	88 (+33) 33% (16%)
1726-1750 N=336	27 8%	30 (+3) 9% (1%)	34 (+4) 10% (1%)	56 (+22) 17% (7%)	84 (+28) 25% (10%)	132 (+48) 39% (19%)
1751-1775 N=308	39 13%	42 (+3) 14% (1%)	49 (+7) 16% (3%)	66 (+17) 21% (6%)	93 (+27) 30% (11%)	152 (+59) 49% (27%)
1776-1795 N=280	6 2%	9 (+3) 3% (1%)	10 (+1) 4% (0,5%)	19 (+9) 7% (3%)	56 (+37) 20% (14%)	97 (+31) 35% (14%)

A = surgeons dying within eight months of departure

B = surgeons dying within ten months of departure (A and B are more or less identical with the sailing time to Batavia)

C = surgeons dying within 12 months of departure

D = surgeons dying within 18 months of departure

E = surgeons dying within 24 months of departure

F = surgeons dying within 36 months of departure

There is also overwhelming evidence, that the longer a European stayed in Asia, the more chance he or she had of dying there, which contradicts the acquisition of immunity theory, and the three-year period excluding the natural cause of dying of old age. It was especially after an uninterrupted stay in Asia of more than 18 months that the dangers of living in Asia began to be felt. At first sight, then, malaria as the main and only cause of death must be reassessed if we bear in mind that, in the case of malaria, there was a reasonable chance of survival during a prolonged stay, if one survived the first couple of months in Batavia. It seems more likely that the extremely high mortality figures among the Batavian population after 1733 were a combination of factors, among which malaria must have been one. Although the search for one determining cause is good medical practice, it does not always produce a satisfactory solution.

The real danger inevitably lay in Asia and this danger continued to rise sharply after 18 months, particularly after 1750 and with a prolonged sojourn of more than 18 months! The longer one lived there, the greater the chances of falling victim to one of the Batavian or Asian diseases. There was a relative decline in mortality rates in the last period of the century, although the rates kept rising the longer a person lived there. There is every chance that these figures may also apply to the rest of the Company's employees coming from the Republic as well. Thus these figures, instead of substantiating Van der Brug's thesis, actually raise more unanswered questions.

After service

In England, many ship's surgeons retired to the countryside. This was made possible by a decision of the House of Lords in 1704 as a result of which anyone licensed by the Society of Apothecaries could prescribe for a patient as well as dispense medicine. Many naval surgeons, upon their retirement from service, obtained an apothecary's licence in order to set up their own general practice.[91] What happened to the Dutch ship's surgeons who survived Company service and retired quietly? The answer to that question is difficult to answer since there are no data mentioned in the Company's pay rolls, unless the surgeons asked to be 'freed' from their contract in one of the African or Asian settlements. Petrus Andreas, the Head of Surgery in Batavia in 1665, for instance, asked to be let go in order to retire to his extensive estates just outside of Batavia, as he suffered from beri-beri.[92] In this sample, some 30 surgeons did indeed ask to be allowed to retire as *burghers*, all, save four of them, in Batavia, and usually they set up a private surgical practice for which the local inhabitants were the cliëntèle as they were not permitted to treat Company servants. Some surgeons asked for permission to be discharged from the Company, particularly during the decade 1740-1750 and after 1780 (which, in light of the unpredictable future one might encounter in Europe, is explainable).

The post-Company careers of those who retired from the Company in the Republic is only incidentally known, such as that of Johan Policarpus Aarholt, born in Naumburg (Saxony-Anhalt). After his one and only voyage as ship's surgeon, Aarholt married Cecilia Swerus, a Dutch woman from the island of Texel. In the Personal Quotes (*Personele Quotisatie*) of 1742, he is listed as a practising surgeon on Texel.[93] As is Gerrit Rottink, born in Delden in the province of Overijssel in 1709, who after his Company career of three voyages, also settled in Texel and married there. His father-in-law, Jan Mazade, was also a surgeon on Texel. Gerrit not only set up a surgical practise on Texel, but he also became a halberdeer (*heilbaardier*) and a fish auctioneer.[94]

George ten Berge, born in Oude Pekela in 1762, was the son of the surgeon and 'obstetrician' (male midwife) Harm Dirks ten Berge. George was, in all probability, trained as a surgeon at the local guild. He rounded off his training as a master surgeon. He married Catharina Pannekoek in 1786 and was employed by the Company Chamber of Enkhuizen in 1793 as a senior surgeon, earning the monthly wage of 40 Dutch guilders. After four years he had still not returned, however. By that time, the Company was practically bankrupt. Ten Berge then left the Company's service in Asia, became a ship's surgeon with the *vrije vaart* (merchant fleet) in 1797 and returned home in the next year to find the Republic in a political uproar. He subsequently found employment as a surgeon in a newly organised Maritime Hospital in Enkhuizen. He died in 1812.[95] Coenraadt Hendrick Otteleben, of Helmstedt in Lower Saxony, was another surgeon who switched to the *vrije vaart* on his third Company contract in 1796, perhaps alerted to the advisability of this move by the political developments, which had as a consequence the temporary break of the shipping connection between the Netherlands and Asia.[96]

Abraham Pourier, born in the village of Dalfsen in Overijssel, found his future in Amsterdam after his two voyages for the Company. In the *Personele Quotisatie* of Amsterdam in 1742, he is listed as a master surgeon, earning 600 Dutch guilders annually, and rented a surgical shop for 325 Dutch guilders a year. Perhaps he had saved enough after his two Company voyages to set up such a shop in Amsterdam.[97]

Dingenis van den Abeele, born in Middelburg in 1739, started his naval surgical career with the Zeeland Admiralty in 1757, and subsequently signed four contracts with the Company, with his last two contracts being as a senior surgeon in 1764 and in 1768. Returning to Middelburg in 1769, he opened a surgeon's shop there, in which he was still practising in 1797.[98] Meanwhile, Johannus Wilhelmus Daman, born in Middelburg in 1735 registered with the surgeon's guild of Middelburg as practising surgeon after five voyages for the Company, and one for the *Middelburgsche Commercie Compagnie* as ship's surgeon. He died in Middelburg in 1783.[99]

After his one trip for the Company, which lasted no less than 12 years, Douwe van Tongeren of Velsen (1711-1740) also returned home to retire. By then, he had probably saved up enough to set up his surgical practise in his native village.[100] And lastly, after his single voyage as Company ship's surgeon between 1737 and 1739, Hermanus van Soest, born in Rotterdam in 1718, became a member of the surgeon's guild of Gouda, and subsequently rose to become a prominent member of the Gouda elite.[101]

Although the evidence is scarce, none of these surgeons retired to a 'life of leisure'. They all went on working as surgeons. Although financially they did not strike it rich, they had had an Asian experience, which had certainly enlarged their medical competence and intellectual horizons.

Conclusion

Recapitulating the evidence, it is quite clear that the Dutch ship's surgeons with the Company came mostly from the Dutch petty bourgeoisie, were schooled and educated at a surgeon's guild, and were not employed by the Company before the age of circa 21 years. By then, they had enjoyed a few years of experience in their profession. These surgeons were examined before employment and/or a promotion within the Company hierarchy. We saw that the prevailing idea that these surgeons were mere quacks and barbers does not hold true upon a closer examination of their educations and careers. Furthermore, although the possible rewards offered by employment with the Company must have influenced their decisions when choosing an employer, in general, the surgeons seldom if ever switched to an administrative career, which would have been far more rewarding, both financially and socially. They tried to build their careers within their own profession as far as this was possible. After 1750, promotion to a more senior surgical position became more difficult to obtain and, moreover, they only had a short period of some four to five years after their first departure in which they could pursue a career. One-third of the sample died within five years of their first departure. Those who did survive the ordeals of the voyage and the prevalent diseases particularly in Batavia, could be relatively certain of a successful career. They must have been given options to be drawn into the administrative side of the Company, which, however, they chose not to follow. Even upon their return to the Republic, they often set up a surgical shop, and did not live as 'gentlemen of leisure'.

Because of the mounting ill health on board the vessels and in Asia, especially after 1750, surgical or rather medical employees became relatively scarce. This situation forced the Council of the Indies to request the Gentlemen XVII to send capable surgeons to Asia, as the training of non-surgical employees for surgery in Asia apparently did not provide satisfactory results. From the very establishment of Batavia, the Head of Surgery, with the support of his surgical colleagues in the *Binnenhospitaal*, had educated and examined prospective surgeons, leading to the creation of a 'surgical school' in Batavia, however shortlived, in the eighteenth century, through which Eurasians were taken into the profession. Tragically, neither the European medical nor the Asian medical/surgical world could offer cures for the myriad of diseases, something that the surgeons came to be blamed for. Even if they had been able to shed the barbering aspects of their profession, the general public had not rid itself of its prejudices.

If they were able to actually accumulate any type of fortune at all in the short time they worked for the Company will be seen in the next chapter.

6. 'Great expectations'!

In the spring of 1769, Christiaan Brauns, from Hannover in Germany, offered his services as a surgeon to the Amsterdam Chamber of the Company. These were gladly accepted for the Company vessel, the *Lycochton*, which sailed on 13 May, 1769, with Brauns on board as first surgeon. Before departing, Brauns visited an Amsterdam notary, Gerardus Wijthof, where he deposited a codicil in which he empowered two of his future fellow crew members to take charge of his belongings in the event of his demise. Indeed, Brauns must have had an uncanny sense of foreboding as he died within some five weeks of sailing, on 20 June, 1769, leaving behind a sizeable number of possessions. After his death, the legally authorized representatives, O. Berg who was the first mate (*onderstuurman*), and A. Stadius van Halm, the second mate (*derde waak*), of the *Lycochton*, listed his possessions, noting each item carefully.

In his cabin, for instance, he kept his clothes, his mattress,[1] two pillows, two blankets, a canister of tobacco, another one for coffee, a German Bible, a mirror, two lacquered serving trays, two books, and his sword. The contents of his cellaret (*kelder*) proved to be some bottles containing distilled waters (Dutch gin, *jenever*). These were served to the crew after his funeral, while the officers were offered the deceased's bottles of red wine, found in a basket.[2] Brauns' representatives listed a number of items related to his professional life including a Chinese box containing a number of surgical instruments, each one of them itemized in the inventory. In preparation for his dealings in the East, Brauns had stored another two 'chests' in the mastergunner's cabin, containing some 20 mirrors, clothes, books, some sealed packages, snuff boxes, tobacco, dozens of buttons and pencils, as well as some invoices for the eight casks of beer and the wine, and some letters addressed to several people in Batavia.[3] Berg and Stadius were bound to keep Brauns' belongings safe and sound in order to pass them on to the person nominated by Brauns at the Cape of Good Hope.

Like all other employees, the Company surgeons were allowed to undertake a little venture of their own, stuffed in *kelders* (cellarets or large chests, used mostly to store bottles) and *kisten* (smaller personal chests), the so-called *voering*. The rank of surgeon (or any other employee) determined the size (and consequently the price) of the chests. The Company initially provided these *kelders* at a cost of three to seven Dutch guilders, which was invariably accurately noted in the Company ship's ledgers (*scheepssoldijboeken*), although, later in the eighteenth century, the employees were permitted to take along more and larger chests. In 1745, for instance, a senior surgeon was permitted to have a chest five feet long by two feet high and wide, as well as two *kelders* each holding a dozen bottles, a smaller chest two-and-a-half feet long by one foot high and wide (which might contain linen and silk), as well as two jars of pickles.[4] Apart from the possible stockage of Dutch gin (*jenever*) or wine, the *kelders* were often filled with pipes, tobacco rolls, books, bric-à-brac, and clothes. As these *kelders* were usually stowed in the holds of the Asia-bound vessel and, therefore, not readily accessible, the contents were not so much intended for personal use during the voyage as for profitable sale upon one's arrival in Cape Town or Asia, which was considered a 'fringe-benefit'. In the Dutch Republic, for instance, one paid 8 *stuivers* for a pound of tobacco. On the Indian Ocean, the price could go for 65 *stuivers* per pound of the very same tobacco.[5] Many employees participated in this trading-on-the-side, and many broke every rule their employer had imposed with respect to quantity, commodity, and cash.

The current historical opinion is that the most common item of private trade was silver coins. In Asia, there was a demand for silver, which the Company exported in the form of coins to Asia in order to pay for products like spices, silk, and porcelain. As J.C. van Leur, the eminent historian of eighteenth-century Asia, wrote: 'Western trade with Asia was always a one-sided movement of goods in the sense that costly merchandise was received in exchange for coin and certain metals in ingot'.[6] The seafarers supplied the Asian market with silver smuggled in the form of *rijksdaalders* (rix dollars) and *ducatons*, which carried a higher value or rate in Batavia, and they took back commodities like pickles and textiles. Whereas the *rijksdaalder* consisted of fifty five-cent pieces (*stuivers*) in the Republic, in Asia the rixdollar was rated at 60 five-cent pieces. The upshot was that it became quite lucrative to deposit money in Batavia, and to collect the given bill of exchange (*wissel*) in the Republic, for the higher rate of Batavia, a handsome interest of some 4 per cent. Besides these rixdollars, there were also *leeuwendaalders*, worth 40 five-cent pieces in the Republic but 48 five-cent pieces in Asia.[7] The Dutch guilder (20 five-cent pieces) was not used as money in Asia. Jacob Berger, a surgeon at the Houghly factory in Bengal, usually bought and sold in Arcat rupees. According to his business agents in Amsterdam, one Arcat rupiah was worth 1.5 Dutch guilders.[8]

As we now know, the Company ship's surgeon, like his fellow seafarers, ran the very real risk of dying during the term of his Company contract, either on board or in an Asian settlement. Therefore, the arrangements Brauns made in Amsterdam were not unusual. Had no such legal provisions been made, the personal possessions of the deceased would be inventoried by a small committee appointed by the captain and his clerk (*assistant*). This committee opened the chests, if any, of the deceased and drew up a list of his possessions. If the chests were stowed in the holds of the vessel and were inaccessible, they were inventoried ashore upon arrival, at the Cape of Good Hope or in Asia. The inventory of possessions was presented to the captain, made public to the crew, and a date was set, weather and circumstances permitting, for the auction of the goods 'before the main mast' as was the custom of the sea.[9] The goods were bid for by the sailors, and the sums given were deducted from the sailors' wages at the end of the voyage. Any outstanding debts the deceased still had with his employer (such as the usual advance on salary upon appointment) were deducted from the proceeds; the net proceeds were noted in the ledger of the vessel and the unsold items were given to the *curator adlites* upon arrival at the Cape or in Batavia; the task of final arrangements with the notary, if any, of the deceased, the deceased's family, and the Company administration were also his responsibility.

Arrangements such as those of Christiaan Brauns were made when a particular crew member had some valuable possessions to call his own or what he was holding for others. They could be made on the spur of the moment and a gravely ill patient might ask some of his fellow seafarers to be his witnesses, for instance, the 'visitor of the sick' (*ziekentrooster*), one of his colleagues, and the captain's clerk (*assistent*). They visited him on his deathbed. There he then revoked all of the previous wills and dictated a new one in the presence of his witnesses appointing his heirs, usually his parents and/or wife and children, although sometimes it was a friend on board, and authorised the witnesses on board to take care of his belongings and to see to it that these belongings or the proceeds thereof would find their way back to his heirs. The witnesses then declared the patient to be ill in body but sound in mind, and that therefore this was a valid last will and testament.

If a surgeon was stationed in a settlement in Asia for several years, he may have been burdened with much more material wealth than his colleagues sailing on board Company vessels. Christoph Godfried Jager for instance, Hospitalier (first surgeon) at the Company's hospital in Macassar, left the following possessions when he died on 19 February 1784: hats, tablecloths, pillowcases, shirts, stocks, shoes, handkerchiefs, gloves, frock coats, mirrors, a saddle, pistols, a musket, settees, Chinese chairs, paintings, spittoons, candles, a trumpet, cutlery, stills, pepper mills, a writing desk, some books, an iron, a violin, tables, surgical instruments, an operating table, medicines, a horse, two Dutch pigs, and seven slaves, among the latter, the mother of his adopted daughter.[10]

A window onto the life of the surgeon opens when these kinds of inventories are read. Even if it is just the mere mention that a surgeon took along some 8,400 corks to Asia.[11] What did he plan to do with them? Only occasionally does the researcher catch a glimpse of the private life of the Company surgeon. Indeed, there are a number of surgeon's journals in the National Archives of The Hague from which we can deduce the tenor of his professional life on board. Sadly, there are practically no such things as personal diaries from which we can get a better idea of his everyday life. The seventeenth-century ship's surgeon Nicolaas de

Graaff, for instance, was more interested in describing the countries and places he visited than in writing an account of his daily routine. The same applies to the diary of the Company surgeon Gijsbert Heeck.[12] Cogently, journals like those of De Graaff were written with a purpose and for an audience.

The financial administration of the Company seafarers, carefully noted in each vessel's musterbook, sometimes offers a wider and more private view of the seafarers' life. Family members are often mentioned as the beneficiaries of a specific Company employee's annual three months salary. As we have already mentioned, in the case of the demise of a seafarer, an inventory of his belongings, the list of sales, and sometimes his last will and testament were noted in the vessel's ledger, which may provide glimpses into the deceased's tastes, interests, and intentions. So does the rarely found letter, such as that of Johan Andreas Muller, and so do the wills drawn up by the Batavian notaries.

The present chapter addresses the question of whether the career of a ship's surgeon in the Company was or could be financially successful. Clearly, the mere wages of a ships' surgeon, 36 Dutch guilders a month maximum, would never suffer him to be rich. If the ship's surgeon fostered any material hopes, he had to turn his hand to Trade or entering into an Advantageous Marriage. These were the only two paths available to him to ultimately avoid financial worries, which the mere pursuing of his surgical profession could never do.

The evidence that the Company surgeon participated in the so-called *morshandel* is hidden away in the archives. It was, after all, a forbidden pastime. However, as will be shown, the surgeon took along products from the Republic to Asia. He participated in trade within Asia and he brought commodities back from the East upon his return. As we have seen in the previous chapter, a number of surgeons from the Enkhuizen Chamber acted as middlemen for traders in the Republic or as traders on their own account: they incurred debts with certain people (traders and/or moneylenders) in the Republic, who made sure that the repatriated surgeon did not receive his wages before he had settled his debts. It is inconceivable that the surgeons did not profit from this arrangement. These Enkhuizen surgeons were surely not unique in their dealings. The surgeon Arnoldus op den Ool, on the pay roll of the Rotterdam Chamber, whom we met in chapter 5, is a prime example of the surgeon-trader who found his niche in Asia. Together with a friend and colleague, whose widow he later married, he bought a small vessel which they fitted out, stuffed with products, and sent to various destinations in Asia. Spreading his network, Op den Ool commissioned friends in the Republic to buy commodities in his name and to send these to Asia to sell there.

In his commercial transactions it was essential that the surgeon-trader had a network of 'friends'. As noted earlier, friends were not friends in the modern sense of the word, but colleagues, acquaintances, acquaintances by correspondence or of other friends, all moving in the same sphere or station of life, all trying to climb to a higher social level and to a more polite society. They wrote to each other; they promoted each other's interests and those of their acquaintances; and they married their acquaintances' widows. It was an extensive network of people pushing and helping each other upwards. As we saw in chapter 5, even a low-ranking surgeon on board (*derde meester*), such as Simon Walmeester, made sure he took the right letters of introduction (to Governor-General Jacob Mossel, not among the least in Batavia) with him on his way out to Asia.[13] Among the possessions of surgeon's mate Jan Dake, who died on 29 November, 1758, three letters and three packages were found, intended for, amongst other recipients, the Head of Surgery in Batavia, J.A. Spenolt.[14] Christiaan Brauns carried six letters with him as well as some packages, all intended for recipients living in Batavia, one of them being Andries Dekker, surgeon-major, a man who belonged to the medical elite of Batavia.[15] Surgeon Jan Roelofs brought two chests intended for the son-in-law of the governor of the Cape of Good Hope as well as five chests for the principal military commander in Batavia.[16] When the German senior surgeon Hendrik Karreman arrived on board the *Oost Capelle* on 16 December 1772, he immediately (because his mattress, blankets and pillows had not yet arrived so that he had to stay awake sitting in his cabin for the rest of the night) wrote to his (unknown) acquaintances that, the moment the ship dropped anchor at the Cape, he would deliver their salmon as requested to the (equally unknown) intended recipients.[17] The surgeons en route profited from an extensive network: it provided the background against which the surgeon-traders operated.

A complete broad canvas of the ship's surgeons' fortunes cannot be painted, however. In all probability, these were modest, even though it was said of Dr Jacobus van der Steege (who introduced variolation – a smallpox treatment – to Batavia) that he had amassed a fortune of 5 million Dutch guilders during his 16 years of residence in Asia.[18] However, the fortunate Dr Van der Steege was a physician, which meant in itself that he enjoyed more protection and influence.[19] Most ship's surgeons could not expect the good fortune which befell Dr Van der Steege. In general, as we will see, even the successful surgeons were small beer compared to the great fortune-makers found higher up in the Company echelon in Asia. Nevertheless, as the pursuit of wealth cannot but have been a co-motive in their acceptance of Company employment, it warrants the query if they succeeded at it. As said, the true extent of their wealth cannot be traced fully, only a vague image can be drawn from the records available in the various archives. Providentially, the nature of these records is such that they offer much more data than purely financial facts, as a result of which their interests, their wives, their children, in short, their joys and their sorrows will also be examined.

This chapter is based on the analysis of 340 legal documents pertaining to surgeons, such as wills and powers of attorney, which were deposited with the Batavian *Weeskamer* (a local institutional board for the administration of the capital of orphans, usually made up of the wardens of the local orphanage and which served as a sort of probate office) by the notaries during the seventeenth and the eighteenth centuries (the 'Batavian Deeds'). These are supplemented by some 90 documents such as lists of possessions and of sales occasionally found in the vessels' ledgers during the eighteenth century. As these documents are concentrated in two archives, namely the Nationaal Archief in The Hague and the Arsip Nasional of Jakarta, it follows that the emphasis of the research will cover those surgeons who tried to make a career with the Company and not on those who settled somewhere in Europe after one or two voyages.[20] May it be concluded, from these wills and inventories, that the surgeon, in pursuit of (material) happiness, did not enter the Company's employ in vain? In short, did he succeed, like Pip, in his expectations?

The laws of inheritance

The law in the Republic was executed either by *Aasdomsrecht* or by *Schependomsrecht*. The *Aasdom* was law north of the Hollandse Ijssel, while *Schependom* was law south of it and in Zeeland, the main differences being that the bailiff had the role of public prosecutor, the *azing* that of counsel, and the neighbours (later men under oath) that of judges in *aasdom* law, while the bailiff and aldermen were the main actors in *Schependom* law.[21]

To draw up a will in the Netherlands is something exceptional: most people do not. Nowadays, only some 15 per cent of the population does so.[22] And so it was in the seventeenth and eighteenth centuries. Most people did not feel the need to do so. The people who did, did so because they had an estate that they wanted to pass down specifically and not according to custom. What happened if an estate was passed down according to local custom? At the time, under both the *Aasdom* system and the *Schependom* system, the property of the deceased passed down equally upon his or her descendants. If there were no surviving children, it was divided equally among the parents. Moreover, under both *Schependom* and *Aasdom* Law, the surviving spouse had no claim on the legacy; unclaimed property would revert to the state. The position of the surviving spouse in the Netherlands only improved in the course of the twentieth century.[23]

In 1580, Holland and Friesland enacted the Political Ordinance, also known as the New *Schependom* Law, which institutionalized traditional *Schependom* Law, privileging collaterals over ascendants and siblings over parents in instances of intestate succession. This ordinance was not popular and failed to win adherents in many of the Holland and Frisian towns and was itself succeeded in Holland by the Edict of 1599, also known as the New *Aasdom* Law. Where *Schependom* demanded that the siblings were the inheritors and *Aasdom* demanded that the surviving parent was the main inheritor, the New *Aasdom* Law split the estate in half: with one-half going to the siblings and the other half to the surviving parent. This edict was a compromise between the principles of *Schependom* law and the *Aasdom* Law, and eventually became the law in Dutch Asia.[24]

The deeds

The seventeenth- and eighteenth century notary in the Republic was an official appointed by local authorities to guard the public interest. It was he who drew up documents which had a probative value. This sort of notary rarely studied law.[25] The notarial documents were more or less standardized in the sense that formulas were used at the beginning and at the end of the deed in which the following data had to be included: the correct date; the personal details of the party(ies); the names of the witnesses; the name of the city or village where the document was drawn up; and the signatures of the party(ies), witnesses, and notary. The notary was obliged to state that he knew the party(ies), and the witnesses had to be truthful people usually over 16 years of age. The documents, thus drawn up, could serve as evidence in court where they had probative value.[26]

As a rule, the opening words of a last will were an *invocatio*. It was essential that the notary stated that the testator was of sound mind, utilising the *compos mentis* formula. Then, the fragility of life was remembered and a recommendation followed recommending the passage of soul into God's hands. Before the naming of an heir, the testator revoked all prior wills, and sometimes bequeathed some legacies, which were always limited by the 'statutory portion' (*legitieme portie* or 'lawful share') of relatives in the direct line (being children of the testator or, in the absence of children, his parent(s), entitled to a specified portion of the estate) and also by the *falcidieke portie*, which required that one-quarter of the legacies go to the executor of the will.[27] An executor of the will was usually named and he, after the demise of the testator, administered the inheritance, paid any debts, and distributed the legacies and the estate amongst the heirs. In Batavia, the executor or the administrator of an estate was entitled to the *veertigste penning* or two and one-half per cent.[28]

It was a common custom for a mutual testament to be made by husband and wife, nowadays no longer possible. In that case, the contents of the will, apart from the formulas with respect to the invocation, being of sound mind, were usually in favour of the survivor and stating that the survivor was bound to give any children of their marriage their lawful share and/or to educate and feed them.[29] This lawful share was sometimes specified as a certain amount of money.

If the children became orphans, without any other family, they became the responsibility of the local authorities and were placed in an orphanage. In the Republic, it was a legal obligation to make an inventory of the estate and this had to be deposited at the *Weeskamer* when there was an issue of guardianship of minors and/or when persons were nominated as executors of the will.[30] Despite this service, it was common practice in the testament to exclude the involvement of the local *weeskamer* (and thus the compiling of an inventory). The *Weeskamer* (not the orphanage!) kept track of, and administered family property, especially that of families in which children had lost their parent(s) and who were still minors. By excluding the *Weeskamer*, it was possible to circumvent the compiling of a household inventory as well as eschew the involvement of local authorities in the guardianship of any minor children (that is, younger than 25 years and unmarried) as the parents usually nominated the survivor as guardian of any children.[31] Whether or not an orphan was involved, if the *Weeskamer* was not excluded by notarial deed, its authorities saw to it that a proper inventory was made of the deceased's estate, and made rulings on intestate succession (in close collaboration with the *curator adlites*). Having dealt with such matters, it handled the passing down of the property in question. In Batavia, a will had to be deposited at the *Weeskamer* within four weeks of the testator's demise, and his (or her) estate had to be probated within three months.

On board, it was the captain's clerk or the captain himself who was authorised to draw up wills for those on board: Leendert van Coopstad, captain of the Company vessel the *Schaegen*, visited his gravely ill senior surgeon, Hendrik Wildermans, in his cabin on 4 September 1772. Van Coopstad wrote down Wildermans' last will, specifying that he, in his function as captain of a Company vessel, was authorised to do so.[32] The clerk on the Company vessel the *Opperdoes* acted as notary for Simon Andeles first surgeon on the ship on 8 November 1725.[33] Notaries did this sort of work in Batavia and at the Cape of Good Hope. At the smaller settlements, the Company clerks or commissionaries were vested with the power to draw up legal documents: Rudolph Florentius van der Niepoort, the first clerk of Semarang wrote down the last will of the senior surgeon, Johannes Munninkhuijsen, who lay ill in the house of the Poorhouse warden of Semarang.[34]

No notary or clerk (nor witnesses) was required if a will was handwritten by the testator and the beneficiaries were the testator's legitimate children. Sometimes even an oral testament was considered valid. On 30 June 1654, council was held at the Company's headquarters in Batavia at the request of Elisabeth van der Leer, the widow of Johannis Grevenraet. Grevenraet had been commissioned by Rijckloff van Goens to inspect and accompany certain vessels of the Company from Surat to Persia. Upon his return to Surat, his ship was attacked by several Portuguese frigates near the city of Damman. After a couple of hours of fighting, the captain of his ship had been forced to surrender and Grevenraet was sent to a prison in Goa where he died on 5 April 1654. Before he died, he told his fellow prisoners that he made his wife the sole beneficiary of his estate, provided that his father received a lawful share (*legitieme portie*) and, if his father had already died, this lawful share would be passed down to his sister. His fellow prisoners were the Company surgeon Johannes

Matthijs Pruijs and Pieter Symonsz Diamantslijper. It was the surgeon, Pruijs, who wrote down this will on behalf of Johannis Grevenraet.[35]

The law in Asia

In the period 1602-1661, the Company experimented with various legal systems, to deal with the problems of (intestate) inheritance. In 1621, Governor-General Jan Pieterszoon Coen received instructions from the *Heeren XVII* that the colonial legal system should simultaneously follow contradictory codes: the Political Ordinance of 1580, which privileged collaterals above ascendants, as well as the Edict of 1599 that gave half to the siblings and half to the surviving parent. The 1642 Statutes of Batavia, promulgated under Governor-General Anthonij van Diemen, brought a semblance of order to the legal world of the Company in Asia. A long section of these statutes (the first attempt to draw up a systematic law code specifically for the Indies) declared that Dutch Asia would base its cases of intestate inheritance on the New *Aasdom* Law. This was countered by the directors of the Company (*Heeren XVII*) who replied that the statute on intestate succession was invalid because the various laws in the respective provinces (from which the employees originated) could be in contradiction to it. As a result, the Company muddled through, trying to apply intestacy law to the deceased based on his or her last place of residence.

Therefore, some surgeons and some surgeons' wives specified that their last will was subject to *Aasdom* law, and that their spouse or husband was allowed only a child's portion (*kindsgedeelte*), as did surgeon Christoffel van Dijk and his wife, Geertruijda van Soest, who decided that their will was subject to *Aasdomversterfrecht* (*Aasdom* inheritance law) in 1760.[36] The spouse of First Surgeon Robert van Waveren, Agita van der Stael, had been married before and had some children by her former marriage. In Agita's and Robert's mutual will in 1681, she decided that her *voorkinderen* (children of a previous marriage) would be the sole beneficiaries, but that her current husband would also count as a child and thus be entitled to a child's portion.[37] Batavia's City Surgeon Andreas Laurentsy made the same provision in 1705 in the mutual will: his children by his former marriage were the sole beneficiaries in the estate, subject to his wife, Abigail Fresel, counting as a child as well.[38] Aaltje Zeeukes, in 1653 wife to Senior Surgeon Lucas Pijl, and her husband made a will in which she made a provision for her current husband to have a child's portion of her estate.[39] First Surgeon Adriaan van der Heuvel specified in his last will that the will was subject to *Schependom* law as his parents lived in Middelburg (Zeeland).[40]

As time passed, it became increasingly necessary to deal with these problems as Batavia grew steadily with an influx of Europeans and indigenous peoples, all residing under Dutch law, in which the Company was supposedly omnipotent but nevertheless struggled to gain a grip on the various legal systems. The founding of Batavia had also given rise to religious, demographic and ethnic issues. At the start of the settlement, some members of the Council of the Indies had plans to colonise Batavia with European settlers on a grand scale, to which end some boatloads full of European women were sent to Asia.[41] The absurdity of these plans, of which the Company was blissfully unaware, is quite obvious given the fact that Asia was already quite densely populated by Asians. Throughout the 1620s, the Company seemed to be searching for both a practical and juridical solution to its demographic problems. Governor-General Coen had envisaged a type of civilization in Batavia that would be teeming with Dutch petty *bourgeoisie*.[42] However, this plan failed to win over the directors at home in the Republic. In 1652, the Company restricted the immigration of Dutch women to Asia. It preferred its employees to be bachelors, and also limited marriage to Asian-born women.[43] The ship's surgeons were also not encouraged by their employer to take their spouses along to Asia, although a few succeeded. Surgeon Mattheus Brauns requested that he be allowed to take his wife and two children to Asia in 1690, which was permitted on the condition that he then fulfilled a tenure of fifteen years in Asia.[44] The same stipulation was made to the Surgeon Francois Scheffens in 1689,[45] to Surgeon Willem Molhuijsen in 1690,[46] and to Surgeon Jacobus de Nijs in 1705.[47] After 1639, no man married to an Asian or part-Asian woman was allowed to repatriate while his wife and children were still alive. Nor could a locally (Asian) born woman accompany her Dutch husband to the Republic in retirement unless special dispensation was given.[48]

It stands to reason that without the company of Dutch women, the initial notion of a homogenous European colony was not realistic and the traditional idea of white marriage and white Christianity ebbed away. Dutch men took long-term Asian mistresses and many children were born within these relationships. These children were often enough acknowledged and/or adopted and/or provided for by their European fathers. To accomplish an adoption and make proper provision for such offspring in a will, a notary was indubitably necessary. Dutch men sometimes even wanted to marry their locally found female-friends, for which they needed the blessings of the Church and of the Company. The Reformed Church Council in Batavia was responsible for registering marriage proclamations until 1632. In 1632, a directive to the College of Aldermen in Batavia instituted the Commissioners of Matrimonial Affairs, which greatly resembled the same institution in the Republic. The 1632 directive required permission from the Governor-General for Company personnel to register a marriage proclamation and required an additional spiritual vow. Asians were not allowed to register a marriage proclamation unless they were furnished with an attestation, granted by the church council, to the effect that they had been substantially instructed in the principles of the Christian faith.

Once married to a European, the Asian-born wife was entitled to inherit his property. According to the American historian J. Gelman Taylor, the locally born and bred women were like spiders in the webs of the Company's privileged positions. In fact, it was these women who provided the gateway for Company employees to establish relationships of connection, protection, and influence, born of the Company's particular policies on immigration and intermarriage.[49] As these Asian wives were entitled by Dutch law and by the will to inherit and retain the property of their deceased husband (perhaps one should say 'husbands' as they often outlasted several), they accumulated great fortunes along the way, and became the objects of desire of career-minded suitors seeking a place among the Company elite.[50]

When a marriage was contracted, the property of the husband and wife was combined and held in common. This community of goods included both assets and liabilities, although marriage settlements (antenuptial contracts) were sometimes made. As a will and/or inventory had to be deposited with the *Weeskamer* of Batavia four weeks after the demise of a person falling under the jurisdiction of the Council of the Indies, the Batavian *Weeskamer* quickly became a powerful financial institution. It had been founded by resolution of the Council of the Indies of 1 October 1624.[51] It also provided for the orphans and minors, many born out of wedlock and of mixed Eur-Asian descent. Children or minors (younger than 25 years of age) were those considered not competent to manage their own affairs. Single women over 25 could represent themselves in court, own and sell property; it was only when they entered into marriage that their 'adult' status was reduced to that of a minor: mothers were not allowed to act as guardians, as married women were themselves under the guardianship of another, although as a widow they could.

Deeds of surgeons in Batavia

In the notarial archives of Jakarta the deeds (consisting mostly of wills) of some 340 ship's surgeons were found, drawn up by 92 different Batavian notaries, clerks or others expressly commissioned to do so between 1643 and 1793 (the 'Batavian Deeds' . They represent a mere 3 per cent of the total number of ship's surgeons employed by the Company during the seventeenth and the eighteenth centuries, bearing in mind that some 10,000 surgeons left the shores of the Republic for those of Asia during these two centuries. Thus the 340 surgeons' deeds in over a period of 150 years may seem small. However, it is not: during the first decades of the Company's existence, there was no question about settlement on a grand scale by Company personnel in Asia and thus the need for notaries and the drawing up of wills was small to non-existent and when the need did arise demand was never very high. This was because European settlement commenced on a small scale; later on, the rising death rates meant large numbers of people died before they even reached Batavia; and those who did only drafted a will if there was an estate that needed to be settled for the survivors. Given these circumstances, most never bothered to draw up a will at all. However, because a senior surgeon or surgeon-trader did not really belong to the general public, it would be reasonable to assume that surgeons usually had their material affairs in order.[52]

There is yet another explanation for the apparently small number of Batavian Deeds. It appears that the surgeons did not immediately seek out a notary upon arrival in Batavia. On the contrary, quite some time passed before they felt the urge to do so. Engel van Tongeren, whose first departure as a third surgeon was in 1702, sought the services of a notary in Batavia in 1730 on his fifth voyage to Batavia in 1729. He was then a first surgeon. Simon Vlaming, a very young surgeon's mate in 1704, saw a notary nearly 25 years later, in 1725. Isaak Baillet, surgeon's mate in 1708, did not request a notary until 1730. Batavia's surgeons only needed a legal deed, be it a will or power of attorney, after some 14 years of acquaintance with Asia. This stretch of time could be filled with voyages back and forth, or by living in some settlement for a period, which allowed these surgeons the time necessary to build up some capital.

When the need for a notary arose, he was requested to wait on his client at home, as notaries did not have offices. Of the 340 Batavian Deeds, there was just the one surgeon who was also a patient at the *Binnenhospitaal*: Johannes Hanevelt. Notary C. Schoute visited him there on 14 May, 1725, depositing Hanevelt's last will at the *Weeskamer* on 6 June 1725.[53] As we mentioned in chapter 3, the *Binnenhospitaal* was not the most conducive place to be when you were ill. Apart from its unhealthy reputation, it was also the place of refuge for the great mass of sick, lower-ranking Company employees. Even the lower ranking third surgeon Jan Takens found another place to be ill (at a burgher's home in Batavia) because decent people died at home, or, in Batavia, at someone else's home. Hanevelt must have been the proverbial exception to the rule.

Surgeons who did not own a house or some rooms in Batavia (or in one of the other settlements) were careful, when *in loco*, to lodge with people residing in Batavia. Sometimes the hosts were friends, sometimes family, and sometimes the surgeons were paying guests. During the illness of surgeon's mate Willem Noordervliet in 1752, he lodged at the home of Company Merchant Groenendijk, in 1752. Noordervliet appointed Groenendijk the executor of his will in the event of his death, for which service the merchant would receive 80 *rijksdaalders*.[54] If a fortieth penny on every estate was an absolute law, this would mean that Groenendijk's estate was worth some 3,200 *rijksdaalders*, an amount not every surgeon's mate working in the Republic could have boasted about. Senior surgeon Jan Baptista Pinket lay ill in the house of burgher Frans van der Duijm in February 1700.[55] Were Pinket to die, Van der Duijm could sell off all his belongings, from the proceeds of which Pinket would posthumously pay for his lodgings. The remainder should then go to his heirs in Europe. Claas Eekel, first surgeon,[56] Jan Takens, third surgeon,[57] Hendrik Stevens, surgeon's mate,[58] and Jan Langsable, surgeon's mate,[59] all sought solace in their last days at a burgher's home. Leopoldus Schrijver, burgher surgeon in Batavia, took patients into his house as a sideline, a service for which he was paid by these patients.[60] Others went to colleagues like Engel van Tongeren, first surgeon, who lay ill at Frans Robbé's home (warden of the *Binnenhospitaal*) in 1730[61]; Gerrit van Groenenberg, surgeon's mate, at the house of his brother and colleague's home[62]; Anthonij Neddermans, surgeon's mate, was cared for at Pieter Kloot's home, who was a senior Company's surgeon, in 1769[63]; surgeon's mate Massener took ill while a guest in Company surgeon Scheffer's home in 1786.[64] Many indeed lodged or shared a house because, apart from the expenses and the responsibility of looking after it, it did not make much sense to own a home in Batavia when people were so much on the move, sailing to other trading posts or back to the Republic.

Of the surgeons who requested the drawing up of a legal document, 62 per cent held a senior rank (*oppermeester*), and some 15 per cent were surgeon's mates; there was only one third surgeon, Jan Takens, who did so. Takens summoned the notary to ratify his testament which had been composed in Amsterdam before he departed for Asia. He added a codicil to his will, leaving a legacy to his cousin, namely all his possessions in Asia, if this cousin took care to see that he was buried properly.[65] Surely, a mere third surgeon could not have been expected to be very prosperous. The fact that he had made a last will in Amsterdam just before boarding as well as bequeathing all his possessions (*goederen*) in Asia to his cousin while in Batavia, arouses suspicions that this third surgeon had other irons in the fire.

A very small number of indigenous surgeons (2.3 per cent), half of whom were in the Company service, also drew up wills. Twelve per cent are referred to as 'surgeon of the Company', specifying no rank but they were definitely of a higher rank than third surgeon. Five per cent were free settled surgeons (burgher surgeons) or European surgeons who had settled in Batavia but no longer worked for the Company, and were thus designated 'free'.

Table T6.1: Ranks of surgeons drawing up a legal deed (1643-1793)

First Surgeon	*Second Surgeon*	*Surgeon (of unknown rank)*	*Third Surgeon*	*Indiginous Surgeon*	*Free settled surgeon*
62% (212)	15% (52)	12% (47)	<1% (1)	2% (7)	5% (18)

The percentages in table T6.1 seem reasonable because it shows first surgeons, who had more capital, make up the bulk of them. They were, financially speaking, more substantial than the others. Nevertheless, a fair number of surgeons and surgeon's mates are represented, meaning that they too had something to dispose of. The drawing up of wills steadily increased over the years, keeping pace with the growth of Batavia as is shown in graph G7.1. The decades 1721-1730 and 1751-1770 were the busiest periods in terms of surgeons drawing up legal documents, the reason for which is not altogether clear. It could have been that during these periods private trading and the accumulation of capital flourished more than in other decades. Having acquired this capital, the owner wanted to have it disposed of properly in the event of his death. If falling ill and a foreboding of imminent death was a reason for doing so, the decade 1721-1730 does not correspond with the explosion of disease-ridden years in Batavia after 1730. Impending death was the motive for drawing up a will for 45 percent (154 cases); of these, more than half succumbed to their illness within three months. Pregnancy is mentioned in four cases; 5 per cent wanted to change their wills as they had become a widow(ers). For 37 per cent, no reason is given, although it seems likely that an impending marriage motivated many of these testators.

Graph G6.1: Number of surgeons whose legal deed was deposited at the Batavian Weeskamer[66]

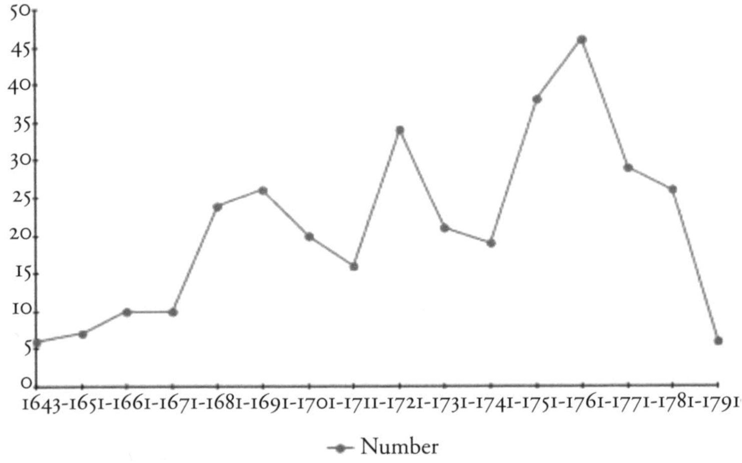

Marriage

The first will made by a surgeon in Batavia was that of the Amsterdam-born first surgeon, Christoffel Dirks, who undertook this step with his bride, Aeltjen Hendriks, in 1643, some twenty years after the foundation of the city.[67] The testament followed the standard Dutch procedure. The notary made it known he was qualified to act in this capacity not only in Holland or in Zeeland but also in Batavia;

he knew the testators, they were sound of mind; former documents were revoked, and their last wishes were that the survivor would inherit the estate provided that this survivor would then take care of any of their under-aged children. After the will was read aloud in front of Christoffel Dirks and Aeltjen Hendriks and the witnesses, the parties acknowledged it as their last will, signed it, and the original document was deposited with the notary.

Of the Company's surgeons sampled (S), it is certain that 16 per cent (470 surgeons) were married while in the service of the Company. Most of them had married in Europe and would have arranged their legal affairs, if any, there. It was established that 1.5 per cent (44 surgeons) got married in Asia. This number is quite small which is understandable as only some 250 surgeons of the sample (8 per cent) remained stationed for any considerable length of time in any one settlement in Asia, which, in their cases, enabled them to marry there.[68] It is advisable to exercise some caution with these numbers and percentages because there must have been surgeons who married and did not feel the need to make a will or make provisions with the Company for their wives.

Table T6.2: Married surgeons

Sampled surgeons (S)	*Those of S married*	*Those of S married in Asia*	*Those of S based in Asia for at least three years*
2988	470	44	250
100%	16% of S	1.5% of S	8% of S

Most surgeons found their wives in Europe. If the surgeons married in Asia, they were usually a bit older. Those surgeons from sample S, whose names are found in the Batavian Deeds, drew up these deeds some 14 years after their first acquaintance with the East.[69] As for some 37 per cent, the reason for the drawing up of a will was an intended marriage. Many of the surgeons were not that young when they married in Asia. Apparently, taking a plunge into matrimony in Asia was even less obvious to the surgeons than such a step would have been in Europe (in total, only 17.5 per cent of all the sampled surgeons married). Perhaps the Company surgeon could not afford to provide for a household and family on his meagre wages. For instance, the minister (*predikant*) of the church of Batavia (whose station in life was perhaps a bit more elevated than that of a senior surgeon) presented the annual costs of his family's household to the Gentlemen XVII, which amounted to some 3,000 Dutch guilders for a household without children (although he did have ten slaves).[70] A senior surgeon with a puny monthly wage of 36 Dutch guilders could not have afforded this kind of household.

Either the (unmarried) surgeons could not afford to marry, or they did not succeed in finding an advantageous party on whose fortune the newlyweds could live or contract an alliance which brought profitable opportunities. In total, among the number of the Batavian Deeds (340), covering both the seventeenth and eighteenth centuries, there were 216 deeds drawn up at the request of a surgeon who was married (44 of them in the sample S). Of the 216 married surgeons in the Batavian Deeds, it was established that 13 per cent of them had European-born wives who were living in Europe; 44 per cent had married in Asia (this does not invariably mean that her parents were Asian, she could have been born of European parents in Asia). Of the 43 percent of surgeons whose wives' descent is not certain, it seems fairly probable that those women had already been living in Batavia before marrying these particular surgeons.

Table T6.3: Wives of surgeons

Population	*European Marriage*	*Asian Marriage*
470 of S	90% (426)	10% (44)
216 of Batavian Deeds	13% (29)	87%(187)

It seems most likely that, if the surgeon did not marry in Europe, and if he did manage to survive and settle somewhere in Asia, he would have married a woman he met there. However, this would have been a false assumption; the number of married surgeons was small, even when we consider that the Batavian Deeds cover both centuries and even though the real number of married surgeons in Asia during the seventeenth and eighteenth centuries may well have been higher (taking into account that not all married couples drew up a will). It must therefore be concluded that the typical Company surgeon was a bachelor. Perhaps he did not feel the need to marry as liaisons not sanctified by Church and Company between Company surgeons and Asian ladies frequently occurred.

Slaves

There were some 19 surgeons who made some particular legal arrangements with respect to a relationship they had with one of their slaves. Sometimes because one child or more had been procreated, sometimes because they maintained special relationships with a female slave. Surgeon's mate Johan Schuts stipulated in his will of 12 December 1687, that after his death his female slave, Sarij of Bougis, should be freed because of the 'services he had enjoyed from her', on the provision that the *Raad van Justitie* judged her to be capable of making her own living.[71] Pieter Kloot, from Amsterdam, having started his career in 1757 as a third surgeon, came to Batavia to settle in 1761. There he met a free Christian woman (*vrije Christenvrouw*, usually the name for a free lady of Eurasian descent), and she had a son by him. Although it was against Company policy, he managed to get her and their son out of Asia. At the time, he drew up his will in Batavia in 1774, bequeathing her a sum of 1,500 rixdollars (*rijksdaalders*). He named his son, at the time living with the mother at Pieter's parents home in Amsterdam, as his sole heir.[72] Senior surgeon Daniel Neuman, from Hirschberg in Silesia, nominated his adopted daughter as the sole heir in 1750. He also bequeathed her the deed of adoption. The girl's mother, Maria of Bengalen, would receive a deed of manumission as well as a sum of 150 *rijksdaalders* and one slave of her choice from his household.[73]

The names of the Asian-born wives are fairly inconspicuous. The 'family' names can be an indication that one or more of their forebears used to be a slave. Or that they descended from families of mixed Asian-Portuguese origins, such as the surgeons' wives Dionisia de Sousa and Anna Adriana Ernesto. Sometimes the women were descended from manumitted slaves as liberated slaves often took their names from their benefactor or from the areas from which they had been transported. This does not mean that these wives themselves were freed slaves, although we do find an 'Annica of Ambon' and an 'Annica of Batavia'. Surgeon Nicolaas Perrera married one of the female slaves of his colleague Quickelenburg, who manumitted her. In their mutual will of 26 November, 1699, she remained grateful to Quickelenburg and bequeathed her former master an amount of 50 *rijksdaalders*.[74] Marriages between the Company's employees and the slave women imported into the Company settlements had to be licensed in writing by the local authorities. The prospective groom was obliged to purchase his bride's freedom and to have her baptised with a new, Christan name. In time, a knowledge of Dutch was also made a formal requirement.[75]

Slaves were a basic fact of life in Asia. Many were household slaves, imported into the Company settlements as the Javanese were not subjected to slavery. Some slaves were paid a small wage in addition to their rations, and a few salaried slaves were able to purchase their manumission while others were released by their owners following the slave's conversion to Christendom or because of a provision in the owner's will. The freed slaves then fell under Company jurisdiction in the same way as burghers.[76] Often enough these manumitted slaves became a burden on the Poorhouse. In 62 surgeons' wills (18 percent of the Batavian Deeds), slaves are mentioned, an indication of a certain degree of wealth, either in relation to a manumission on the testators' death or in relation to a bequest. Two-thirds of these surgeons did indeed provide for the liberation of at least some of their household slaves. Usually, they also bequeathed a sum of money to the liberated slave, which could vary from 20 to 2,000 *rijksdaalders*. This served a practical purpose as well as it meant that the manumitted slave would not lapse into poverty. If the testator had children, he usually stipulated that the manumitted slave had to serve with his children until these children were adults or married. One surgeon's wife made sure that the manumitted slaves working in her children's houses would be paid a monthly *rijksdaalder*. Such were the wishes of Maria Rodrip, wife to the Company surgeon David Pasqualsen in 1687.[77]

An advantageous marriage?

Not only was it quite common to mingle in the existing (mixed) Asian population, it was also the done thing to marry the widow of a colleague. As we saw earlier, Arnoldus op den Ool married the widow of his colleague; Cornelis Provo, a surgeon from Breda, who first married in the Republic in 1699. After the death of his own wife, he sailed as a first surgeon (*opperchirurgijn*) to Asia in 1720, where he married Cornelia Smits in Batavia.[78] As Provo was now rather advanced in years, she soon became his widow in early 1746. She remarried Johannes Keil, born in Wesel in Germany, who had sailed to Asia as a senior surgeon; he had become warden of the *Binnenhospitaal* in Batavia in 1745.[79] Cornelis van den Berg, also born in Germany, sailed in 1766 as a surgeon's mate. In Batavia, he married Anna Maria Holtman and died in 1780.[80] Within three years she had remarried Andreas Auerbach, surgeon in Batavia.[81] The Rotterdam-born Pieter Hogewoning (1708-1745) was not to return to the Republic after his second voyage as surgeon's mate. He married Lidia van der Leen in Batavia, drawing up a will with her in 1745, just before he died.[82] She remarried Hendrik Radermacher, of Amsterdam, whom she must have met through her former husband, as both of them started to work as surgeon's mates in Batavia at the same time, climbing the ranks over the years.[83] Jan Adam Spenolt married Petronella Stellingwerf in 1765, widow of the surgeon J. Hinneville. Spenold, at the time Head of Surgery,[84] was also survived by Petronella. Sybrand Schouten, surgeon of the Company, married the widow of surgeon Johannes Vegnerus. Within one year of their marriage Schouten died.[85] And, finally, surgeon Jan Munt married his colleague's wife Margaretha Molanus, who had been married to surgeon Mathijs Voskuil.[86] As these (partly) Asian-born girls married quite young, often enough in their early teens, it was natural enough that they outlasted a husband or two.

If the surgeons did marry in Asia, they tended to marry 'in the profession' as it were. They must have felt that this was a realistic option and advantageous to their careers. The parties concerned already moved in the same social circles and it was easy anough to become acquainted with each other. While marrying 'in the profession', Spenold also entered into a fortunate marriage. Whereas Spenold's estate was not worth more than 2,000 *rijksdaalders*, his wife's far surpassed this amount. In her last will, she changed the antenuptial contracts and nominated Spenold as sole legatee. Alas, but that he could have been able to have enjoyed it.

If a surgeon did have a spouse, European or otherwise, she was usually the beneficiary of his will, as he was of hers. These, mostly mutual, wills provided for the children procreated in their marriage, born or unborn, at least with a legal share, and if the marriage had not been blessed with any offspring, that share would usually go to one of his parents. It is remarkable that this lawful portion did not invariably go to one of her parents. The reason for this could be that she had no surviving parents or that she did not bring any possessions or capital into the marriage. The moment she did, one of her parents would also be provided for in the absence of children.

For some 19 (Eur-)Asian ladies and for some eleven surgeons, it was a second marriage. In cases of a second marriage, children born of the former marriage were provided for. These children were called *voorkinderen* or 'before-children'. Although the *Weeskamer* was usually excluded from these wills, nominating the survivor executor and guardian, it did happen that in the case of a second marriage there was the stipulation to put the lawful share of the *voorkinderen* under the trusteeship of the *Weeskamer*. Apparently, these newlyweds did not trust a stepmother or a stepfather to deal scrupulously with their children's inheritance, a stepfather being perhaps even worse as he would have guardianship over the natural mother. Even though it did occur, this remained a rare stipulation, occurring in only four instances.[87]

Rich or poor

Lawful portions (usually being half of the entire estate to be passed along to the children), coming on top of the children's schooling, clothing, and food, were stipulated by 80 surgeons and their wives and ranged from 20 rixdollars to some portion of 8,000 rixdollars: Marcus Andriesz was only able to bequeath 20 *rijksdaalders* (amounting to circa 50 Dutch guilders) to his daughter, although this did not stop him from donating some additional money to the Poorhouse in Batavia and the leprosy hospital on the island of Purmerend. Martinus Troef struck it rich and was able to leave each of his three children some 8,000 *rijksdaalders* in 1693, something he had not been able to do some 30 years earlier in his first will of 1663. By 1693, Martinus Troef was medical inspector of Batavia (*visitateur ter rheede*), had remarried and had produced two sons and one daughter.[88] The Company surgeon Johan Schopper and his wife, Anna van Esten, were also relatively well off. Although they only donated some 20 *rijksdaalders* to the Batavia Poorhouse (*diaconie*), and stipulated a parentally lawful share of 3,000 *rijksdaalders* in their mutual testament, their estate was estimated to be worth some 18,000 *rijksdaalders*.[89] Quite an achievement for the son of a City and Plague surgeon from Nörenberg in Prussia!

Ten surgeons left their (eventual) offspring a portion under 100 rixdollars. Forty-two left an amount of between 100 and 1,000 rixdollars, of which 11 specified 200 *rijksdaalders*. Twenty-eight lawful portions ranged between the 1,000 and

8,000, of which 11 shares were 1,000, four were 1,500 and five were portions of 2,000 *rijksdaalders*.

Table T6.4: Sums of lawful shares stipulated by 80 ship's surgeons in the Batavian Deeds

<100 *Rijksdaalders*	100 – <1,000 *Rijksdaalders*	1,000–<2,000 *Rijksdaalders*	2,000 – 8,000 *Rijksdaalders*
10 (12.5%)	42 (53%)	17 (21%)	11 (14%)

Most of the surgeons in Asia were able to reserve a capital of between 100 and 1,000 *rijksdaalders* for the children. Usually, the lawful portion for children was half of the estate, the other half being reserved for the widow. Seventy-five surgeons (21 per cent of the Batavian Deeds) mentioned that their estates were worth less than 2,000 rixdollars. 10 per cent (34 surgeons) stated that it was more. Only one told the notary that it was more or less exact. The others do not mention it at all. While some felt they were able to stipulate lawful shares of more than 2,000 *rijksdaalders* and/or to bequeath sums of more than 1,000 *rijksdaalders*, it may have been quite possible that those who failed to mention it had estates worth over 2,000 *rijksdaalders*. It does seem that the financial position of a Company surgeon was somewhat more fortunate than that of his colleagues practising in the Republic. More than 80 per cent of the master surgeons in Amsterdam left an estate worth less than 2,000 Dutch guilders (800 *rijksdaalders*) during the period of 1741-1750. Although their financial positions brightened somewhat over the course of the century, 71 per cent of the master surgeons did not have an estate of more than 2,000 Dutch guilders in the period of 1776-1780.[90]

The surgeons' wives did remarry slightly more often than their husbands. However, those who struck it rich or fell into extreme poverty were rare: Elisabeth Anna van Driel, widow of the warden and surgeon of the Chinese Hospital, Jan Liesthout, manumitted 14 slaves, one of whom also received 500 *rijksdaalders* and bequeathed some 8,000 *rijksdaalders* to some seven lady friends in Batavia, as well as a house and a slave in her last will of April 1746. Her nephews were to be her sole beneficiaries of the (remainder of the) estate.[91] Taking account of the fact that a physician's fee (not a surgeon's) for a visit to a patient in Batavia was one *rijksdaalder* (twice that of a physician in Amsterdam), these sums are large indeed.[92] At the other end of the scale, are widows like Pieter Jansz's. She mentioned in her will of 1728 that her husband had died some three years previously, and had left her very poor indeed. Now, three years later, she did not have enough money to be buried properly and pleaded for her godmother to take care of that.[93] Petronella van den Vijver, widow of Abraham Morell (surgeon with the Company), also stated in her will of 1728 that she was extremely poor. She only had one slave, the proceeds of whose sale would not be sufficient to cover the costs of her burial.[94]

The funeral

This preoccupation with a proper burial was a feminine trait.[95] It was mostly the wives of the surgeons who took precautions in their wills for the proper disposal of their dead bodies, perhaps because these wives ran an additional risk of an untimely death the moment they married. From then on their lives would be preoccupied with the bearing of children, the labour of which was a real danger to the mother. For instance, the average age of the 'Company's' woman who died on the Coast of Coromandel was between 20 and 30 years; fairly often the newborn child would be buried with the deceased mother.[96]

Liesthout's widow, Anna, the one who bequeathed some 8,000 *rijksdaalders* to her lady friends, also asked those friends to properly take care of her body. The wife of surgeon Isaak Baillet would receive a silver spittoon if she laid out the body of Johanna van der Burg (widow of Christoffel de la Marre).[97] Alida Coster, the widow of surgeon Petrus Alma, stipulated that someone was supposed to wash and lay out her body to whom she would donate 40 *rijksdaalders*.[98] Susanna de Feijter arranged not only the laying-out of her body, but also the payment of her pallbearers and the meal after the funeral.[99] Angila van den Berge, the widow of Gerrit van Broekhuijs, bequeathed those who had prepared her body for burial each 10 *rijksdaalders*.[100] Aletta Taas, widow of J.J. Cogh, donated her future pallbearers each six *ducaten*.[101] Perhaps, these ladies wanted to look their best on the bier and were slightly more aware than their husbands of the social distinctions and opportunities a funeral could offer. With the body cleansed and shrouded, and placed in an open coffin, and the house, its furniture, and its inhabitants draped in black shrouds, friends and family paid their final respects to the deceased, after which the coffin was taken to the cemetery in cortège. In 1743, it became obligatory to hire the official bearers from the Batavia garrison. They consisted of a corporal and some 12 soldiers, who had to be paid.

The funeral could be a costly event. The Hospitalier Christoph Godfried Jager in Macassar had to spend some 370 Dutch guilders posthumously on the affair: the surgeon's mate and his assistant had to be paid for the laying-out of his body; the pallbearers, no fewer then 20 men, had to be paid; the purchase of cloth and the making of the shroud, funeral trousers and the coffin as well as its lining (some 200 copper nails were needed for the coffin); 24 candles for the vigil during the night before the interment; arak was needed for the cleansing of the body although the carpenters and smiths and sailors also liked to drink it; the gravediggers; the city mason; the Poorhouse for the hiring of the bier's shroud; the composition and delivery of the invitations; the hiring of eight boy slaves and eight girl slaves; some ham; cheese; 40 pounds of flour for the pastry; some Dutch gin; 24 bottles of red wine; some eight pounds of tobacco and six pipes.[102] It was not only costly but it was also an important social event, in which everyone wanted to participate, looking at his (or her) best, walking in an impressive cortège, or, even better, riding in a carriage draped in black, and having the 'best' place in the cortège, which was a reflection of a person's status in town.[103]

Occasionally, the Batavian Deeds offer an insight into a family tragedy. First surgeon Leendert Bollekeus had lived and worked at the Company settlement on Taiwan since 1656, where he married and raised a family of two children, a son Joost and a daughter Dieuwertje.[104] When he died in 1663, his estate needed to be settled. In the will, it appears that the family Bollekeus had incurred many debts in Taiwan, especially among the Chinese population. Upon Bollekeus's inability to repay, these Chinese had subsequently kidnapped his son, Joost. When the will was opened, it was still hoped that Joost was alive somewhere along the shores of China as the family did take into account that perhaps in the future a ransom for Joost would have to be paid.[105]

There were 108 surgeons (33 per cent of the Batavian Deeds) who felt they were able to bequeath something. In about one-eighth of the wills (42) of the ship's surgeons, the poorhouse and the leprosy hospital of Batavia were often remembered. The legacies these institutions received ranged from 3 to 200 *rijksdaalders*. However, the common amount was some 20 *rijksdaalders*. Surgeon's mate Abraham Rombouts, who nominated a soldier as his sole beneficiary, bequeathed the capital sum of three Dutch guilders to each of his sisters, this being the sum of his fraternal love.[106] Slaves were bequeathed to friends and offspring, and so were money, clothes, furniture, jewelery, *port d'épée*'s (swords), surgical instruments and books. First surgeon Hendrik Oldenzeel, for instance, left all of his books and surgical instruments to the surgeon's mate, Middeldijk, upon his death in 1689. Surgeon's mate David Heijn, born in Bantam, besides a sum of 200 *rijksdaalders*, bequeathed one *port d'épée* with a silver grip, one cane with a silver mount, all his surgical instruments, a silver travelling writing box, and one big chest filled with books to the senior surgeon, Jan August Oostwalt.[107] Such bequests of books and medical instruments were also made by surgeons Croon, Koedijk, and Weidner.[108]

Books

The wills of prominent sixteenth-century English surgeons reveal that these men accumulated considerable libraries ranging from classical literature to medical treatises.[109] The seventeenth-century German surgeon, Gijsbert van Imbrock, who worked for the Dutch West India Company in New Amsterdam possessed several anatomical and medical books by Christoph Wirtsung, Ambrosius Paré, Johannes de Vigo, and Nicolaas Tulp. Besides these he owned quite an extensive collection of schoolbooks; religious books (one on the Catholic faith, one each by Jean Taffin (theologian, 1529-1602), Albertus Arnoldus Huttenus (1587-1663), Johan Sarcharson, Jacobus Borstius (Protestant theologian, 1612-1680)), and some historical studies such as the Dutch translation of Livy; the *History of Van Meteren*; *Frederick Henry* by Caspar Commelin (1636-1693), and a chronicle of the life of the English kings by Richard Bakers.[110]

Ringoir claims that not much is known about the ownership of books among Dutch surgeons.[111] Nonetheless, Rotterdam surgeon Joost Pietersz. Helburgh, who died in 1666, needed not to be ashamed of his library. In his estate, he left some 153 books of which at least 20 were of a surgical nature.[112] The well-read Helburgh possessed an extensive and typical library on surgery of the seventeenth century. However, he practised in Rotterdam, where books were easier to acquire than in Asia. The data found in the financial records of the Company clearly show that most ship's surgeons carried a Bible in their sea chests. More interesting for our purposes would be to know whether they possessed medical or classical literature, although it should be remembered that most (sea)surgeons had not enjoyed the benefits of a classical education, so that most of them could not read Latin.

Physicians read Latin easily because it was a prerequisite for a university education. Batavia's licentiate-physician Andries Cleijer's scholarly and literary interests spanned far and wide. Besides books on medicine, his collection varied from theology to politics, and from law (such as intestate succession) to philosophy. The following books were found in his library, arranged according to size as was custom:[113]

- Ludovici Vlasblom, *De nature ofte cort begrijp der sienlijcke dingen*[114]
- *Opera Calvini tot Amsterdam gedrukt* (printed in Amsterdam)[115]
- J.A. Comenij, *Didactica opera omnia*[116]

In Quatro:

- Joan. Strauchy: *Amoenitatum Juris canonici, semestria duo*[117]
- Joan Christian Fromay, *De Fascinatione*[118]
- A. Kircheri, *Domus Joannia Siloe Archetypou politiacum*[119]
- Joan Hiskia Cardiluci, *Officina Sanitatis etc*[120]
- Joannis Stalcy, *Dissertatio Theologo-politica*[121]
- Thomae Bartholonii, *Actorium medicorum pars 3- 7*[122]
- Eliae Schnegassi, *De jure successionis ab intestato!*[123]
- Francisi de le Boe Sylvi, *Opera Omnia*[124]
- Miscellanea, Curios. Annuss. Octava et noni[125]
- Athanas Kircheri, *Scrutinium Physico-medicum sive de peste etc.*

In Octavo :

- *Fortunatus Fidelis de Relationibus medicorum*[126]

- Benedics, *De Bacquere Ismen medicq.*[127]
- Ferdinandi Francisi, *Jachi Syntaxis Latino-Germanica*[128]
- *Goosen Vreeswijcks alle chirurgische Werken*[129]
- Anthony le Grand, *Justituio Philosophia Secundum Carthesium*[130]
- Thomae Bartholinii, *Opuscula Sacra* and *Euisd. Disputator Hafnicuf benovat. Et autum*
- Benjamin Scharly, *Toxicologia*[131]
- Franscisi Bayle, *Dissertationus Physica*[132]

In Duodecimo :

- Theod. Graswinkeli, *Strictua ad Censura Joannis a Felden*[133]
- Israeli Conradi, *Dissertatio medicophysica de Frigoris natura, etc.*[134]
- *Matthaei Compani Horologium solo naturo motu etc.*[135]
- Hugo Grotius, *De Imperio summa potestat. Circa sacra sui recedant Blandellq*[136]
- *Lampas Vita et Plortifs*, printed in Leiden 1678. Authore: G.F.M.D.C.S.[137]

It is interesting to note that Cleijer not only read the works of Calvin but also studied Cartesian philosophy. As did Johannes Groeneveldt, the Amsterdam doctor who had left some 38 books in the care of friends, most of them medical, when he left for England. He too was influenced by René Descartes.[138] Amongst Cleijer's rather meagre collection of medical textbooks, Kircher is certainly worth mentioning as he was the first to express the doctrine that contagious diseases were spread by small living animals, invisible to the naked eye. The book written by Schnegas probably means that the ambitious Cleijer was interested in inheritances and how to procure them. Cleijer liked to trade in contraband so much that the Japanese authorities deported him from Nagasaki to Batavia, under pain of death should he ever return.

Although surgeons usually enjoyed a less extensive education and lower status than physicians, they too were expected to be able to read and write. This had become a necessity in their profession over time. Thus, one would expect them to have the obligatory Bible, but also some professional literature, especially as so many books had by that time been translated from Latin into the vernacular; and indeed many of them did. Orphans from Middelburg (Zeeland) who were placed on a Company vessel as third surgeons were given textbooks by the orphanage to suit their future profession: Cornelis Herls,[139] Helvetius,[140] Cornelis van de Voorde,[141] and Abraham Titsing[142] are some of the authors of the books with which these orphans were burdened.[143] Some surgeons borrowed books. The Pattna surgeon Andries Thuinzaad borrowed Jan Hoogvliet's book *De Konst om Wonde te Schouwen*[144] from his colleaque Jacob Berger at the Hooghly settlement in Bengal (near Chinsura) in exchange for his *herbarium vivum*.[145] Others bought books. Surgical works were less expensive than Bibles, even more so when they were bought second-hand at auctions on board of the deceased estate of a ship's surgeon, for instance.

Table T6.5: Prices of surgical books in the Dutch Republic[146]

Year	*Title*	*Price in Dutch guilders*
Circa 1680	Battum Medicijnboek	3.-.-
	Willis Anatomica	1.-.-
	Bartholini Anatomica	2.10.-
Circa 1710	Ambroisius Paré Chirurgie	-.18.-
	Beverwijkse Werken	1.5.-
	Aquapendente Chirurgie	-.14,-

If the books of a ship's surgeon were auctioned off on board, the titles or authors of the books auctioned were not always listed. Christiaan Brauns's list only mentions that he possessed two books and one *octavo* Bible in German.[147] The possessions of surgeon's mate Bernardus Scharl were listed as 'several books', which brought in the capital sum of six guilders.[148] So it is listed for Wijnand Worms ('several old books');[149] Pieter van der Sande ('several books');[150] while the books of surgeon's mate Jacob Curvemaker were sold on board for the meagre sum of 1.4 guilders in 1752;[151] surgeon's mate Hendrik van der Kemp possessed 'some books';[152] third surgeon Claas Boom, who died in April 1763, had 15 books that sold for a total of three Dutch guilders;[153] senior surgeon Bernardus ten Cate also owned 'some books';[154] while senior surgeon Johan Stilzer had a 'chest of books written in High German'.[155] First surgeon Georg Veltjes[156] had 'several books'; and first surgeon Weemeijer possessed 'two'.[157] Sometimes these books are specified as 'surgical books' (*chirurgijnsboeken*), as was the case with the inventory of Pieter Everhard Hink's belongings;[158] the 'surgical books' of Jan Gouwenaar, surgeon's mate on the *Orangezaal*, were sold for two-and-a-half Dutch guilders after he died on 16 August, 1752;[159] and the inventory of third surgeon Mathijs Weijers's listed 'surgical books' that had been found among his belongings.[160] In his will, first surgeon Jacob Neiman bequeathed some *geestelijke* (religious) books to a minister (*dominee*) of his acquaintance,[161] while surgeon's mate Johannes van Willemsvaart possessed more than 30 books[162] and senior surgeon M. Ulman possessed some 58 books.[163] Chief surgeon Jan Abbing, who died in 1728 had one big Bible and a smaller one with silver mounts for which the sum of 64(!) Dutch guilders was paid at the auction on board.[164] Third surgeon J. van Mellingen possessed 'three books'.[165] From these lists of possessions found during the research of the financial records, one may safely conclude that the ship's surgeon had at least some interest in books. In this connection, I also refer to appendix 6.2.

Some inventories are more detailed, for instance, that of Cornelis van Sorgen (1731-1754). Born in Stavenisse (province of Zeeland), he became employed as a surgeon's mate by the Company at the age of 20. Returning to the Republic two years later, after spending seven months on shore, he set sail again as a first surgeon in February 1754. Two months after his departure, he died on 7 April 1754.[166] Amongst his belongings, various books were found, namely:

In Quatro: Laurens Heijsters[167]
Cornelis van Solingen[169]
Petrus Nijland[171]

In Octavo: Paulus Barbette[168]
Hendrik van Rhoonhuijse[170]
Job van Meekeren[172]
Johannes Gorter, I[173]
Jan van Kouwenburgh[174]
Twee delen disteleerkunst[175]
Arend Blankert[176]
D'Amsterdamsche Apotheek[177]

Van Sorgen's reading interests were pretty seventeenth century, conservative, and confined to surgery. His was a library to be expected of a surgeon, as the authors of these books wrote particularly for surgeons. Christoph Godfried Jager, of Schlauwen, whose funeral was so expensive, was more widely read. He was employed by the Company Chamber of Enkhuizen as surgeon's mate in 1776. In 1779, he was settled in Macassar and worked there in the hospital as Hospitalier. Amongst the inventory of his belongings upon his death on 19 February 1789, was a bookcase containing the following books:[178]

- Octavo Statesbible
- Johannes Jacob Woijth (MD), *Schatzkammer medicinischer und natürlicher Dinger*, with plates, Leipzig, 1755[179]
- Justus Auldus, *Thuijspostille*, Amsterdam, 1618
- Richard Steele, *The Guardian of de Britse Zedenmeester*, I, III, Rotterdam, 1734[180]
- Richard Steele, *De Spectator of de verrezene Socrates*, I-VIII, Amsterdam, 1743
- Richard Steele, *The Snapper of de Britse Tuchtmeester*, I, Amsterdam, 1733
- Richard Steele, *Urbana Cerri, De Staat der rooms-katholijcke religie*, Amsterdam, 1715
- August Gotlieb Richter (MD), *Chirurgische Bibliotheek*, I, II, Göttingen, 1771[181]
- Albrecht von Haller (MD), *Umrisz der Geschäfte des Körperlichen Lebens*, Berlin, 1770[182]
- Samuel Schaarsmidt (MD), *Physiologie*, I, Berlin, 1751[183]
- David Samuel Madai, *Kort bericht van de nuttigheid en het gebruik van enige beproefde geneesmiddelen*, Amsterdam, 1760[184]
- Guliemus Harveum (MD), *Anatomische Oefeningen*, Amsterdam, 1650[185]
- Percival Pott (MD), *Abhandlung des Mastdarmfistel*, Wien, 1768[186]
- As well as various other old books.

This German surgeon obviously preferred modern eighteenth-century writers. Woijt, for instance, had even been translated into Japanese and was also widely read by Dutch surgeons. Haller was a very up-to-date physician. The same is true of Schaarsmidt, while Percival Pott was the leading man in surgery in eighteenth-century England.

If the possession of books was an indication of whether someone belonged to the literate elite, the ship's surgeons could have claimed to have done so. But their tastes were mostly pragmatic. The classics by authors like Virgil or modern poetry did not seem to interest them. The bulk of their possessions consisted of textbooks related to their own field so that they were able to keep apprised of developments in their profession. They would buy each other's surgical books and surgical instruments when one of them died. Half of the surgeons took along their own *instrumentarium*, other than what the Company provided (appendix 6.3). The fact that they bought surgical books and instruments indicates the professional quality of the Company's ship's surgeons.

Company surgeons were not poetically inclined, nor were they musically so. Analysing the lists of possessions and/or auctions we can only conclude that the Company ship's surgeons were anything but musical. Only four surgeons' inventories mention a musical instrument. Bernardus Scharl had a side-blown flute, and so did Lambert Elikman. Among hospitalier Jager's many household possessions were found a trumpet and a violin. First surgeon Werner August Mester brought along his own bed on board as well as two flutes.[187] Besides music, Mester liked a smoke. He was the proud owner of 25 pounds of tobacco, 9 rolls of tobacco, 100 linen pouches (*cardoes*) of tobacco, and 23 parcels of snuff. This extraordinary amount can hardly have been solely for his own consumption, however.

The surgeon-trader

Given the cramped space on board, we might expect that most surgeons would take along only a few personal belongings and everyday necessities like knives and forks; some surgical instruments; perhaps some medicines; a book or two; two or three pairs of breeches; two or three camisoles; four or five shirts; a writing desk, pens and paper, as letters had to be written; some food, wine, and tobacco. However, Werner Mester's chests were stuffed to the brim with tobacco. Surgeon's mate Wessel Meijer brought along 111 breadknives as well as 36 hats.[188] Third surgeon Jan Bovet possessed 12 hats and 14 pairs of stockings;[189] Johan Spies, third surgeon, was the proud owner of 24 knives as well as a big chest full of *glaslampen* (lamps);[190] Jan van Mellingen, third surgeon, had four dozen razors.[191] Surgeon S.H. Twent took along seven boxes of beer glasses, 28 dozen chisels, and seven dozen locks![192] Hille Swart, third surgeon, possessed eight boxes filled with watch glasses.[193] Jan Dake, surgeon's mate, had no less than 57 hats;[194] Jacob Curvemaker, surgeon's mate, had 36 hats and 175 pounds(!) of tobacco;[195] If Christiaan Nasbij was not a trader then he was certainly a thirsty third surgeon as he possessed 123 bottles of red wine.[196] Charles-Ghislain Wilmet, whom we met earlier, nagged his family in Belgium (Gembloux) to give him 10,000 Dutch guilders to invest in contraband to be sold at the Cape or in Batavia. He reminded his family on 6 September, 1790, that *qu'il achète des marchandise de contrabande que l'on ne peut avoir sans argent contant* and also *qu'il prendra encore pour 10.000 florins de marchandises car j'ai de Bons Marchands avec lesquelles je commerce ce qui me permettrai de gagner 10.000 florins supplémentaires.*[197] He had plenty of experience in trading as he had written earlier, in 1786, from the Cape to his family that it was possible to make huge profits selling rolled tobacco (*Pour le tabac en rolle [...] on y gagne un capitale*) and that the products which sold best at the Cape were shiny, cheap things for the handyman as well as Parisian trinkets (... *très brillantes et bon marché, de la quincaillerie, des colifichets de Paris*).[198]

Thus, there seems to have been a great deal more to the surgeons than meets the eye: apparently, these surgeons were involved in numerous other non-surgical pursuits. When Arnoldus op den Ool sailed as a third surgeon in 1747, he could not have known that 15 years later he would (as a senior surgeon) own 11 slaves whom he used as security in the financing of a small vessel and crew. Furthermore, in conjunction with a colleague Michiel Reijn, he financed, *inter alia*, in the purchase of five chests of red wine; one chest filled with pipes; 50 hams; 60 cow tongues; 50 cheeses; 600 dozen knifes; 50 glasses; 60 barrels of butter; 400 bottles of 'spirits'; 100 blankets; 30 barrels of Haarlem water; all to be sold in Batavia.[199]

How did a ship's surgeon get involved in something so entirely different from his own line of work, and how could he afford to finance these investments on his meagre wages? If surgeon Jacob Berger (Dokkum 1711–Hougly 1752) had still been alive in Houghly in 1753, he would have received a letter from Peter Bolten, employee of the Amsterdam brewery, the 'Hooijbergse Princesse Royal'.[200] In his letter, Bolten proposed sending Berger (who was unknown to Bolten but recommended to him by others) some barrels of Hooijbergs beer in order to explore the possibilities of trade in Bengal. Indeed, so wrote Bolten, the brewery had excellent experiences with the sale of Hooijberg's beer in Batavia and in Ceylon, although, in India, they feared competition from English beers. Transport was not a problem, Bolten insisted, because it was the brewery's practice to buy the *voering* of some Company officers (the amount of trading goods allowed for each sea-faring employee working for the Company). The barrels of beer (all 21 of them) would be delivered to the Company Chamber in Amsterdam (the East India House), where the officers would claim the barrels as their permitted *voering*. Subsequently, the barrels would be marked with the initials of said officers and transported from Amsterdam to the vessels on which the officers sailed and stowed in the holds. The officers accompanied the beer to Asia, and the representative in Batavia, Ceylon, or, in this case, Berger in Hougly, would sell it and send the proceeds thereof to the Republic by means of a bill of exchange.[201]

This was a practice well known to Jacob Berger. Did he not himself follow the same principle, he and his business agents in Amsterdam, David d'Arnaud and Steven Dissel? Even more than that, his business agents, acting simultaneously as his bankers, sent him, Berger, bills of exchange taken along by various sea-faring officers on a regular basis. These bills invariably amounted to sums of over 1,000 guilders. Often enough, the *voering* of these officers would be purchased as well. Surgeon Willem Mazee had stated in a notarial deed on 15 November 1752 in Amsterdam that he, first surgeon on the *Kasteel van Tilburg* and soon to leave for Asia, had sold his two chests of permitted *voering* to Steven Dissel for the amount of 44 Dutch guilders. Mazee had undertaken to deliver the chests to Jacob Berger in Hougly.

Mazee was not the only one involved in Berger's trading network. The cost of the contents of the chests (officially belonging to senior surgeon Frans Puthuijs) was 10,042 Dutch guilders, in which Berger had invested 50 per cent. The investment in Indian linen stuffed into the chests of surgeon Gerrit van Geel was worth 2,000 Arcat rupiahs (3,000 Dutch guilders), which Berger had financed. Van Geel's sale of the linen in Rotterdam was not spectacular; he made a profit of only 800 guilders. However, he was able to repay his colleague with a 400-guilder profit. This colleague, Joseph Berggo, surgeon on the island of Onrust, was able to sell Berger's goods at a 30 per cent profit. The revenues for the contents of the chests of Simon Ang (bought by Berger) was a 'mere' 7,993 Dutch guilders, and as these were sold by the Company (the chests having been detected by Company authorities and marked as contraband), 20 per cent went to the Company. The chests of surgeon Puthuijs had also been detected by the Company: Berger's business agents wrote that the revenue from these was only some 9,000 guilders, of which 20 per cent had to go to the Company. Batavia-based surgeon Albert Nack sent Berger sums of rupiahs concealed and wrapped in cloth. Berger's trading business was mainly served by his colleagues, although occasionally a captain, a first mate or another non-surgical seafaring officer also participated in his network.

Berger's chief purchase was Indian chintz (which was certainly not permitted by the Company) and Indian linen, for which he chartered, assistants such as his colleague Andries Thuinzaad. Thuinzaad was stationed at Pattna as the Company's surgeon and was the one who sent Berger a *herbarium vivum* in exchange for a surgical book. Thuinzaad saw to it that the textiles were sent to Chinsura (Houghly), and there Berger would ask for a repatriating acquaintance to take these along as his permitted *voering*. Upon his arrival in the Republic, D'Arnaud and Dissel would have a little boat ready on Texel to evade Company authorities (which was not always successful), and the commodities were then sold. Furthermore, 'Berger & Co.' participated in bottomry transactions (*bodemerij*), a practice already known in Antiquity as *foenus nauticum* and *pecunia traiectitia*: Berger financed cargoes on vessels by way of a financial agreement drawn up by a notary, which stated that Berger would supply a sum of money against a certain percentage of interest for which a vessel or the cargo on the vessel would serve as a guarantee. Op den Ool also financed these kinds of transactions. He empowered the Company merchant at Surat, R. van Hedin, to demand the products covered by the bottomry contract, which were sent on the *Rebecca Jacoba* in 1763.

Jacob Berger also sent bills of exchange from Bengal to his business agents. He would deposit a certain amount with the Company at Houghly, for which he received a letter (bill of exchange); this letter was subsequently taken by a returning friend. Captain Pieter Jongedijk, for instance, took along a bill of exchange worth 6,190 Dutch guilders, for which service he received no less than 1,630 guilders(!). The amount of 4,560 Dutch guilders was credited to Berger's account by D'Arnaud and Dissel. Besides this, Berger ordered D'Arnaud and Dissel to buy English bills of exchange in London, then send them to Houghly, where they were subsequently sold by Berger for cash, which he deposited with the cashier of the Company's offices in Bengal. These were collected and cashed by D'Arnaud and Dissel in Amsterdam. As everyone was making a profit on these financial transactions, it must have been one of those rare 'win-win' situations in life. Although Berger died young in 1752, his Hougly representatives did receive 21 barrels of Princesse Royale beer, the profits of which the accompanying officer was entitled to one-third.[202] One could say that, in all probability, this was the first appearance of Heineken Beer in Asia, as it was Heineken who bought the Hooijbergse brewery in the nineteenth century.[203]

Another example of a surgeon-trader was Frederick Kruijs, who was born on 7 July 1754 in Amsterdam. After his schooling as a surgeon at the Amsterdam guild, he was employed as a third surgeon by the Company in 1777. He made two voyages to the Cape of Good Hope and four to Asia in the service of the Company.

Table T6.6: Kruijs' voyages for the Company

From	*Until*	*Capacity*
21/1/1777	9/6/1778	Third Surgeon
6/1/1779	24/1/1780	Surgeon's Mate
15/8/1780	21/11/1784	First Surgeon
9/9/1785	27/8/1787	First Surgeon
25/11/1788	25/11/1788 to China	First Surgeon
11/7/1792	11/7/1792	First Surgeon

How did he operate? The first two voyages served as a reconnaisance mission to learn more about the employer's environment. His trading ventures started with his third voyage, when he was employed as a senior surgeon. His financial operations are summarised in table T6.7:

Table T6.7: The debts (investments?) incurred by Frederik Kruijs [204]

Date	*Debt in Dutch guilders*	*Where*	*Paid*	*Where*
24/2/1784	1500	Batavia		
11/8/1785	223.15	Republic	18/2/1786	Cape of Good Hope
30/8/1785	Chest filled with silk and gauze, etc. amounting to 1,704.40	Republic	25/2/1786	Cape of Good Hope
01/09/1785	45.10	Republic	24/6/1786	Batavia
1/09/1785	266.50	Republic	24/7/1786	Batavia
1/09/1785	1065.10	Republic	24/6/1786	Batavia
1/09/1785	182.00	Republic	24/6/1786	Batavia
1/09/1785	96.00	Republic	01/01/1789	Republic
12/9/1785	206.00	Republic		
13/9/1785	300.00	Republic		Cape of Good Hope
13/10/1788	743.00	Republic	10/8/1790	Republic?
16/10/1788	1,300 (products in boxes, in commission for L.D. Kreps)	Republic		
16/10/1788	325.00 (interest on 1,300)	Republic		Batavia
17/10/1788	3740	Republic	25/6/1792	
20/10/1788	2,540.00 products such as stockings, clocks, watch glasses, cotton, surgeon's chest with contents, knifes, etc.	Republic	30/10/1788	Republic
30/10/1788	320.00	Republic	July 1789	Batavia
30/10/1788	355.00	Republic	July 1789	Batavia
30/10/1788	1184	Republic	July 1789	Batavia
30/10/1788	1067	Republic	July 1789	Batavia

Date	Debt in Dutch guilders	Where	Paid	Where
1/11/1788	181.00	Republic	22/9/1790	Canton?
5/11/1788	140.00	Republic	20/8/1791	
7/11/1788	300.00	Republic	2/9/1789	Batavia
24/8/1789	67.00 for pickles, candied fruits, lemon, sirups, etc.	Batavia		
30/10/1789	650.00	Republic	15/8/1789	Batavia
14/6/1792	212.60	Republic		
20/6/1792	128.00 for 4 half barrels beer	Republic		Batavia

From these financial transactions, of which the exact details remain rather unclear (for instance, did he act for himself or on the behalf of others), it should be obvious, that Frederick Kruijs was a surgeon-trader if ever there was one. He borrowed sums of money in the Republic, which he invested in commodities before setting sail. In all probability, his monthly Company wages served as security by way of a pledge drawn up by a notary, in which the lender assumed the risk as it could not be guaranteed that the borrower would live long enough to earn the borrowed sum. With fortune on his side, Kruijs sold his trading products the moment he arrived in Cape Town or in Asia and he could repay the sum immediately. This was a widespread practice, and a number of such agreements are found in the local notarial archives in the Republic. To mention a few examples: Evert de Leegh, master surgeon, borrowed from Maria van Snellenberg some 600 Dutch guilders before sailing for which he pledged his Company salary.[205] Jacobus van Buren (not a Company surgeon but a Company's steward), borrowed some 300 Dutch guilders from the widow Cornelia van Outhoorn under the same conditions.[206] On his last voyage, on which he died in 1762, Anthonij Werick, first surgeon to the Company, took along not only five chests of wine; three chests of Dutch gin; 48 smoked tongues; 36 hats; 58 pieces of smoked meat; 69 hams and 124 cheeses; but he was also the bearer of a piece of paper addressed to surgeon Van Nier at the Cape asking Van Nier to declare he had received 400 rixdollars (each of 40 five-cent pieces), which were minted in the Republic (*uitgaande penningen*).[207]

Sometimes it is clear that Kruijs was operating on a commission, for instance, for surgeon L.D. Kreps, who worked in Batavia as the warden and surgeon of the *Binnenhospitaal* (see table T6.7: 1,300 guilders for various products in boxes). We find that Kruijs, too, exported beer to Batavia, although it has not been possible to ascertain if this was *Princesse Royal* beer. Besides this, watches, stockings, gauze, clocks, and general household necessities were apparently needed in Asia, and when he returned, his chests were filled with Asian delicacies such as candied fruit (*confijten*) and pickles. To profit substantially from the opportunities offered by the Company, Kruijs borrowed sums of money which he sometimes invested in products and sometimes in bills of exchange.

The German first surgeon, Bernardus Johannes Engelbert (Lingen ? – Batavia 1788), perhaps tops them all, although his career at the Company started modestly enough:

Table T6.8: The career of Bernardus Johannes Engelbert

Departure Republic	*Rank*	*Monthly salary*	*Return Republic*
05 June 1769	Third surgeon	14.00	07 July 1771
22 August 1771	Surgeon's mate	22.00	26 June 1773
14 Dec. 1773	First surgeon	36.00	3 August 1775
11 May 1776	First surgeon	40.00	25 May 1778
06 Jan. 1779	First surgeon	45.00	11 June 1780
05 Dec. 1780	First surgeon	50.00	23 July 1784
12 Dec. 1784	First surgeon	50.00	Free burgher Batavia on 8 Nov. 1785, dying there on 2 Jan. 1788

His sixth voyage for the Company was a risky one, because the Fourth Anglo-Dutch War had just broken out. The vessel on which he was employed, the *Held Woltemade*, was bound for Ceylon. On 1 July 1781, it was captured off the Cape of Good Hope by two English frigates under the command of Commodore Johnstone, and the *Held Woltemade* was forced to sail to Plymouth. In Plymouth, the crew and contents of the vessel were listed. The English clerk needed seven quarto-pages to list all of Engelbert's commodities, which were noted as 'purchased at Amsterdam and were on board said ship at the time of capture and seizure thereof as his own private adventure consisting as undermentioned'. They comprised the following: 12 pear-shaped drop-earrings set with a total of 642 rose diamonds; hairpins; rings and bracelets set with 501 rose diamonds; gold thread and silver thread weighing 25 pounds; 120 yards of gold-flowered lace; 442 yards of gold and silver satin and lace; 36 golden and silver pairs of buttons; 194 dozen looking-glasses; 96 gilt-edged books; two table clocks; some 500 rolls of tobacco; fine glassware; bolts of velvet; dozens of knives, forks and spoons; cruets in ivory, enamel and silver; chocolate; butter; circa 5,000 bottles of red wine. The total value amounted to 31,400 Dutch guilders, a sum on which, in those days, one could possibly retire on and spend the rest of one's life as a 'gentleman of leisure'.[208]

Clearly, Engelbert's goods had been purchased for purposes of commerce, but he had either had to take out loans to buy them, or fork up the cash out of his own pocket. As any loan would have required some collateral, one thing that Engelbert was not was poor.

Meanwhile, although surgeon Marcus Ulman may not be accused of private trading, he may have been a trifle foppish because never was there a seafaring surgeon with such a wardrobe. He possessed seven waistcoats of black velvet, red velvet, blue silk, yellow silk, and three in cotton. Furthermore, he had nine white shirts without frills compensated by 17 shirts with frills. Moreover, he possessed black velvet breeches, black satin breeches and black sayette breeches, and 13 pairs of stockings: black silk, white, clocked, black sayette, among others. His chests were filled to the brim with ribbons and bows, whilst two mirrors would have allowed him to inspect the allure of his toilette. For his leisure time, he also possessed an old damast dressing gown and camisole.[209]

Concluding observations

When we once again examine the question of whether a ship's surgeon in the Company could be and was financially successful, we cannot but conclude that he could and that he occasionally was. Any expectations he might have fostered before sailing were therefore justified. The data in the Batavian Deeds, as well as those of the inventories, reveal this in glaring detail. Martinus Troeff and Johan Schopper, for example, were both able to bestow a very substantial amount of money on their heirs. In general, however, the fortunes made by the Company's surgeons were modest. Table T6.4 showed that 42 per cent of the ship's surgeons in Asia were able to leave their offspring a legal amount of between 100 and 1,000 *rijksdaalders*.

As no comparison could be made between surgeons with the Company and those surgeons practising in the Republic (the data concerning the master surgeons practising in Amsterdam offering only an indication), one is inclined to think that, however modest their fortunes were, their way of life, with slaves and all, was not unsuccessful, at least from a financial point of view. The ship's surgeons were not burdened by investment costs for a surgical shop, for instance, which they would have needed in Europe. Only one-fifth of the surgeons recorded in the Batavian Deeds declared that their estate was worth less than 2,000 *rijksdaalders*, leaving us to wonder whether four-fifths of the surgeons who appear in the Batavian Deeds' indeed had a more substantial estate. Jacob Berger and Fredrick Kruijs, for instance, are examples of the active and successful surgeon-traders. Why did not all of the surgeons succeed in this area, which would lead, if not to fame, then certainly to riches?

There were a number of conditions that limited the surgeons' financial opportunities-. First they had to survive for a certain length of time in order to be able to explore their material possibilities. This might mean taking some voyages to and from Asia, like Frederick Kruijs did. Or, like others, spend some time in a settlement in Asia. As shown in chapter 5, only one-third of the ship's surgeons in the sample were still alive three years after their first departure. On average, they needed an acquaintanceship with Asia of more than a decade before they could engage a notary to draw up their wills and, basically, it were 'surgeons of means' who did so. However, a decade after the surgeons' first voyages, their number had depleted to some 15 per cent. If they proved to be resilient enough to deal with the diseases they encountered, the most important hurdle had been successfully leapt.

Physical health and vigour alone were not enough. A quick eye and mind, eager to engage in new opportunities, was also a requirement. Dr Gelman Taylor's main condition for the beginning of a successful career in Asia (or rather in Batavia) was marriage to an influential Asian-born woman. She (the Asian lady) and her connections would then see to it that her husband was pointed in the right direction towards fulfilling his goals, usually involving employment in the Company's administrative department. If we grant that a surgeon was *a priori* not in the right profession when it comes to government functions in Batavia and/or Asia, he was also certainly not part of the general mass of anonymous seafarers employed by the Company. It is obvious that the ambitious surgeon would have been wise to follow the advice of Dr Gelman-Taylor, had he only known it.

It would seem that most of them chose not to follow this trajectory. As has already been shown, they tended to marry 'into the profession', or rather into their own network of friends. If Berger had not died in April 1752, besides receiving 21 barrels of *Princesse Royal* beer, he would have married a daughter of a rich shipowner (*groot reders dochter*), to whom his brother Marten, also a surgeon[210] in Dokkum (Friesland) had already betrothed him. However, to marry her, he would have had to have returned. When surgeons married, which not many of them had the chance to do, they did so mainly in Europe. Most of them never got married, perhaps the main reason being that they died at such an early age and that there was no need to marry. It was quite possible to maintain a relationship in Asia without the blessings of either one's employer or the Church. Even the fact that children were begotten as a result of these friendships did not always convince the fathers to marry the mothers, as the legal system made it possible to provide for these children and their mothers upon the demise of the fathers, on the condition that there was sufficient capital.

If they failed to profit from an Advantageous Marriage, they could and did profit from Trade, as long as the first condition (surviving long enough) was fulfilled. Sometimes they sold their permitted space on board (in the form of chests); sometimes they participated more directly and engaged in trade themselves: silver coins and household necessities were shipped to Asia, bills of exchange and textiles to the Republic. Of course, the ship's surgeons were not the only ones, from steward to captain, the vessel was literally filled with a crew of 'merchants', something the Company could do very little about. The ships' surgeons, like their fellow-seafarers, used every opportunity as well as every friendship to enhance their incomes, from which everyone profited, probably the Company as well.

Conclusion: The surgeon's legacy

We have come to the conclusion of our surgeon's tale, or, more particularly, our ship surgeon's tale. We have traced his professional origins and found them to be rooted in the Middle Ages, when the emerging universities in Europe began to separate surgery from medicine. The foundation of the universities was closely linked to the rediscovery of texts from Antiquity, and the sort of medicine taught by the medical faculties was very much influenced by Hippocrates, Aristotle, and Galen. Consequently, the university-schooled physicians learned to argue and debate logically, and diagnosed the (internal) diseases of mankind according to Galen's system. The empirically-trained barber surgeons found themselves authorised – besides shaving beards – to set bones, to extract teeth, and to treat people's skin. The physicians' prescriptions usually consisted of dietary measures through which the humoral balance of man, according to his age, sex, and environment, should be re-established. The use of other therapies, such as bloodletting, purging, or clystering, increasingly fell within the professional scope of the barber surgeons.

During the late Middle Ages, the barber surgeons organised themselves into guilds to protect their craft, to regulate competition, and to maintain the standards of quality of their work. These guilds became institutionalised bodies and were granted certain rights by the municipal authorities. Within the guilds, the barber surgeons slowly raised the standards of their surgery by setting ever stricter and higher criteria for the obtaining of a master's certificate. First, they separated barbering from surgery. The shaving of beards and the letting of blood became only a preliminary step towards the full mastery of surgery. To obtain the latter, theoretical knowledge based on Guy de Chauliac's *Chirurgia Magna*, Vesalius' *De humani*, and Paracelcus' *Wundartzeney* became obligatory reading. From what had first been merely the sharpening of pieces of iron into lancets and the probing of the lancets into the veins, the surgeon-master's examination in the larger cities of northwestern Europe of the eighteenth century had expanded to include extirpation, trepanation, the treatment of contusions, bandaging, and a theoretical examination on anatomy and the *materia chirurgica*.

This was certainly true in the Dutch Republic where an interested trainee surgeon could receive an excellent surgical education, although this tended to be concentrated in cities such as Amsterdam and Middelburg. Indeed, surgical guilds were only found in the cities of the Republic. The villages, the countryside, and even some of the smaller cities did not have 'structured' medical/surgical provisions, which could offer surgical training. In the larger surgical centres, bandaging lessons in the local *gasthuizen* were obligatory, as well as the sessions on the composition of ointments and identifying herbs in botanical gardens, the lectures given by the *praelectores*, and witnessing the dissection of corpses. Surgical catechisms were written for apprentices, in which the views of contemporary anatomical literature were included. Some medical faculties offered special education to surgeons as physicians and surgeons grew more interested in each other's discipline. In the eighteenth century, this meant that it could take ten to 12 years of surgical training before a candidate passed his master's examination, a trajectory which used to take only five to seven years.

By that time the European maritime world had witnessed several interesting developments. For instance, the voyages of discovery of the fifteenth century and the consequent development of world trade had a tremendous impact on the various participants in these commercial voyages. Europeans suddenly encountered completely different disease environments, of which they had had no previous experience and to which they had no immunity or resistance. By fits and starts, the profession of the ship's surgeon came into being, but it was only with the emergence of the Dutch and English trading empires that this function emerged into the full light of day. Each vessel sailing under the flag of the Dutch or the English East India Company employed surgeons for the benefit of the entire ship's company; these surgeons did not restrict their skills to the physical care of one or two important officials as had been the early Spanish custom. They did not serve the church, the viceroy or the captain, which had been the practice in the early Hispano-Portuguese maritime-medical experience. What had commenced as a vague sense of responsibility towards the members of a crew as expressed in the medieval Oléron Rolls would now grow into a full-fledged maritime medical service, under the specific auspices of the Dutch East India Company.

This maritime medical service was mainly staffed by ship's surgeons. They were needed on board and in the settlements of the Cape of Good Hope and those in Asia. These surgeons have been the main subject of this book. From the very beginning of their existence, they received an extraordinary amount of bad press. The charges laid at their door, such as incompetence, opportunism, ignorance, being 'half-grown stunted apprentices' or mere village barbers, have been examined to see if these approached the truth in any way when applied to the Company's surgeons. In order to do this, nearly 3,000 surgeons from the financial records of the Company were sampled. As far as was possible, we traced their geographical origins; we tracked down their birthdates; we investigated their motives for enlisting with the Company; we examined their surgical education; followed their careers; sought their extra-curricular activities; we calculated their life expectancies; and we described the contents of their last wills. To give greater depth, the background against which the Company surgeon worked, namely the medical health service as provided by the Dutch East India Company, was analysed. As a result of the material extant in the archives, the surgeons sampled were nearly all eighteenth-century men. They constitute between one-quarter and one-third of the total number that the Company employed during its entire existence of nearly 200 years.

Besides providing ship's surgeons on its vessels and settlements, the Company also developed a highly organized medical department and system. Right from the start, the Company directors sought counsel concerning the contents of the medical chests needed on board. Each chamber sought local advice among the various apothecaries in the cities where that particular chamber was located. Later, the Amsterdam Chamber employed a pharmacist on a full-time basis for preparing the medical chests needed on board, as well as for dispensing the medicines needed in Asia. The Amsterdam and Zeeland Chambers each recruited a physician, who, in collaboration with the pharmacist, standardised the list of medicines for use on board and in Asia. Keeping pace with the growth of knowledge, the Company regularly updated the contents of the medical chests; these were constantly adjusted and tested against the prevailing 'pharmaceutical' theories. Advice on medicines given by the medical faculty of Leiden University (Boerhaave!) in 1737 was valued. Under these circumstances, the ship's surgeon was provided with the most 'modern' medicines. The fact that these medicines did not cure the diseases most prevalent in the tropics nor those that were contracted in the overcrowded environment on board is not relevant to this context.

As early as 1618, the Company drew up a scale of compensation for disabilities sustained during Company service. This in itself was quite extraordinary because the Company was not obliged to do so. The uniqueness of all this also holds true for the other services the Company provided for the health care of its employees. With the exception of the Oléron Rolls, there was no historical precedent that could have served as a blueprint for the directors of the Company and no comparable development was found in other East Indian companies during the seventeenth century.

The Company stocked surgical instruments at both the chambers and the settlements. In Asia, the *Medicinale Winkel* functioned as the central entrepôt for medicines and surgical instruments. These instruments could be borrowed by the ship's surgeons. The Company chambers also examined the prospective ship's surgeons on their knowledge. In Amsterdam and Middelburg the chamber's own medical department took care of this examination; while the smaller chambers outsourced this duty to the proper authorities in the cities.

In 1695, spurred to action by the prevalence of diseases and the high mortality rates on the outward-bound vessels in the years 1690-1695, the Company laid down specific regulations concerning the duties of the ship's surgeons. These regulations do not differ much from what might have been expected from a surgeon of those times: Visit patients and treat them. What does stand out in contrast to those surgeons employed by other maritime employers is the fact that the Company surgeon was never obliged to provide any shaving services during his tenure; he, a surgeon of the Dutch East India Company, was employed solely to treat ill or injured Company employees. This was a sign of great progress because the formulation and regulation of the Company surgical duties may be seen as a step towards greater efficiency and modernisation.

To help the ship's surgeons in Asia, the Company recruited the physician J. Bontius and sent him to Batavia to set up a medical system there. All Company surgeons serving in Asia were subject to the Head of Surgery, of which function Bontius was – as well as being the creator – the first occupant. The Head of Surgery, posted in Batavia, headed the Asian medical/surgical hierarchy.

To accommodate its ill employees, the Company built and staffed hospitals in Asia. These hospitals were meant solely for the benefit of Company employees, and as such, had broken away entirely from the traditional, usually Christian, European multifunctional hospitals (*gasthuizen*). Although high-ranking officials in the employ of the Company were not found among the patients at the City Hospital of Batavia, this Company hospital was never at any time an institution of 'refuse-heap relief', and, more strongly, it had never been intended to function as such. If the ailing Company sailor or soldier was not exactly a highly valued employee, he did have sufficient value to his employer to warrant an efficient health-care service. And despite appearances to the contrary, the patients of the Batavian City Hospital (or any other Company hospital) did benefit from the medical services provided. Away from home, family and friends, the hospital functioned as a medical substitute for the Company employee, which at least, however ineptly, tried to cure him of his ailment.

During its existence, the Council of the Indies in Batavia (the governing body of the Company in Asia) satisfied most of the expectations which might have been entertained regarding a pre-modern institution faced with medical challenges, which, in the final analysis, could not always be successfully met. Everything possible was done to cure the indisposed Company employee. In light of the fact that there was a lack of surgeons in Asia, local people were often trained right on the spot. Because of the high mortality rates in the hospitals, special courses were offered to surgeons and even more hospitals were eventually built. The diseases most prevalent on the overcrowded vessels and in the often crammed Asian hospitals ended up being a significant part of the agendas of the Council of the Indies in Batavia. This body was very much aware of the problems of keeping its employees healthy, without which the pursuit of successful trade was simply impossible. It was directly and permanently involved in all current medical issues, and during the second half of the eighteenth century it included the entire top brass of the Batavian medical/surgical establishment in the decision-making process concerning health care.

During the eighteenth century, however, it was the Gentlemen XVII who were unable to fulfill their obligations towards the running of a profit-oriented company, which is, given the constant decline in the financial viability of the Company itself and the directors confined traditional paradigms perhaps understandable. When in the eighteenth century, the Company empire became so large that it reached from the Cape of Good Hope to Deshima in Japan, it needed to hire thousands of men to maintain the Company's possessions and trade interests in the East. These men had to be shipped to Asia on vessels already manned by a crew and filled with trade-worthy products. It was quite ordinary for 300 men or more to be shipped to Asia on one Company vessel. However, the Republic could not fulfil this demand for men adequately and consequently many foreigners (read Germans) were recruited. Modern historiography teaches us that these new recruits were not used to the ways of the sea and that their health was often not so robust. The upshot was the infection and contamination of the fewer and fewer healthy sailors on board.

Overcrowding was certainly one of the complicating factors of the eighteenth century. This automatically meant that conditions on board were less hygienic. The structural poor health of many of the seafarers, although unproven, may have been another one. If blame has to be meted out, it has to be said that, as far as the Gentlemen XVII are concerned, preventive measures which could have been taken and which would have made a difference to the high mortality rates on the outward-bound vessels, such as those suggested by the Company physician De Famars in 1773, were not followed up as they were considered to be too expensive. The medical examination of the prospective crews prior to embarkation, the delousing of these crews, and the providing of new clothes, all of these recommendations were deemed not feasible given the budgetary limitations even though had they been put into practice the mortality rates might have been significantly reduced. This lack of constructive action was exacerbated by the high demand for employees needed in Asia, as a result of which the Company could not afford to be too selective in their employment of any willing candidate. Eighteenth-century recruitment became a 'Catch 22' situation, where increasingly potentially less-than healthy crews were almost certainly crammed onto the Company vessels and they, in their turn, infected their colleagues on board. The inevitable consequence was the steady draining of the resilience of the Company's economic strength. This, indeed, was a serious flaw in the Company's recruitment practices, which should not be underestimated as the consequences were disastrous to the employer and fatal to many an employee.

How did this all affect the Company surgeon? No less than one-third of the surgeons sampled died within five years of their having taken Company employment. Of this one-third, the surgeons had a five-year life expectancy only in the first half of that century; this detoriated to three years in the second half of the century. Turning to the entire sample (of 2,988 surgeons), at the beginning of the eighteenth century the surgeon had a 50 per cent chance of surviving ten years of tenureship; at the end of the century, this 50 per cent chance was also reduced to three years. Those surgeons who were more resilient and who were able to make several voyages could look forward to reaching the age of 38 in the first half of the century; after 1750, this 'fine old age' dropped to 33 years. Those who remained permanently in a settlement in Asia reached the average age of 27 years, all of whom fell dramatically short of the ages they might have been expected to reach in Europe. There, one could at least look forward to almost reaching the age of 50 had he or she, as the Company surgeon had done, not died in infancy. In short, most of the ship's surgeons died fairly early on in their employment with the Company. One shudders to think of the life expectancy of most of the other seafarers on board, which must have been at least the same, if not worse.

In view of these figures, it is an extraordinary fact that there were still surgeons willing to enlist with the Company. As we saw in chapters 4, 5, and 6, there were a few conspicuous motives for the ship's surgeon to choose the Company as his employer. One of them was simply to earn a living in a profession, the choice of which had often enough been determined by tradition as his father, uncle, and/or grandfather had probably practised the same profession and/or had worked for the same employer. Most ship's surgeons were raised in the (petty) bourgeoise households. Their families were respectable and neither wealthy nor poor. As such, the sons were encouraged to learn a profession for which the training required some (relatively small) investment to be made by the parents when the child started his training around his 14th year. The networks of their families offered the prospective surgeons some degree of influence in the cities where they sought employment. This facilitated their chances of finding work. After all, when all is said and done, the function of a Company's ship's surgeon was not one for which all candidates who presented themselves were accepted. The candidate Company surgeon needed to show his certificates and his letters of introduction; he was examined on his abilities before being offered employment; and let us not forget that there were more candidates than vacancies.

The Company could offer an ambitious surgeon a career and financial gain, but these opportunities were found mostly in Asia. As we saw in chapter 3, the hospitals in Asia were not run as charities but were managed by the members of the Company's trading *elite*, usually in close collaboration with the medical/surgical *elite*. As a surgeon, to be given the function of warden or trustee of the City Hospital in Batavia was tantamount to being accepted into the Batavian elite. The management of these hospitals meant in itself that the Company hospitals were more 'modern' (than European hospitals) in the sense of efficiency for both staff and patients, since additional motives such as charity were eliminated. Consequently, these hospitals focused mainly on curing the patient and offered a wider range of medical practices to its staff. There were more opportunities for a surgeon to climb the career ladder (which was also related to the high turnover of personnel), as well as more social status for the hospital staff. To be employed as a surgeon in a Company hospital meant one could rise to the rank of *praktizijn* (medical practitioner), a formal recognition that the Company surgeon worked on a level equal to that of the physician. This official recognition was only accorded in 1752, but the title had already become common parlance by the end of the seventeenth century. Similar attempts by the surgeons in the Dutch Republic, as seen, for instance, by those employees who worked on the hospital ship that lay anchored between Den Helder and Texel, and who began using the title practitioner in the 1770s, were was very much frowned upon and in the Republic any such claim was generally seen as uppishness of a 'mere' surgeon.

There were other opportunities for a surgeon to improve his status which he, however, did not choose to act upon. The Company surgeon rose mostly on his own merits and not, as was common practice in Batavia, by marriage. He tended to marry within the profession; surgeon's widows were favourite.

Yet another motive was the advancement of the surgeon's own education. Many apprentices seized the opportunity to fulfil their journeymanship with the Company in order to prepare for their master's examination, although many died along the way before they ever reached this final step. As there were more candidates than surgical vacancies, many a ship's surgeon ended up employed in a lesser rank than his stature and education would have entitled him to. The Company could take its pick of surgical employees: apprentices in the possession of the *leerbrief* usually found themselves employed as third surgeons (*derde meester*) even though they could already boast of some six years acquaintance with their profession, while the surgeon's mates in general had enjoyed a surgical training period of nine years, and a first surgeon had some 13 years surgical experience before being hired on as such by the Company. This senior surgeon had by then reached the age of 30 years. This clearly demonstrates that the surgeons' contemporaries lived under the misunderstanding that there were no experienced and qualified surgeons to be found. This dearth had resulted in the employing younger and less-experienced surgeons, which consequently led to higher mortality rates, both on board and in Asia. In fact, this notion is completely groundless, as the practice was non-existent, which is so overwhelmingly shown by the Amsterdam and Enkhuizen recruitment practices and further substantiated by the data in table T5.5. In general, any shortage of surgeons was only experienced in the early eighteenth century.

Moreover, a voyage or two for the Company offered the surgeon a unique experience not found in Europe, professionally speaking, which in terms of investment money and medical/surgical knowledge could set him up for life. A significant number of surgeons (at least 12 per cent of the sample) must have seen the Company's tenureship as such. They had gone on their one unique voyage before returning to Europe. Some of them then disappeared to enjoy the rustic delights of a country practice; others took their master's examination and set up a practice in town, enriched by their experiences and adventures.

There was also the chance to make a fortune, and it appears that many of them did participate in the forbidden activity of private trading. The networks which had helped them to find a position on the Company payroll, also assisted them to pursue their commercial ventures; they took along many products to trade in Asia and brought many Asian commodities back to the Republic. However, making a successful trading career alongwith one's surgical profession was the fate of only a happy few, as most of them died long before it came to pass. As shown in chapter 6, the successful surgeon-trader needed to be acquainted with Asia for at least ten years' before he knew enough about the trading ins and outs to amass some capital to bequeath. By then, very few of these surgeons were still alive.

The analysis of the employment motives of the Company surgeons cogently established that these were strongly linked to urbanisation, population growth, and economic prosperity. The Company surgeon came from an urban environment (where surgical guilds existed), whether in the Dutch Republic or in other countries. The Company recruitment areas of Dutch surgeons were mostly the densely populated coastal province of Holland (where five of the six chambers of the Company were located), the cities of the eastern region (Gelderland and Overijssel), and those of the coastal province of Zeeland (mainly Middelburg). The northern (Drenthe, Friesland, Groningen), southern (States Brabant and Limburg) and central (Utrecht) regions were insignificant as recruitment areas.

At first sight, this recruitment pattern seems to have been a more or less normal practice as far as the coastal provinces were concerned. It is a pattern that we can see in the other groups of seafarers in the Company as well. After all, the traditional view of Company recruitment is that the easterly provinces and countries gradually became more significant as recruitment areas at the expense of the recruitment in the coastal provinces of Holland and Zeeland. The intense recruitment of ship's surgeons from Gelderland and Overijssel in the period 1700-1750 was more promising precisely because these landlocked provinces had little direct connection with life and work at sea. That it faded away after 1750 is even more interesting in its deviation from the traditional pattern, which would have led us to assume that the easterly provinces would have become *more* significant as recruitment areas in the course of the eighteenth century.

If we dig even deeper into the analysis of surgical recruitment, it reveals that the de-urbanisation of the Dutch Republic was glaringly obvious in the Company's recruitment of Dutch surgeons. Between 1680 and 1750, the industrial cities of Holland (Delft, Haarlem, Leiden) experienced major population shrinkage, to which we may safely attribute the sharp fall in Dutch surgeons recruited from these cities, which probably set in after 1725, if not earlier. Although population growth returned to some agrarian areas of the Republic after 1750, the major cities (except for Amsterdam and Rotterdam) declined even further. The Company's Dutch surgical recruitment efforts enjoyed a period of stabilisation after 1750, and some areas even showed a slow (although insufficient) recovery, although the provinces of Gelderland, Overijssel, and Zeeland disappeared completely as recruitment areas. The recovery of the recruitment from the province of Holland was mainly attributable to the Chamber cities of Amsterdam (from 40 per cent to 70 per cent) and Rotterdam (from 28 per cent to 44 per cent), which grew in significance after 1750 as suppliers of surgeons to the Company. The other cities of this province, certainly in the northern part of Holland became even more depopulated; consequently, Dutch surgical recruitment from those cities continued to decline. The geographical concentration of surgeons recruited became more and more dependent on those born (in the vicinity of) in Amsterdam and Rotterdam at the expense of the smaller Chamber cities of Hoorn, Enkhuizen, and Delft. For those Chambers, the recruitment grew more geographically diverse. The Enkhuizen Chamber in particular lost its appeal to native-bred surgeons (from 32 per cent to 6 per cent).

The Chamber city of Rotterdam in the southern part of Holland demonstrates the significance of economic and population growth. After 1750, the Rotterdam Chamber gradually attracted more Rotterdam-born ship's surgeons, a process which went hand in hand with the economic prosperity of that area and the emergence of the city of Rotterdam as a major recruitment city. The cities of the eastern area (Gelderland and Overijssel) were fairly well represented in the first half of the century, when that area enjoyed economic prosperity and population growth. After 1750, this growth declined, and consequently the participation of surgeons from this area in the Company's surgical labour market diminished as well. The peculiarity of the other maritime province, namely that of Zeeland, where the Middelburg Chamber was located, is that surgeons from this province all but disappeared after the 1760's which is completely inexplicable. Admittedly, Zeeland was never a recruitment city like Amsterdam or Rotterdam, but this in itself is not a sufficient explanation. The prosperity of Zeeland did not decline as of 1760 either; in fact, for years this province had been suffering from a long-term depression both economically and in terms of population growth. The surgical guild of Middelburg did not disappear in 1760. The reason why Zeeland's surgeons lost interest in employment with the Company at that particular time must, for the moment, be left unresolved.

There is every indication that the same factors were at work for the non-Dutch surgeons that drove these surgeons into the arms of the Company. They came from urban backgrounds; the economic prosperity of their native areas influenced their decisions to work for the Company; and their employment by the Company was motivated by professional interest and financial opportunities. Most non-Dutch surgeons were German. Scandinavia, the Austrian Netherlands (Belgium), and France were insignificant as recruitment areas. In 1731, when the Prussian King Frederick William I passed the Trade Edict, in Germany, stricter criteria were also established for the surgical examinations, which may have had an influence on the German *Wanderburschen* to seek employment with the Company.

During the first half of the eighteenth century, the German ship's surgeons mainly hailed from the traditional labour migration areas of Westphalia and the coastal region of Lower Saxony. After 1750, this coastal region followed the example set by the provinces of Gelderland and Overijssel and disappeared as a Company surgical recruitment area. This was not true for the city of Hamburg, which enjoyed a thriving economy and explosive population growth. The decline in number of Hamburg's surgeons applying for employment with the Company coincided with the economic depression that afflicted the city at the end of the Seven Years' War (1756-1763). During the second half of the eighteenth century, the region of Westphalia remained a strong surgical recruitment area, while those of Saxony, Saxony-Anhalt and Thuringia emerged. Surgical recruitment then shows a broad belt that sweeps across from the province of Holland (particularly Amsterdam and Rotterdam) and penetrates deep into Germany, and sometimes even into Russia.

The scope of the research does not extend to an in-depth study of these (East) German regions. Consequently, one can only postulate the motives why the German recruitment patterns changed. Was the interactive relationship beween demography and economy as seen in the Republic and in western Germany also valid for these eastern German states? Or, was it because these eastern German states did not enjoy the same economic and political developments as the western part and thus remained rather impoverished and largely feudal, that this relationship became reversed? In other words, does the historiographical idea of poor, illiterate, even desperate individuals seeking employment with the Company, really hold true for these particularly underdeveloped areas of the disintegrating Holy Roman Empire?

To recapitulate, this study provides a contrast to the prevailing besmirched image of the ship's surgeon because what we discover is that he was not an illiterate barber but had undergone a formal and lengthy training within the guild system; he did not come from the lowest strata of society but came from an educated and a respected family; he was interested in his craft and considered a professional career and professional experience important. He did not originate from the countryside but had an urban background, and, as far as he was Dutch, he came mostly from the province of Holland. In theory, the Company could fulfil the dreams of many an apprentice. By being employed as a ship's surgeon, he gained far more professional experience than he would have ashore in Europe in his master's shop, and, at the same time, he enjoyed many financial opportunities for private trading, which certainly must have played a role, since the surgeon, as a rule did participate in trade transactions. On the other hand, his life expectancy while employed by the Company was not particularly encouraging. In fact, his life was at stake the moment he set foot on board.

Medical reality on board and in the settlements in the tropics confronted the ship's surgeon with a reality that was completely different from what he had learnt to expect on the basis of his traditional conditioning in the guild. Was he not supposed to wield the knife and lancet, the saw and tongs, to exercise the curative *artisanat* as he had done in former ages? His empirical education had essentially remained the same for centuries. If it had changed at all, it was in the sense that it had become more gruelling and difficult as a result of stricter criteria set by his guild and by the medical discoveries of the fifteenth and sixteenth centuries. The tasks for which he was trained were still basically to set bones, to extract teeth and treat the skin. But besides wounds, fractures, abscesses of all sorts, limb amputation and teeth extraction, the ship's surgeon was suddenly faced with fevers of all sorts, gastro-intestinal disorders, deficiency diseases, malaria, leprosy, and a host of other infectious diseases; in short, he faced a systemic rather than a more localised pathology. From South Africa to the island of Deshima in Japan, the Company surgeon must have initially been bewildered by what he encountered professionally; he was not trained to cure internal diseases, moreover, most of those he encountered were unknown to Europeans. The surgeon thus used trial and error, learned how to cope with these challenges and his empirical training must have come in handy here. Indeed, empirical surgical training was probably more valuable than any academic education. While this may have been so, the ship's surgeon continued to often treat his patients using old Galenic therapies because neither surgeon nor physician could escape the Galenic brainwashing they encountered, despite the heavy criticism Galenism already had in Europe. The dogma of *saignare, purgare et clisterium donare* was embedded deep down in the collective memory of northwestern Europe, and most of the ship's surgeon's prescriptions ran along these lines.

In the absence of the medical breakthroughs which finally occurred in the nineteenth century, when cellular pathology replaced humoral pathology, most of the diseases the Company surgeon dealt with remained *a priori* incurable. That is the material point in the conceptualisation of the Company surgeon in the seventeenth and eighteenth centuries. As he, unwittingly, laboured under various medical misapprehensions, the results of these cannot but have influenced his reputation. It was particularly in the eighteenth century when the overcrowded Company fleets were occasionally severely infected by raging diseases, sometimes to such an extent that the fleets could not even set sail, that criticism of the ship's surgeons and their skills became commonplace and can only be explained by the sociological need of people to have a scape-goat on whom to put the blame.

The Company's medical system was unavoidably constrained by the lack of modern medical knowledge and its inability (or unwillingness) to provide a sufficient level of funding which meant that this service was unable to cope with the problems with which it was confronted. Although the Company was a major power with a standing army and territorial possessions far larger than those of the country which gave it birth, by the end of the eighteenth century, it was also a trading company of quite shaky solvency which made investments in its health-care system a rather scarce commodity. Nevertheless, the Company's health-care services were truly 'revolutionary' in the sense that it was set up to *cure*. Alas, this revolutionary seventeenth-century development, could not cope with the altered physical circumstances of the eighteenth century, as expressed in the mass migration of vulnerable crews from Europe to a Batavia stricken by epidemics. It is really a shame that, next to his patients, the schooled and experienced ship's surgeon of the Company drew the short straw of it all.

Appendices

Appendix 1. Methods, statistical account, graphs and tables pertaining to chapters 4-6

The sample (S)

A host of questions confront the historian who ponders the possibilities by which to characterise the Company ship's surgeons as a (social and professional) group. Delineation of such a group requires the detection of elements shared by the majority of the group's members. Before launching such an exploration of the possibilities, it is essential to question whether the promise of homogeneity of that group is *a priori* a plausible one. It is very possible that a multiplicity of individual chance events ultimately generated the growth of a heterogeneous surgically skilled labour force. Such an analysis may be the equivalent of an attempt to detect a common denominator within a group of, say, today's Army physicians. However it is viewed, history is the ultimate outcome of the interactive behaviour of the constituent elementary particles of society, namely the human individuals.

The analysis presented in chapters 4, 5, and 6 was beset by a number of pitfalls. The surgeon, upon signing his five-year contract with the Dutch East India Company, had his first name and surname as well as his rank on board and his place of geographic origin recorded in the ship's financial administrative records (*scheepssoldijboek*). This was the policy and the routine for everyone else on board as well. This is precisely where the researcher encounters his or her first problems: the surgeon might correctly state his birthplace in reply to the question 'Where do you come from?' (instead of 'Where were you born?'), but he might as well state the most recent place he had lived, either abroad or in the Republic, or he may have lied about his place of origin. For example, the ship's surgeon Cornelis Mouthaan offered his services at the Amsterdam Chamber of the Company, where he told the clerks that he came from Haarlem. However, the surgeon's guild archives of Haarlem revealed that, although he did learn his craft in Haarlem, he was born in Medemblik. Arnoldus de Reus, who sailed for the Enkhuizer Chamber, told the clerks that he came from Enkhuizen, but the next time he said he was from Dunkirk. Jan Brusekom told the Company's clerk that he came from Meppel in Drenthe; however, when he came to work for the Middelburgsche Commercie Compagnie, he stated that he was from Lingen in Germany. In all probability, Jan Brusekom came from Meppen – not Meppel – a place not far from Lingen, and if so, Jan Brusekom was part of the travelling tradition of migrant workers from Lower Saxony who arrived in the Republic via Lingen. The only way to verify the statements with respect to the surgeons' geographical origin was to go to the various municipal archives to check the baptismal registers.

To complicate matters further, the Chamber's clerk, who recorded the data, perhaps sometimes did not understand what was said (i.e., Meppe*l*-Meppe*n*) because the name or place was unknown to the clerk, or did not know how to spell it (there was no standardised spelling at the time), or he was unfamiliar with the surgeon's dialect or language. The clerk then might simply have written down what he thought he heard, or, to simplify matters, dream up some place or make a wild guess to get things over with. But this is not the end of the acrobatics: the clerk's handwriting could well fall shy of legibility, taxing the researcher's eyes, imagination, and patience in the efforts to verify all the possible variants of the place's name in geographic dictionaries two to three centuries later. More often than one would expect, the place named turns out to appear numerous times on a map of the country of origin (e.g. the Company surgeon Johan David Saltsman came from Ostheim but there are seven places named Ostheim in Germany) as well as in several countries, or the name as stated simply does not appear in eighteenth-century atlases and dictionaires, or the surgeon came from a small village near a large city and simply used the city's name instead. In this context, research of the 134 listed 'Delft' surgeons showed that the recorded place 'Delft' was indeed the place of birth for 75 per cent (101 dates of baptismals have been found in the Delft archive) of the surgeons. However, for Leeuwarden only 24 per cent actually appear in the baptismal registers. The province of Friesland is extremely difficult to research for primary data prior to 1811, as family names were rarely mentioned in the registers because children took the patronym as their surname. The *Naamsaanneming* (1811) was introduced during the Napoleonic period, in which it became obligatory to have a surname. In addition, over 5 per cent of the names analysed, the one and same surgeon's name was recorded repeatedly in many variants by various clerks. Moreover, the clerks at the different chambers did not work consistently. The Rotterdam Chamber's clerks were the most accurate; their recorded birthplaces proved to be correct most often, whereas the clerks of the chambers of Hoorn and Enkhuizen were the most sloppy.

At the Amsterdam Chamber, where nearly 1,000 names of ship's surgeons were extracted, one finds many German sounding names among them but listed as being from Amsterdam which, of course, was a 'pull area', and attracted many of the surgeons at the time. In all cities, the turnover among urban dwellers was high. Many migrant apprentices and rural-born servants came for a temporary period of time, and people also passed through smaller towns to arrive in the larger ones.[1] Cities in the pre-modern period could not grow without migration. Although one is inclined to disbelieve *a priori* the recorded places of origin noted by the Amsterdam Chamber clerks, research at the baptismal registers of Amsterdam for the period 1760-1795 showed that most of them (78 per cent: 182 verified of

233 surgeons who stated that they came from Amsterdam, and served as surgeons for the Amsterdam Chamber after 31 December 1769) were indeed born in Amsterdam, as descendants from foreigners who had migrated to Amsterdam. The chamber in Zeeland has its own problems with regards to research as practically no primary records (baptismal registers) are available to research. And those that survived, for instance the birth registers of Vlissingen, yielded 0 per cent results. It was impossible to trace the 'Vlissingen' surgeons in the Vlissingen surgeon guild's archives because these archives are non-existent.

Clearly, there are numerous possibilities to hinder the clarification process, which deters researchers from examining their subject. Mostly, research done on the geographic origins of Company employees simply took the recorded place as factually true, and did not check the baptismal registers of local parishes to cross-reference the recorded places of origin. The historian P. Boon encountered the same problems in his research on seventeenth-century seafarers of the Westfrisian area on the Baltic Sea. His thesis showed that more than 50 per cent of the places noted as domiciles by the masters (*schippers*) of Baltic Sea trade were definitely not where they were born or had ever lived.[2] Such hurdles and pitfalls prove to be higher and steeper when the surgeon is a foreigner, as he is as likely as not to be.

The only way to overcome these obstacles is to engage in a process of systematic checking by consulting available sources in order to verify what has been recorded, – most significantly in this context are the baptismal registers and surgeon's guild archives – and to retain a high measure of suspicion. A method was developed to yield, if not fool-proof, then at least fairly reliable results. It started with reading through the ships' financial books. These books ('muster rolls') are the administrative records of the ships in which the names, birthplaces, and ranks of all those on board in the service of the Company are listed, including their wages, the dates from the moment of setting sail, the subsequent course of their service with the Company until their return to the Republic or demise during their contract; sometimes the names of their parents and/or wives were listed as well.

As noted, a financial book existed for each ship that included the entire company on board. These books are preserved in the National Archives in The Hague. The task to make abstracts of every surgeon's data would defy the most intrepid among us, because the Company throughout its existence had in general three surgeons on board each ship which sailed to Asia (ratio ship/surgeons = 1:3) and sent those ships to Asia on some 4,720 voyages during the seventeenth and eighteenth centuries. Sometimes, there was only one surgeon on board if it was a small ship, for instance, a mail ship (*pakket-boot*). In times of war, only two surgeons were sent on board. After 1770, due to the Batavian demand for surgeons, vessels had five to seven surgeons, if that many were found who were willing to be recruited.

Theoretically, assuming that generally three surgeons boarded a Dutch East Indiaman that sailed for Asia (this was common prior to 1770), this would mean that the data of 4,720 ship's financial-books multiplied by three = 14,160 surgeons would have to be recorded and checked. However, as researcher's 'luck' has it, the financial records covering the activities of the seventeenth century are largely lost, leaving the practically complete collection of 2,996 muster books (3,185 voyages to the East were made in the eighteenth century) available for investigation. That is still too many for one lonesome researcher. Because the chambers in Amsterdam and Zeeland had the bulk of these financial books, it was decided to check a 25 per cent sample from these Chambers: of the financial books, which are largely arranged chronologically, every one out of four was used (book 1, 5, 9, etc.) and the names of its surgeons were noted and were entered into a database. For the other chambers, all of the pertinent data were abstracted from all of the available books. This yielded the following table (TA.1):

Table TA.1: Financial books and number of sampled surgeons

Chamber	*Number of Financial books*	*Number of surgeons' first departures in eighteenth century*
Amsterdam (sample) Total of 1,376 books	357	977
Delft (complete)	205	347
Enkhuizen (complete)	206	418
Hoorn (complete)	183	396
Middelburg (sample) Total of 631 books	149	410
Rotterdam (complete)	195	440
Total	1295	2,988 = S

The remaining 75 per cent of the rolls of Middelburg and Amsterdam Chambers were checked for the surgeons who figured in the initial 25 per cent sample to see if these ship's surgeons undertook second or more voyages; if they did, their data were added to those already obtained. This meant that a certain bias did enter the database, namely for those surgeons whose names were found in the financial books prior to their first appearance in the sample. However, by the running of queries it turned out that this bias was so slight that it made no difference to the outcomes of the queries.

The names of the surgeons, constituting the entry to the fully collected material, were cross-checked by a run through the database and in quite a few instances the various spellings of a certain name were reduced to a single standardised spelling, identifying a single surgeon. By this procedure, a total of 2,988 surgeons were obtained (S), of whom 2,176 the recorded place of origin was Dutch (73 per cent); 716 were found to be foreign (24 per cent), and 96 places of origin were illegible or not stated at all and as such unidentifiable (3 per cent). Among the numbers with altogether unidentifiable birthplaces, there must have been many a foreigner. The question of the veracity of the recorded places of birth has to be tackled first because any attempt at correlation with labour streams within and to the Republic would be futile without this ascertained data.

Baptismal records and surgeon's guilds

The next step consisted of a systematic check of the baptismal records and surgeon's guild archives deposited in provincial or municipal archives. This task encountered its own limitations: apart from the rather extensive expense of time in travel and searching, in a number of instances, the registers are unavailable, for instance, in the city of Middelburg where all of them were lost in a fire as well as the archives of Middelburg's surgeons guild. Furthermore, a substantial portion of the baptismal records available are not indexed, a detail that necessitated resisting any attempts that promised to turn out to be too time-consuming.

Personal research has been done in a number of provincial state archives such as Amsterdam (baptismal records and surgeon's guild archives), Haarlem (baptismal records and surgeon's guild archives), Hoorn (baptismal records and surgeon's guild archives, these latter containing virtually no data). This was enhanced by requests for help from amateur and (semi-) professional genealogists; archivists at regional archives; provincial genealogical club centres (Twente, Utrecht); the genealogical database of The Church of Jesus Christ of Latter-day Saints (the Mormons, Salt Lake City); Internet searches of municipal archives (such as Delfshaven, Rotterdam, Delft) and ISIS Gens Data. Moreover, the site *Digitale Bronbewerkingen* by Herman de Wit turned out to be a nearly ideal search engine as it gives weekly updates of the inventory of newly available genealogical and archival sources on the web.[3] Using this approach, any verified 'variable' instances (or discovered birthplaces) were retained and added to the gradually increasing collection of verified variables.

At the moment that I terminated my search, the method described above as applied to the population of 'Dutch ship's surgeons on their first voyage to Asia' (N=2,176) with the specific aim of detecting how many Recorded Places of Birth ('POB.r') agree(d) with the Verified, or correct, Places of Birth ('POB.v') resulted in POB.r = 882 (882 birthplaces of surgeons were checked, 40% of the Dutch ship's surgeons) with POB.v = 776. However, of these 776 found birthplaces, 22 POB.rs (table A.4) were indeed proven to be incorrect (and were corrected) and should be deducted from the POB.vs total, resulting in 754 POB.vs.[4] The implication of the result (being a 'veracity of recording') is then 82%. For the other variables, no attempts at verification were done because their primary records (baptismal) were not easily retrievable for various reasons.

Table AT.2: Verified birthplaces

Chamber	*number surgeons first departure*	*POB.v*
Amsterdam	977; Dutch: 646	196 (30%)
Hoorn	396; Dutch: 272	82 (30%)
Enkhuizen	418; Dutch: 302	51 (17%)
Delft	347; Dutch: 285	173 (61%)
Rotterdam	440; Dutch: 345	204 (59%)
Middelburg	410; Dutch: 326	43 (13%)
Of which non-Dutch or unknown	812	27 (3%)

Can we justifiably extrapolate the correlation factor between POB.r and POB.v (as approximated above on the basis of 754 instances to the remaining 2,176-754= 1,422 variables? One could say that the chances of diminishing correlation for the remaining lot increases *a pari passu* the number of variables with the perfect correlation-factor of 1: if one takes out the good apples from a basket containing a mixed quantity of good and bad apples, the number of bad apples in the basket increases in relation to the quantity remaining in the basket. However, it may be that the other apples are mostly good as well although not always easy to prove. Aldert Strantvliet, for instance, came from Alkmaar. He can be found in the primary records but only with his patronym and not with his family name. Second, there remains a number of variables that have not been researched because the POB.rs defy archival tracing from a cost-benefit point of view. A certain number of these POB.rs are so obscure (little villages) that they are probably correct because neither the recording clerk nor the surgeon making the statement could have dreamt up such obscure POB.rs. This is backed up by the experience of research done for these little villages, which usually tends to correspond with the stated place of origin (100% at the baptismal registers), while the chances are that the POB.rs of cities are more likely to contain 'rotten apples'. The veracity of 82% encourages one to extrapolate the remaining POB.rs as long as one keeps the limitations (brought to light by the research done) in mind.

The database

All of the birthplaces thus collected and checked were entered into a database, enabling one to set up spreadsheets and to carry out other simple statistical analyses (if necessary) in order to establish relationships between places of origin and the Company chamber of service, between places of origin and period of time (in 25-year tables), between places of origin divided into six areas (North-Holland, South-Holland, Zeeland, the northeastern provinces, the eastern provinces, and the south-central provinces) as well as abroad, and the number of surgeons per Chamber and for all of the Chambers together in order to detect factors that determine labour streams. The results are presented in tables.

The non-Dutch surgeons deserve some attention as well. One fundamental factor that should be kept in mind, is namely that the primary data of the material of the non-Dutch ship's surgeons in general have not been checked and are as such not entirely reliable. Collection and verification of biographical details concerning those foreigners would have required an inordinate input of time, travel, energy and money, and accordingly, remains illusory from a cost/benefit point of view.

Because Amsterdam, as centre of activity, remained a focus of attraction of (international) labour throughout the century, labour migration toward its chamber may be expected to show more diversity in biographical detail than the other chambers. Therefore, the Amsterdam Chamber was subjected to a separate analysis where results were compared, as much as possible, with known data notably such as from S. Hart's study on the migration to Amsterdam.[5] According to Hart, people left their own villages and cities mainly for economic reasons. His study is based on the registers of intended (first) marriages between 1578 and 1810. The clerk at the Town Hall or church noted not only the names of the intended partners, but also the places and years of birth. There are two drawbacks to his study, however. The recorded places of birth were not checked in baptismal registers, nor was the immigration from the eastern German countries included.

Table TA.3: Number of surgeons and birthplaces

BOP.r's and BOP.v's of Company surgeons		*Verified birthplaces*
Total number of surgeons	2988	776 (26%)
Dutch	2176	749 (34%)
Non-Dutch	716	27 (3%)
Unknown	96	0 (0%)

The tables and graphics that are presented in chapters 4- 6 are based on the *first journeys* the surgeons made for the Company to the East, in order to avoid duplicates and triplicates (the second or third voyages) or, for that matter, even ten-doubles.

Finally, I have assumed that if there were less than three surgeons on an East Indiaman's outward journey, this meant that not enough surgeons could be found and that a certain amount of tension prevailed in the recruitment areas. Contrariwise, if there were more than three, one may infer an abundance of surgeons who were available to serve on the Company's vessels.

Financial books

Hereunder follow the tables on which the graphs presented in chapter 4 are based. The numbers in the tables are based on the data derived from the following financial books, which are kept in the National Archives in The Hague (NA, VOC collection 1.04.02):

- the Company Chamber of Delft, numbers VOC 13.876 up to and including VOC 14.079;
- the Company Chamber of Rotterdam, numbers VOC 14.102 up to and including 14.296;
- the Company Chamber of Hoorn, numbers VOC 14.348 up to and including 14.527;
- the Company Chamber of Enkhuizen, numbers VOC 14.640 up to and including 14.842.

The sample of the financial books of the Amsterdam-Chamber which range largely from VOC 5470 up to and including 6842 were made up of the following:

VOC 5471, 5474, 5477, 5484, 5485, 5488, 5494, 5498, 5502, 5492, 5493, 5510, 5515, 5517, 5519, 5528, 5534, 5531, 5548, 5543, 5551, 5552, 5555, 5559, 5563, 5564, 5568, 5575, 5580, 5586, 5587, 5591, 5594, 5598, 5609, 5613, 5614, 5618, 5619, 5626, 5627, 5630l, 5637, 5640, 5642, 5647, 5644, 5654, 5656, 5660, 5665, 5672, 5669, 5683, 5679, 5680, 5682, 5697, 5701, 5693, 5706, 5718, 5712, 5714, 5717, 5732, 5726, 5729, 5738, 5742, 5746, 5754, 5756, 5758, 5769, 5772, 5776, 5763, 5767, 5782, 5785, 5794, 5789, 5795, 5799, 5810, 5804, 5806, 5818, 5825, 5828, 5832, 5821, 5842,5846, 5839, 5850, 5852, 5861, 5865, 5867, 5877, 5871, 5873, 5874, 5894, 5911, 5914, 5908, 5926, 5929, 5924, 5925, 5939, 5942, 5938, 5950, 5958, 5961, 5953, 5966, 5970, 5972, 5974, 5981, 5985, 5995, 5990, 5994, 6001, 6005, 6014, 6011, 6017, 6021, 6025, 6029, 6047, 6036, 6039, 6043, 6049, 6053, 6060, 6063, 6066, 6069, 6073, 6077, 6081, 6086, 6085, 6092, 6096, 6100, 6105, 6109, 6113, 6122, 6123, 6125, 6129, 6138, 6134, 6141, 6149, 6151, 6153, 6157, 6164, 6165, 6173, 6170, 6186, 6180, 6183, 6193, 6192, 6197, 6201, 6207, 6206, 6213, 6217, 6220, 6223, 6228, 6232, 6233, 6241, 6245, 6249, 6255, 6257, 6252, 6265, 6272, 6271, 6277, 6281, 6287, 6289, 6292, 6296, 6300, 6304, 6308, 6312, 6316, 6320, 6324,

6328, 6332, 6336, 6339, 6344, 6348, 6350, 6355, 6358, 6366, 6368, 6372, 6379, 6378, 6386, 6392, 6401, 6396, 6400, 6408, 6410, 6416, 6423, 6425, 6428, 6457, 6435, 6443, 6447, 6451, 6458, 6460, 6464, 6468, 6471, 6475, 6487, 6483, 6489, 6492, 6496, 6500, 6507, 6508, 6512, 6516, 6520, 6524, 6528, 6532, 6536, 6540, 6547, 6549, 6552, 6556, 6560, 6565, 6564, 6571, 6576, 6580, 6584, 6588, 6592, 6596, 6600, 6604, 6608, 6612, 6616, 6620, 6628, 6627, 6632, 6636, 6640, 6644, 6648, 6652, 6656, 6660, 6664, 6668, 6672, 6676, 6680, 6684, 6688, 6692, 6696, 6700, 6705, 6708, 6712, 6716, 6720, 6724, 6725, 6728, 6732, 6735, 6740, 6744, 6748, 6752, 6760, 6764, 6768, 6772, 6776, 6780, 6784, 6789, 6792, 6796, 6800, 6804, 6808, 6813, 6818, 6822, 6825, 6826, 6832, 6835, and 6840.

The sample of the financial records of the Company Chamber of Zeeland which range largely from VOC 12.674 up to and including VOC 13.307 consisted of the following financial books:

VOC 12.674, 12.678, 12.681, 12.685, 12.691, 12.688, 12.697, 12.702, 12.705, 12.709, 12.714, 12.720, 12.723, 12.726, 12.735, 12.733, 12.739. 12.743, 12.747, 12.749, 12.755, 12.758, 12.761, 12.767, 12.773, 12.780, 12.781, 12.783, 12.790, 12.789, 12.796, 12.794, 12.803, 12.806, 12.811, 12.815, 12.819, 12.828, 12.824, 12.826, 12.835, 12.839, 12.847, 12.843, 12.851, 12.853, 12.859, 12.862, 12.867, 12.871, 12.875, 12.879, 12.883, 12.887, 12.890, 12.895, 12.9999, 12.902, 12.909, 12.911, 12.915, 12.919, 12.923, 12.927, 12.931, 12.935, 12.939, 12.943, 12.947, 12.951, 12.957, 12.955, 12.963, 12.967, 12.970, 12.975, 12.979, 12.983, 12.987, 12.992, 12.995, 13.000, 13.003, 13.007, 13.010, 13.015, 13.019, 13.023, 13.027, 13.141, 13.035, 13.038, 13.043, 13.046, 13.050, 13.053, 13.058, 13.062, 13.066, 13.070, 13.074, 13.078, 13.083, 13.086, 13.090, 13.097, 13.095, 13.102, 13.106, 13.110, 13.114, 13.118, 13.123, 13.126, 13.130, 13.133, 13.138, 13.143, 13.147, 13.151, 13.155, 13.159, 13.162, 13.167, 13.171, 13.175, 13.179, 13.182, 13.187, 13.191, 13.195, 13.199, 13.203, 13.207, 13.211, 13.215, 13.219, 13.223, 13.226, 13.231, 13.235, 13.239, 13.243, 13.246, 13.251, 13.255, 13.260, 13.264, 13.268, 13.272, 12.276, 13.280, 13.284, 13.288, 13.292, 13.295, 13.299, and VOC 13.305.

The percentages listed in table T4.4 are based on the absolute numbers presented in table TA4:

Table TA.4: Geographic origin of VOC surgeons

	1700	*1710*	*1720*	*1730*	*1740*	*1750*	*1760*	*1770*	*1780*	*1790*
Republic	33 (87%)	29 (97%)	27 (93%)	30 (85%)	20 (71%)	25 (53%)	15 (100%)	19 (61%)	14 (67%)	24 (55%)
Abroad	5 (13%)	1 (3%)	2 (7%)	5 (14%)	8 (29%)	20 (43%)	0	11 (35%)	7 (33%)	18 (41%)
Unknown	0	0	0	1	1	2	0	1	0	2

To check the places of origin as stated by the surgeons, a number of sources were consulted. Table TA.4 presents the places and sources that have been researched.

Table TA.5: Researched sources

Place in Republic	*Number*	*Found*	*Percentage*	*Particulars*
Aalten	3	3	100%	Via research by H. Schutte.
Alkmaar	17	6	35%	Only Catholic baptismals indexed.
Almelo	1	0	0%	Not researched.
Alphen a/d Rijn	6	0	0%	Not researched.
Ameide	1	0	0%	Not researched.
Amersfoort	6	1	17%	Source: the genealogical database of the Church of Jesus Christ of Latter-day Saints (the Mormons, Salt Lake City).
Amsterdam	399	86	77%	Please note that only the period 1760-1795 is indexed (in this period, 112 Amsterdam born surgeons were employed by the Company).
Amsterdam* (Engel van Tongere)	1	0	0	The wife of this 'Amsterdam-born' surgeon lived in De Rijp north of Amsterdam. In all probability, so did her husband.
Appingedam	1	0	0%	Not researched.
Arnhem	11	6	55%	F. van Langen has researched these in the Arnhem archives; 45 percent was not found.
Axel	1	0	0%	Not researched.
Beijerland	1	0	0%	Not researched.
Bemmel	1	0	0%	Not researched.
Bennebroek	1	0	0%	Not researched.
Bergen op Zoom	8	5	63%	Research via ISIS on which, however, only the protestant baptismals are listed.

Place in Republic	*Number*	*Found*	*Percentage*	*Particulars*
Bodegraven	2	0	0%	Not researched.
Bolsward	3	0	0%	Not researched.
Bommel	6	0	0%	Not researched.
Borculo	1	1	100%	Via research by D. van Zuidam.
Borne	1	1	100%	Via research by D. van Zuidam.
Boskoop	1	0	0%	Not researched.
Bovenkarspel	2	0	0%	Not researched.
Breda	8	0	0%	Not researched.
Breda*	2	1	50%	The two who stated Breda as their place of origin, probably came from Luiksgestel and from Delft.
Bredevoort	7	0	0%	Not researched.
Breskens	1	0	0%	Not researched.
Breukelen	3	1	33%	Data received from A. Mesman.
Bronkhorst	1	0	0%	Not researched.
Brummen	1	0	0%	Not researched.
Buiksloot	1	0	0%	Not researched.
Buren	2	0	0%	Not researched.
Cadzand	3	0	0%	Not researched.
Capelle	1	0	0%	Not researched.
Charlois	1	1	100%	Rotterdam archives
Coevorden	2	0	0%	Not researched.
Colijnsplaat	1	1	100%	Data received from P. Poortvliet
Culumborg	3	1	33%	From Burrows, E.H., *A history of medicine in South Africa up to the end of the nineteenth century* (Cape Town and Amsterdam, 1958).
Dalfsen	3	3	100%	Researched by D. van Zuidam.
De Klundert	1	0	0%	Not researched.
De Lier	1	0	0%	Not researched.
De Oude Tonge	1	0	0%	Not researched.
De Rijp	2	0	0%	Not researched.

Place in Republic	*Number*	*Found*	*Percentage*	*Particulars*
Delden	3	3*	100%*	Researched by D. van Zuidam.
Delfshaven	17	11	65%	Rotterdam archives
Delft	133	97	73%	Delft archives
Delft*	5	0	0%	Probably not born in Delft, as their baptismal dates were not found in the Delft archives; one probably came from Delden, which the Company's clerk wrote down as Delft.
Delfzijl	2	0	0%	Nor researched.
Den Bosch	9	4	44%	Data received from J.H.M, Verhagen (†).
Den Briel	18	13	72%	Data from ISIS Gensdata.
Den Haag/ The Hague	56	22	39%	Data received from J.C. van Woggelum.
Den Ham (1*)	4	1	25%	Source: genealogical database of the Church of Jesus Christ of Latter-day Saints (the Mormons, Salt Lake City); the Company's clerk wrote down Zwolle which is the nearest city to Den Ham.
Den Hoof	1	0	0%	Not researched.
Deventer	10	8	80%	Data received from T. Kloosterboer.
Dieverden	1	1	100%	Data received from A. Hummel.
Dinxperlo	3	3	100%	Data received from G. Rijsdorp.
Dirksland	1	0	0%	Not researched.
Doesburg	11	3	27%	Data received from Giessen, the municipal archivist of Doesburg archive.
Doetinchem	2	0	0%	Not researched.
Dokkum	4	2	50%	Data received from Meerema.
Domburg	1	0	0%	Not researched.
Dordrecht	25	1	4%	Source: genealogical database of The Church of Jesus Christ of Latter-day Saints (the Mormons, Salt Lake City)

Place in Republic	*Number*	*Found*	*Percentage*	*Particulars*
Dordrecht*	1	0	0%	Not found; could also originate from Middelburg.
Dreischor	1	0	0%	Not researched.
Edam	2	0	0%	Not researched.
Eede	1	0	0%	Not researched.
Eibergen	1	1	100%	Data received from D. van Zuidam
Elburg	9	8	89%	Data received from D. van Zuidam (1 was not found).
Elsen	1	0	0%	Not researched.
Enkhuizen	187	0	0%	Not researched, as not indexed.
Enkhuizen* (Johan C. Coenraardi, Arnoldus de Reus, and Pieter Appelboom)	3	0	0%	One probably came from Dunkirk, while the other came in reality from Germany and the last one also stated Hoorn as his place of birth.
Franeker	3	0	0%	Not researched.
Geldre (Jan Klute and Pieter ter Steegh)	2	0	0%	These two surgeons merely stated the province they came from.
Gendringen	2	0	0%	Not researched.
Goedereede	1	0	0%	Not researched.
Goes	9	0	0%	Not researched.
Goes*	1	1	100%	Source: genealogical database of The Church of Jesus Christ of Latter-day Saints (the Mormons, Salt Lake City), which lists Wolphaarsdijk as place of birth.
Gogh/Haarlem	1	0	0%	Not researched.
Goor	1	0	0%	Not researched.
Gorinchem	6	1	17%	Source: the genealogical database of The Church of Jesus Christ of Latter-day Saints (the Mormons, Salt Lake City).

Place in Republic	*Number*	*Found*	*Percentage*	*Particulars*
Gouda	7	2	29%	Source: for one surgeon, the genealogical database of the Church of Jesus Christ of Latter-day Saints (the Mormons, Salt Lake City); the other was found among the Lutheran baptismals of Gouda.
Grave	2	0	0%	Not researched.
Grijpskerke	1	0	0%	Not researched.
Groede	1	0	0%	Not researched.
Groenlo	6	2	33%	Data received by D. van Zuidam
Grol	1	0	0%	Not researched.
Groningen	21	4	19%	Data received from A. Doornbos.
Haaksbergen	2	2	100%	Data received from the Centre of Genealogy of Twente.
Haamstede	1	1	100%	Data received from J.F. Stoutjesdijk.
Haan	1	0	0%	Not researched.
Haarlem	20	10	50%	Kennemerland Archive in Haarlem, index baptismal dates.
Harderwijk	3	3	100%	Data received from D. van Zuidam.
Harlingen	6	0	0%	Not researched.
Harreveld	1	0	0%	Unidentified.
Hasselt	8	4	50%	Data received from D. van Zuidam who found 50 percent of the stated Hasselt surgeons.
Hattem	2	1	50%	Source: for one surgeon, the genealogical database of The Church of Jesus Christ of Latter-day Saints (the Mormons, Salt Lake City).
Heemstede	2	0	0%	Not researched.
Heesch	1	0	0%	Not researched.
Hellevoetsluis	3	0	0%	Not researched.

Place in Republic	*Number*	*Found*	*Percentage*	*Particulars*
Hengstdijk	1	0	0%	Not researched.
Het Loo	1	0	0%	Not researched.
Heusden	2	0	0%	Not researched.
Hilversum	1	0	0%	Not researched.
Hoge Zwaluwe	1	0	0%	Not researched.
Hoogziel	1	0	0%	Not researched.
Hoorn	132	44	33%	Westfrisian archives, archive Hoorn. 67 percent not found there.
Horne	1	0	0%	Not researched.
Huizen	2	0	0%	Not researched.
Hulst	3	0	0%	Not researched.
IJsselstein	1	0	0%	Not researched.
IJzendijke	1	1	100%	Source: for one surgeon, genealogical database of The Church of Jesus Christ of Latter-day Saints (the Mormons, Salt Lake City).
Kampen	31	22	71%	Data received by D. van Zuidam.
Kantens	1	0	0%	Not researched.
Kortenoort	1	0	0%	Not researched.
Kortgene	1	0	0%	Not researched.
Koudekerke	1	1	100%	Data from 'Zeeuwsche Stam'. The Company's clerk stated Middelburg as place of origin.
Kralingen	1	1	100%	Source: genealogical database of the Church of Jesus Christ of Latter-day Saints (the Mormons, Salt Lake City).
Krimpen	1	0	0%	Not researched.
Kruijningen	1	0	0%	Not researched.
Kuilenburg	1	0	0%	Not researched.
Langstraat	1	0	0%	Not researched.
Leerdam	2	1	50%	Data received from the Genealogy group South-Holland.

Place in Republic	*Number*	*Found*	*Percentage*	*Particulars*
Leeuwarden	16	3	19%	Just protestant baptismals on municipality site of Groningen.
Leiden	34	18	53%	Data received from research by J. Renema.
Leiden*	2	1	50%	Of these two surgeons, one came from the island of Texel, and the other from Alphen aan den Rijn, although he did receive his surgical training in Leiden.
Leidschendam	1	0	0%	Not researched.
Lemmer	1	0	0%	Not researched.
Leusden	2	0	0%	Not researched.
Lichtenvoorde	1	1	100%	Data received from H. Schutte.
Limburg	1	0	0%	This surgeon only stated the province he came from, which made research impossible.
Lochem	2	2	100%	Data received from D.van Zuidam.
Loevestein	1	0	0%	Not researched.
Loon-op-Zand	1	1	100%	ISIS Gensdate site.
Lumen	1	0	0%	Not researched.
Maasland	1	0	0%	Not researched.
Maassluis	5	1	20%	Source: genealogical database of The Church of Jesus Christ of Latter-day Saints (the Mormons, Salt Lake City).
Maastricht	12	0	0%	Not researched.
Medemblik (*)	9	1	11%	Kennemerland archive, surgeons archive.
Meppel (*)	10	0	0%	Not researched; one surgeon probably came from Lingen.
Middelburg	167	9	5%	Source: genealogical database of The Church of Jesus Christ of Latter-day Saints (the Mormons, Salt Lake City).
Monnikendam	4	3	75%	Data received from C.A.E. Groot.
Montfoort	1	1	100%	Gensdata ISIS internet

Place in Republic	*Number*	*Found*	*Percentage*	*Particulars*
Moordrecht	1	1	100%	Source: genealogical database of The Church of Jesus Christ of Latter-day Saints (the Mormons, Salt Lake City).
Muiden	2	0	0%	Not researched.
Naaldwijk (*)	4	1	25%	Source: the genealogical database of The Church of Jesus Christ of Latter-day Saints (the Mormons, Salt Lake City); the Company's clerk had stated as from Rijswijk.
Naarden	3	1	0%	Not researched.
Nieuwenhoorn	1	1	100%	Gensdata ISIS internet
Nieuwkerk	3	0	0%	Not researched.
Nieuwkoop	1	0	0%	Not researched.
Nieuwpoort	3	0	0%	Not researched.
Nieuwveen	1	0	0%	Not researched.
Nijmegen	9	9	100%	Data received from Ms. Mieke van Veen.
Nijmegen*	6	1	17%	Source: the genealogical database of The Church of Jesus Christ of Latter-day Saints (the Mormons, Salt Lake City); the Company's clerk had stated as from De Gester
Noordwijk*	1	0	0%	The Company's clerk wrote down as from Haarlem. However, in the Haarlem (Kennemerlandarchief) surgeons' archives it proved that his place of origin was Noordwijk although he received his surgical training in Haarlem.
Nordwolde	1	0	0%	Not researched.
Nieuw Bijerland	1	1	100%	Source: the genealogical database of The Church of Jesus Christ of Latter-day Saints (the Mormons, Salt Lake City).
Odink near Brevoort	1	0	0%	Not researched.

Place in Republic	*Number*	*Found*	*Percentage*	*Particulars*
Oldenzaal	6	2	33%	Data received from Davina.
Ooltgensplaat	1	1	100%	Data received from L. Akershoek.
Oosterwijk	0	0	0%	Not researched.
Ootmarsum	3	0	0%	Not researched.
Oud Beijerland	4	0	0%	Not researched.
Oud Vossemeer	1	1	100%	Data received from N. Boevé from the Genealogy group of Zeeland.
Oude Pekela	2	1	50%	Data received from Ms. M. Teunis.
Oudshoorn	1	0	0%	Not researched.
Overschie	5	2	40%	Source: genealogical database of The Church of Jesus Christ of Latter-day Saints (the Mormons, Salt Lake City).
Paterswolde	1	0	0%	Not researched.
Pijnacker	1	1	100%	Delft municipality archive (on internet).
Pingjum	1	1	100%	Source: genealogical database of The Church of Jesus Christ of Latter-day Saints (the Mormons, Salt Lake City).
Prinseland	2	1	50%	Source: genealogical database of The Church of Jesus Christ of Latter-day Saints (the Mormons, Salt Lake City).
Purmerend	6	0	0%	Not researched.
Rheden	1	0	0%	Not researched.
Rhenen	1	0	0%	Not researched.
Rijswijk	6	0	0%	Not researched.
Roden	1	0	0%	Not researched.
Roermond	2	0	0%	Not researched.
Roosendaal	1	1	100%	Data received from M. A. Mulder.
Rotterdam	222	143	64%	Municipal archive Rotterdam (on internet).

Place in Republic	*Number*	*Found*	*Percentage*	*Particulars*
Sardam	1	0	0%	Could be Zaandam?
Sas van Gent	1	0	0%	Not researched.
Schagen	1	0	0%	Not researched.
Scherpenisse	1	0	0%	Not researched.
Scherpenzeel	1	0	0%	Not researched.
Scheveningen	2	0	0%	Not researched.
Schiedam	15	12	80%	Data received from research done by J. Leenderts.
Schoonderloo*	1	1	100%	Municipal archive Rotterdam on internet.
Schoonhoven	4	3	75%	Source: genealogical database of The Church of Jesus Christ of Latter-day Saints (the Mormons, Salt Lake City).
Serooskerke	2	0	0%	Not researched.
Sloten	1	0	0%	Not researched.
Sluis	6	0	0%	Not researched.
Sneek	2	0	0%	Not researched.
Sommelsdijk	1	0	0%	Not researched.
Spaarndam	1	1	100%	Data received from Van der Veen.
Spanbroek	1	0	0%	Not researched.
Stavenisse	1	1	100%	Source: genealogical database of the Church of Jesus Christ of Latter-day Saints (the Mormons, Salt Lake City); the Company's clerk just mentioned the island of Tholen in Zeeland.
Steenwijk	3	2	33%	Data received by Dick van Zuidam.
Stolwijk	1	0	0%	Not researched.
Streefkerk	1	0	0%	Not researched.
St.Philipsland	1	0	0%	Not researched.
St.Jacobsparochie	1	0	0%	Not researched.
St. Maartendijk	3	1	33%	'Van Zeeuwsche Stam'

Place in Republic	*Number*	*Found*	*Percentage*	*Particulars*
Swaanshals*	1	0	0%	The Company's clerk mentioned Rotterdam; he did marry in Rotterdam, but he came from Swaanshals.
Ter Apel	1	0	0%	Not researched.
Terborg	1	0	0%	Not researched.
Terschelling	1	0	0%	Not researched.
Tholen	6	0	0%	Not researched.
Tholen	1	1	100%	Source: genealogical database of the Church of Jesus Christ of Latter-day Saints (the Mormons, Salt Lake City). Although the Company's clerk wrote down Tholen, the Mormons specified this in Axel.
Tiel	4	3	75%	Data received from P. Hanry.
Tilligte	1	0	0%	Not researched.
Tongeren	2	0	0%	Not researched.
Uithoorn	1	0	0%	Not researched.
Uithuizen	1	0	0%	Not researched.
Ulft	1	0	0%	Not researched.
Urk	2	0	5	Not researched.
Utrecht	42	22	52%	Municipal archive Utrecht
Veenendaal*	2	2	100%	Data received from P. Menso.
Veenhuizen	1	0	0%	Not researched.
Veere	10	0	0%	Not researched.
Velsen	2	2	100%	Gensdata ISIS internet.
Venlo	1	0	0%	Not researched.
Vianen	2	1	50%	Source: genealogical database of the Church of Jesus Christ of Latter-day Saints (the Mormons, Salt Lake City).
Vinkeveen	1	0	0%	Not researched.
Vlaardingen	5	3	60%	Data received from J. Odijk.
Vleuten	1	0	0%	Not researched.

Place in Republic	*Number*	*Found*	*Percentage*	*Particulars*
Vlissingen	13	0	0%	None of them found at Gensdata ISIS internet.
Vollenhoven	1	0	0%	Not researched.
Voorburg	6	0	0%	Not researched.
Voorschoten	1	0	0%	Not researched.
Vreeswijk	1	0	0%	Not researched.
Vrieseveen	1	1	100%	Data received from A. Idzinga.
Waalwijk*	1	1	100%	Source: genealogical database of the Church of Jesus Christ of Latter-day Saints (the Mormons, Salt Lake City). In that database city of origin stated as Naaldwijk!
Waddingscha	1	0	0%	Not researched.
Waddinxveen	1	0	0%	Not researched.
Wageningen	1	0	0%	Not researched.
Warmetten	1	0	0%	Not researched.
Wedde	1	0	0%	Not researched.
Weert	1	0	0%	Not researched.
Weerts/Weesp	1	0	0%	Not researched.
Westkapelle	1	0	0%	Not researched.
Westzanen	1	0	0%	Not researched.
Weutersdijk	1	0	0%	Not researched.
Wijhe	1	1	100%	Data received from J.H. Wissink.
Wijk bij Duurstede	3	0	0%	Not researched.
Wildervank	1	0	0%	Not researched.
Willemstad	1	0	0%	Not researched.
Winterswijk	7	6	86%	Data received from H. Schutte.
Wissekerke	1	0	0%	Not researched.
Woerden	2	0	0%	Not researched.
Worckum	1	0	0%	Not researched.
Zaamslag	2	0	0%	Not researched.
Zaandam	1	0	0%	Not researched.

Place in Republic	*Number*	*Found*	*Percentage*	*Particulars*
Zaltbommel	4	1	25%	Data received by genealogical database
Zevenaar	1	1	100%	Data received from Giessen, the municipal archivist of Doesburg.
Zevenhuizen	2	0	0%	Not researched.
Zierikzee	7	0	0%	Not researched.
Zoetermeer	2	1	50%	Source: genealogical database of the Church of Jesus Christ of Latter-day Saints (the Mormons, Salt Lake City).
Zutphen	12	0	0%	Not researched.
Zwammerdam	2	1	50%	Source: genealogical database of The Church of Jesus Christ of Latter-day Saints (the Mormons, Salt Lake City).
Zwijndrecht	2	0	0%	Not researched.
Zwolle	25	25	100%	Data received from D. van Zuidam.
s-Gravenzande	1	1	100%	Source: genealogical database of The Church of Jesus Christ of Latter-day Saints (the Mormons, Salt Lake City).
's-Heer Arendskerke	1	0	0%	Not researched.

To answer the questions posed in chapter 5, use was made of the sample ('S') of 2,988 ship's surgeons. However, not all of the surgeons in S meet the criteria of each query. Therefore, groups and subgroups are made in order to answer each specific question. According to the query, I distinguish:

Group S: the total population (100%) of the sample of 2,988 ship's surgeons. S was analysed to answer queries regarding the number of departures (contracts) a surgeon made; the total time of employment at the Company.

Group A: consists of those ship's surgeons of S of whom the dates of birth have been found to be able to address the question of age and rank upon first contract with the Company (the ship's surgeon's first departure to Asia). Within this group A, there are three sub-groups, according to the surgeons' rank: first surgeon (I), second surgeon (II), and third surgeon (III). This group A consists of 776 ship's surgeons, a large 25 per cent of the total sample S.

Group B: the population of the sample (S), which departed just once (one contract) and did not repatriate to the Republic within five years after first (and only) departure. I have drawn the line at five years, as the minimum tenure was five years.

Group C: This group consists of those surgeons who made more than one departure from the Republic to Asia, and were thus in a position to be promoted along the ranks. C consists of 1,112 ship's surgeons. There were two ways of making a career: by making numerous voyages, or by staying in a settlement.

Group D1: the population of those surgeons of S who only made the one voyage for the Company and who repatriated within five years and never to be employed again by the Company (390 ship's surgeons, 13 per cent of S).

Group D2: that part of S who died within five years after the first departure (1,059 or 35 per cent of S). Consequently, these men (D1 and D2, 1,449 surgeons) could or did not consider a further career with the Company and will not be analysed.

Group E: as the surgeons of Group D1 and D2 could or would not make a career with the Company, we have to subtract those from the sample S (2,988-1,449), which leaves us a group of 1,539 surgeons fit for analysis on points of career.

Group F: the population of the sample (S) of whom facts on education or schooling (entry at local surgical guilds and/or the passing of examinations at the local surgical guilds) are known in order to establish the level of the surgeons' education at first contract. F consists of 152 ship's surgeons. Also F is divided into subgroups (such as rank and per period), one of which is that the population of F of whom the birthdates are known (F1). F1 consists of 72 ship's surgeons. The facts of schooling are derived from the archives of surgeon guilds in the cities Amsterdam, Haarlem, Leiden and Schiedam.

Group G: that part of S which only made the one departure and did not repatriate to the Republic and consists of 1,375 ship's surgeons.

Group H: that part of S, of which the birth data and the death data are known and consists of 509 surgeons.

Group I: that part of S, for whom death data are known, consisting of 1,900 surgeons.

Appendix 2. Maps

Map A2.1: Surgical recruitment from the northern area

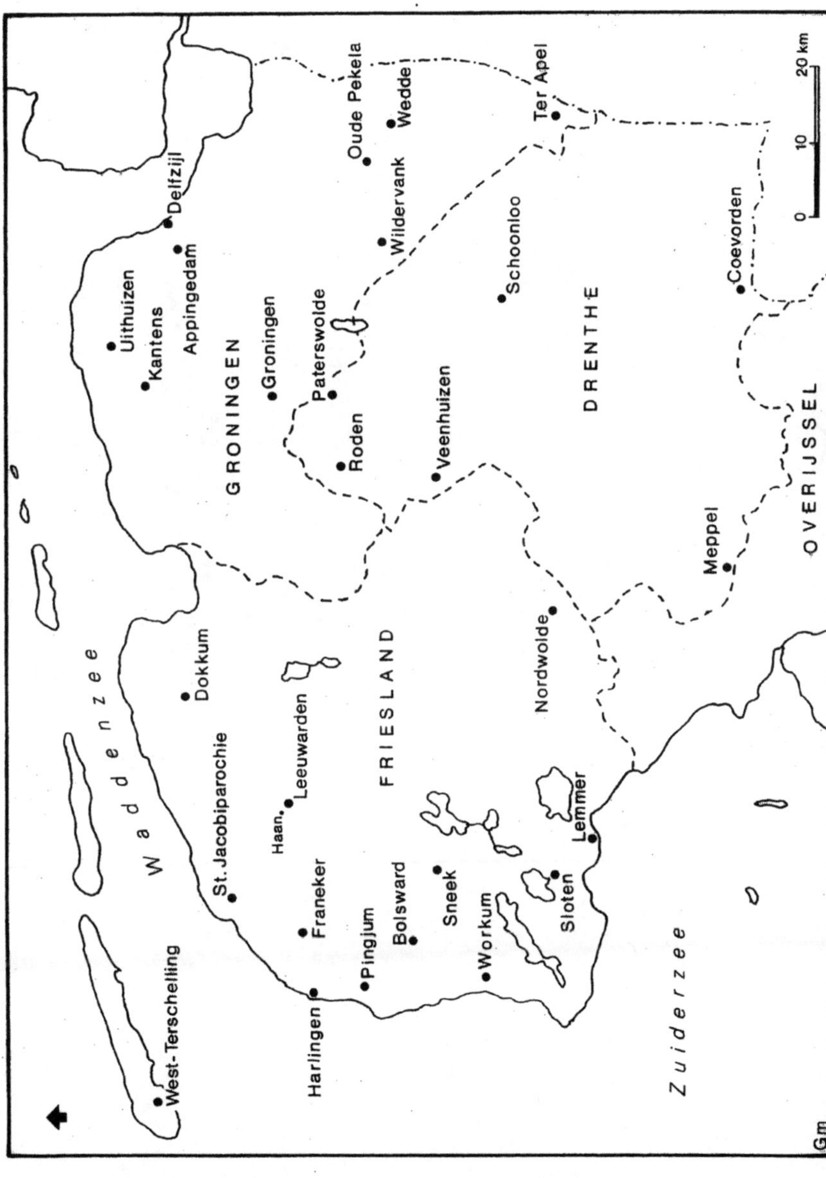

Map A2.2: Surgical recruitment from the eastern and central areas

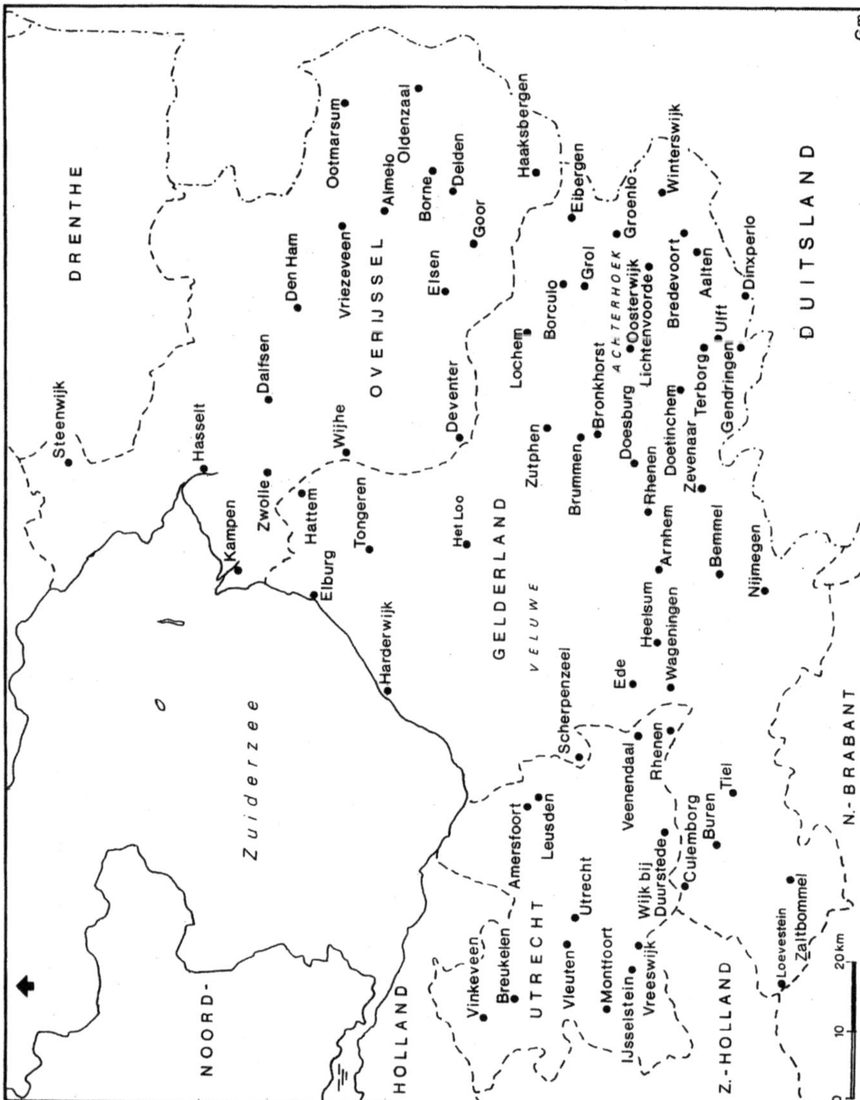

Map A2.3: Surgical recruitment from the southern area

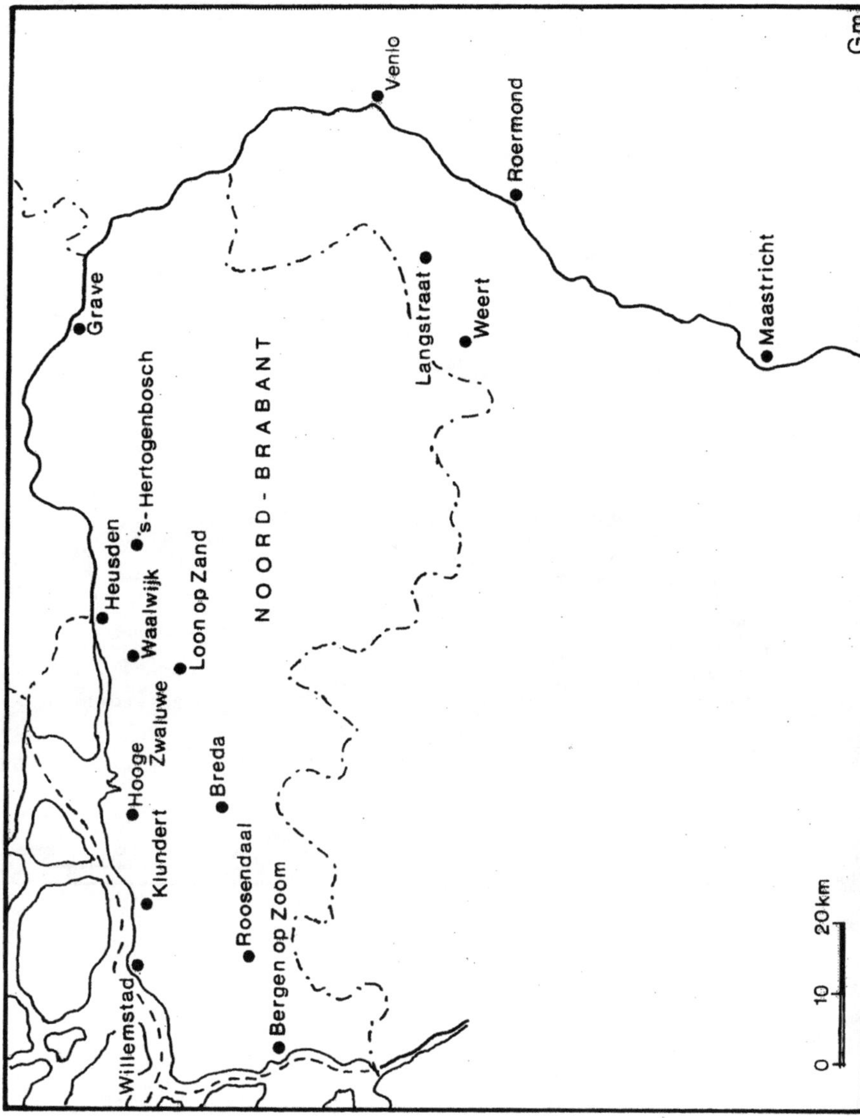

Map A2.4: Surgical recruitment from North Holland

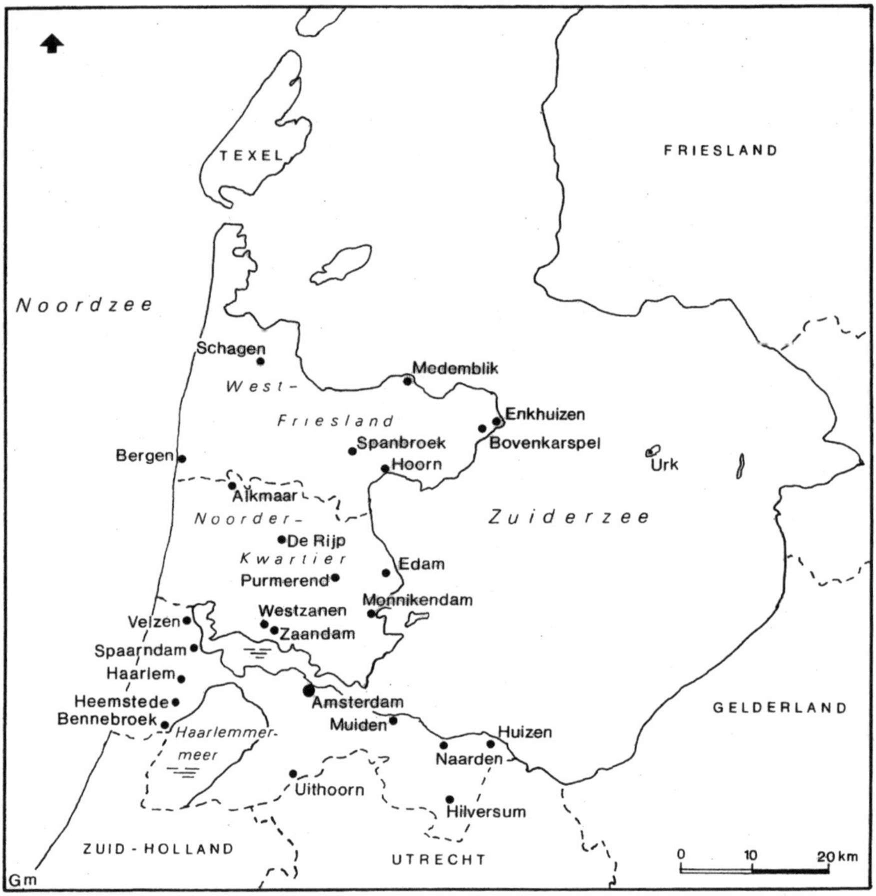

Map A2.5: Surgical recruitment from South Holland

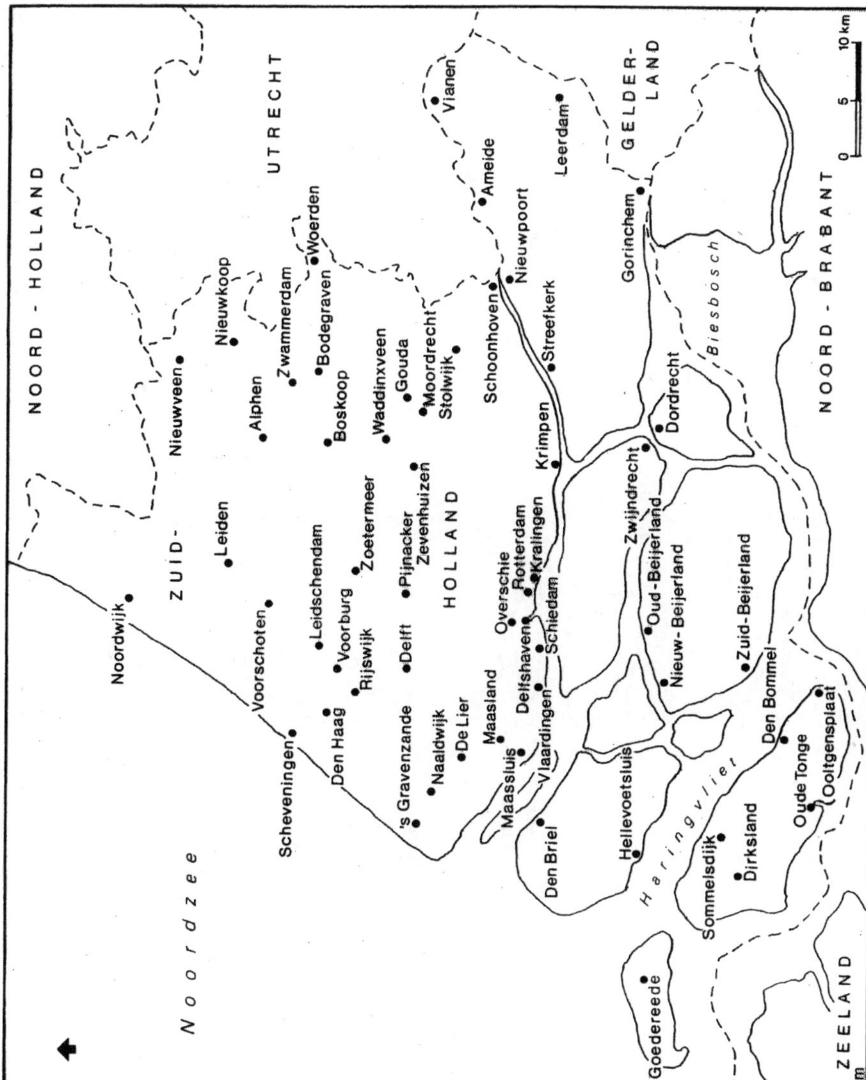

Map A2.6: Surgical recruitment from Zeeland

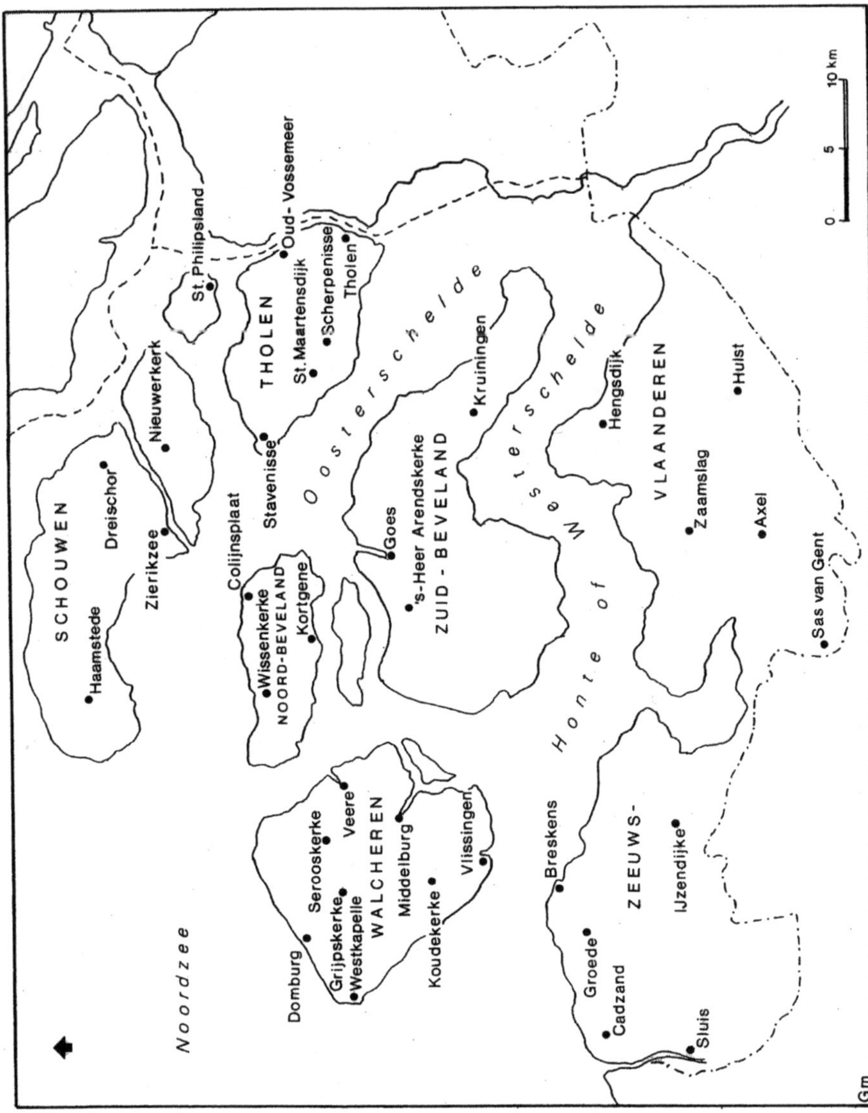

Map A2.7a-b: Surgical recruitment in the Dutch Republic 1700-1750

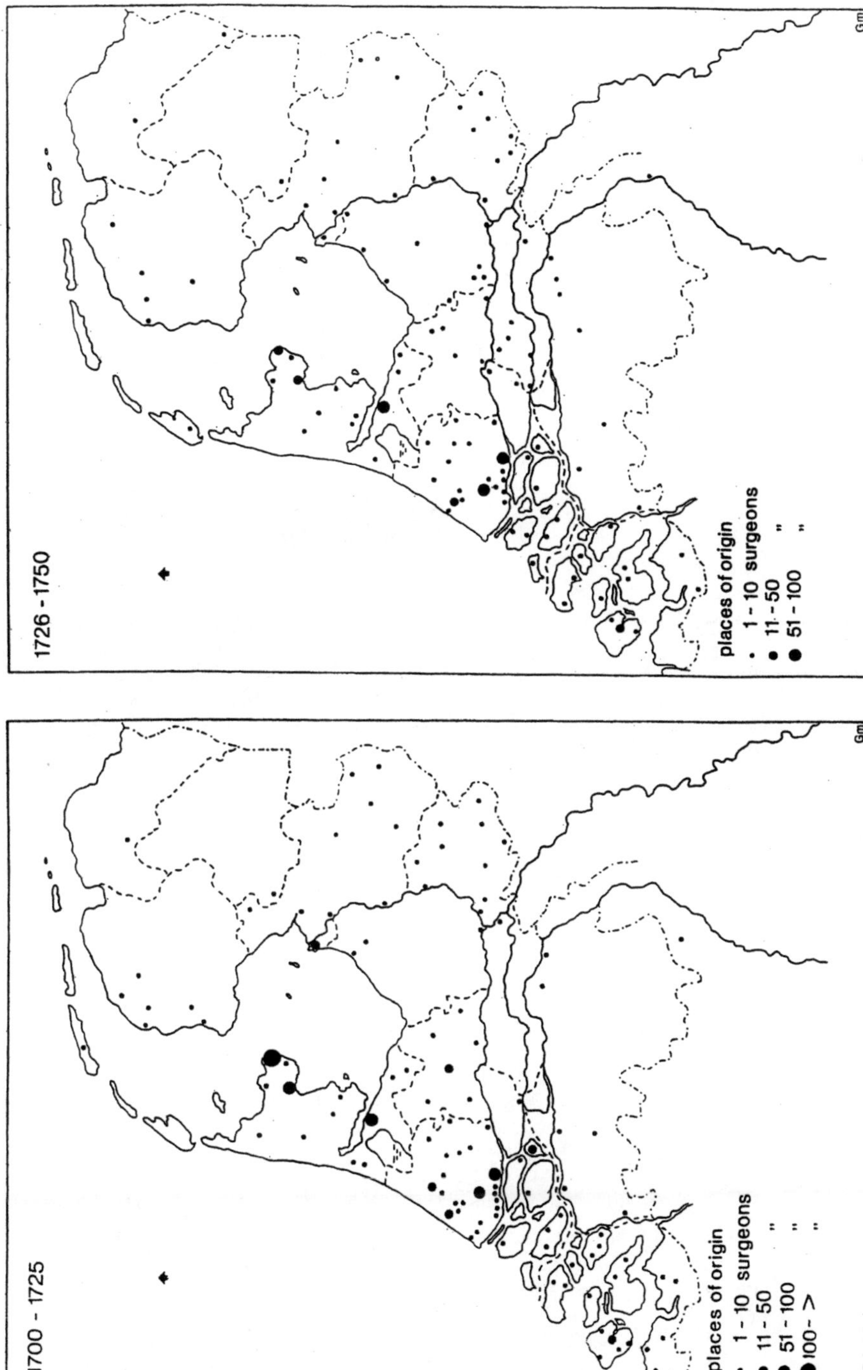

Map A2.7c-d: Surgical recruitment in the Dutch Republic 1751-1795

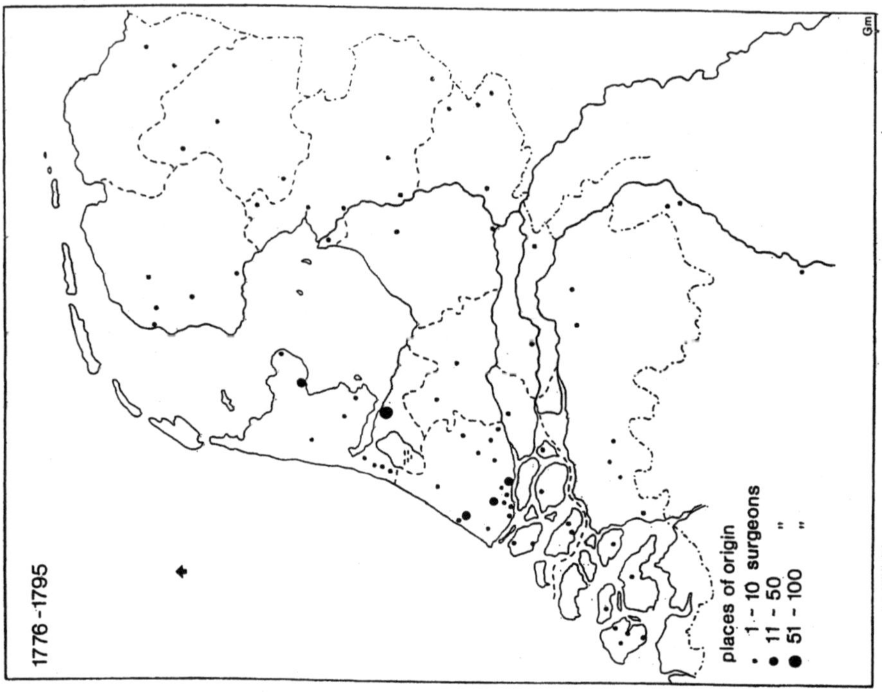

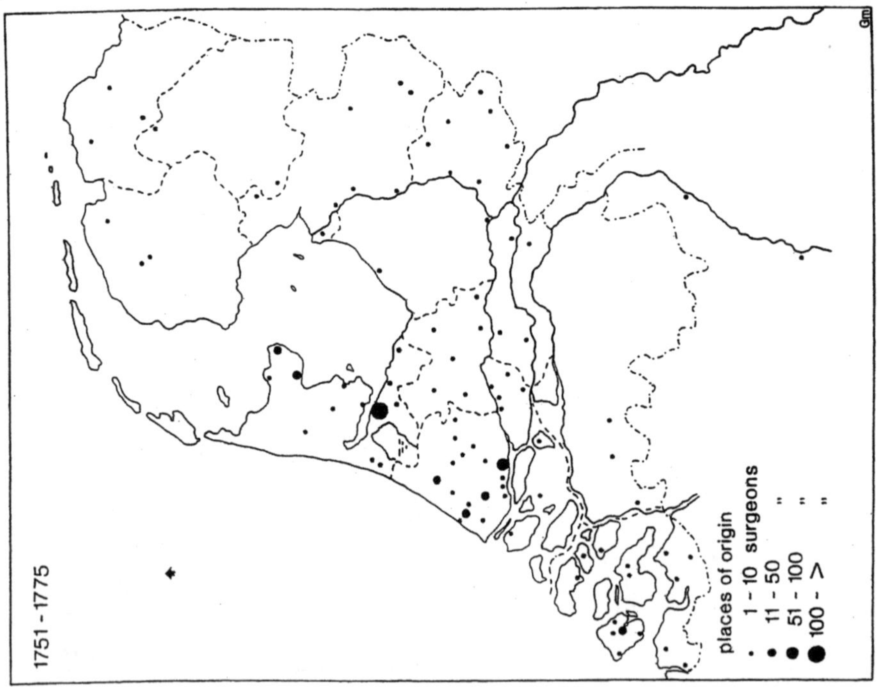

Map A2.8a-b: German surgical recruitment 1700-1750

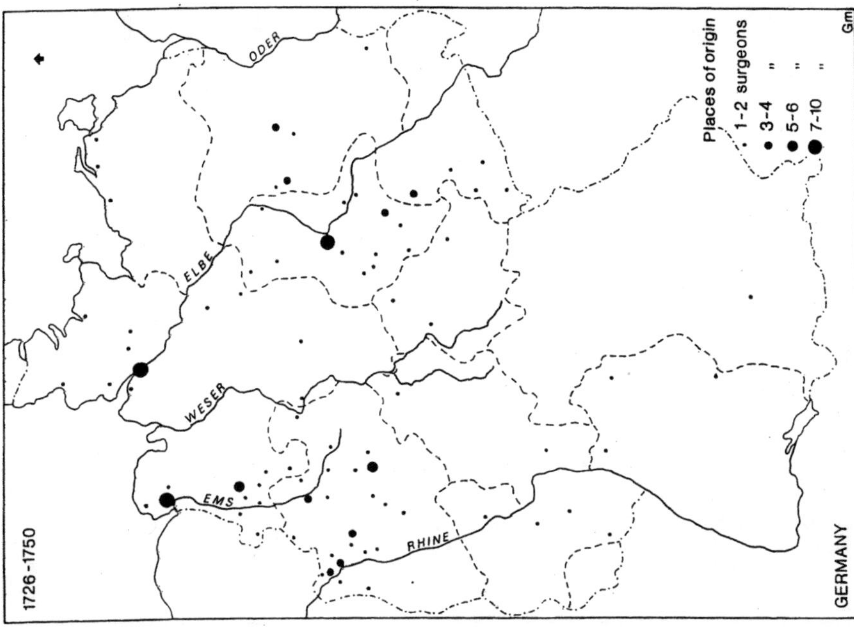

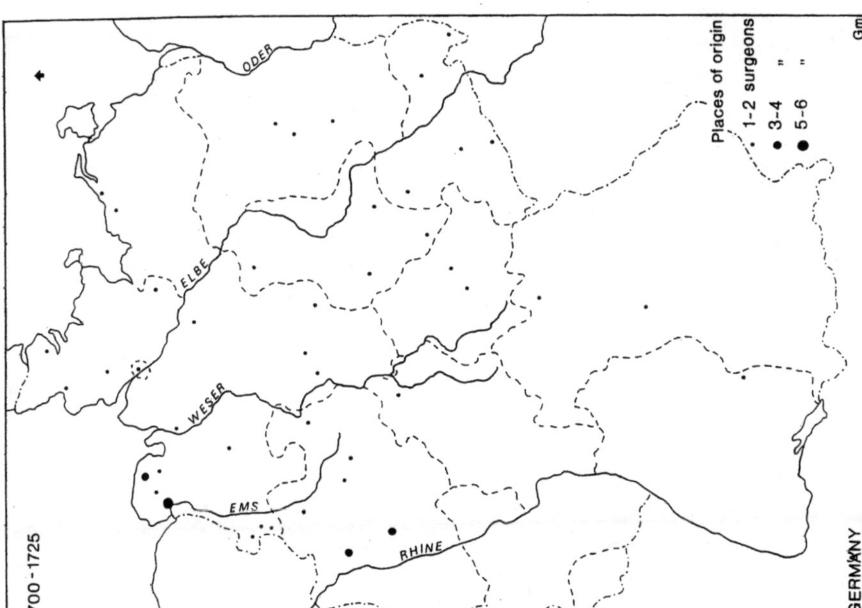

Map A2.8c-d: German surgical recruitment 1751-1795

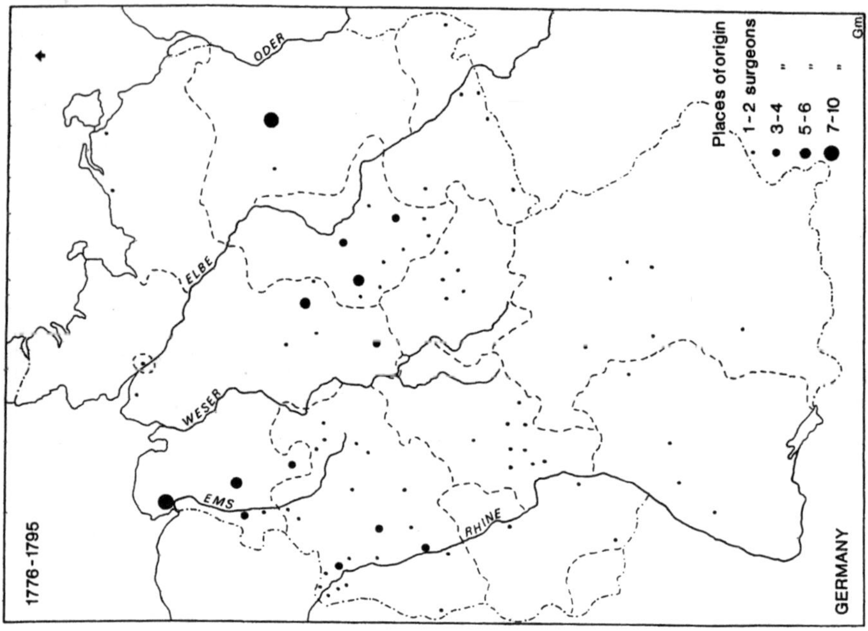

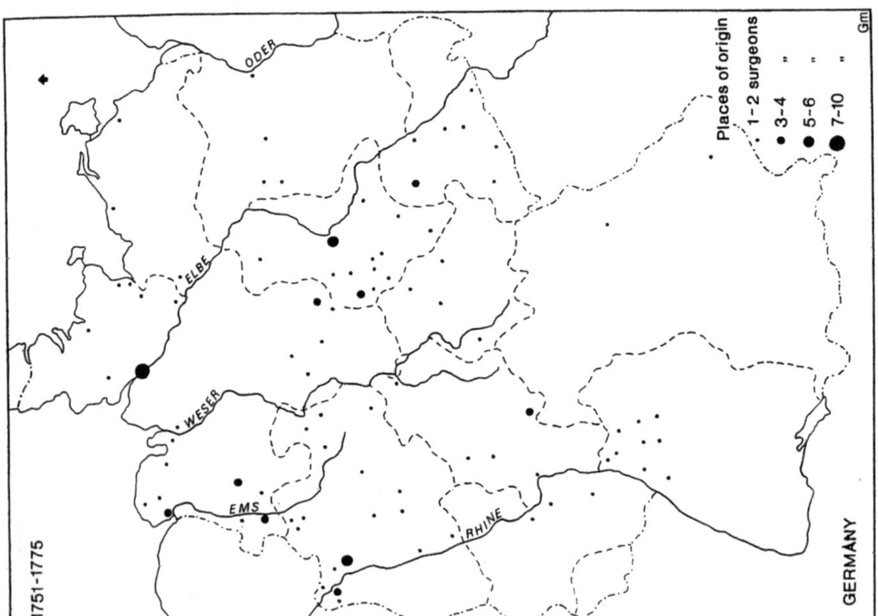

Map A2.9: Surgical recruitment from Lower Saxony

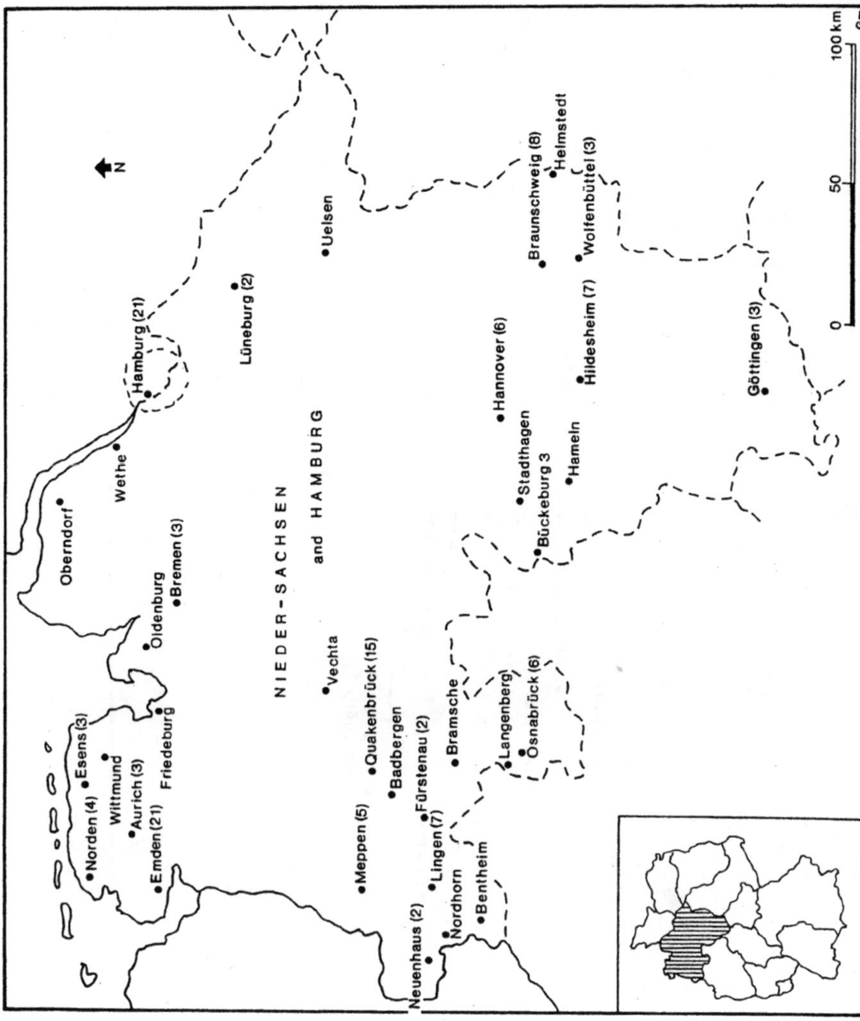

Map A2.10: Surgical recruitment from Saxony

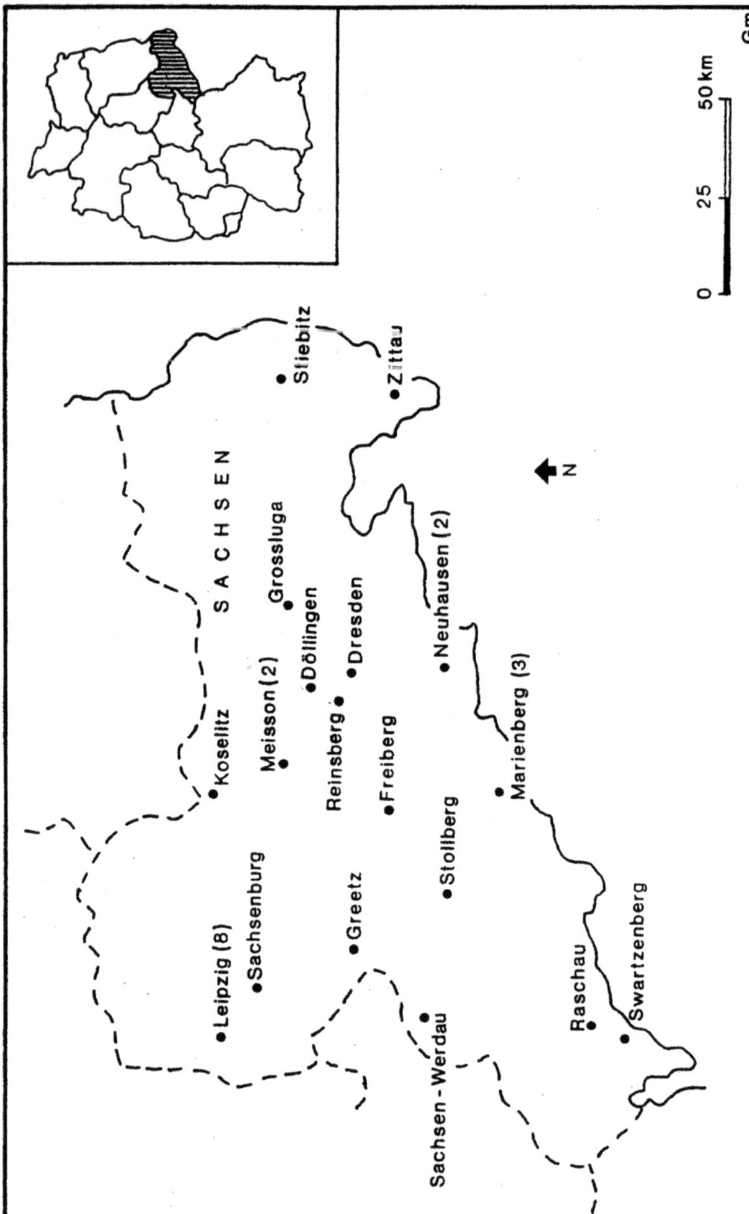

Map A2.11: Surgical recruitment from Saxony-Anhalt

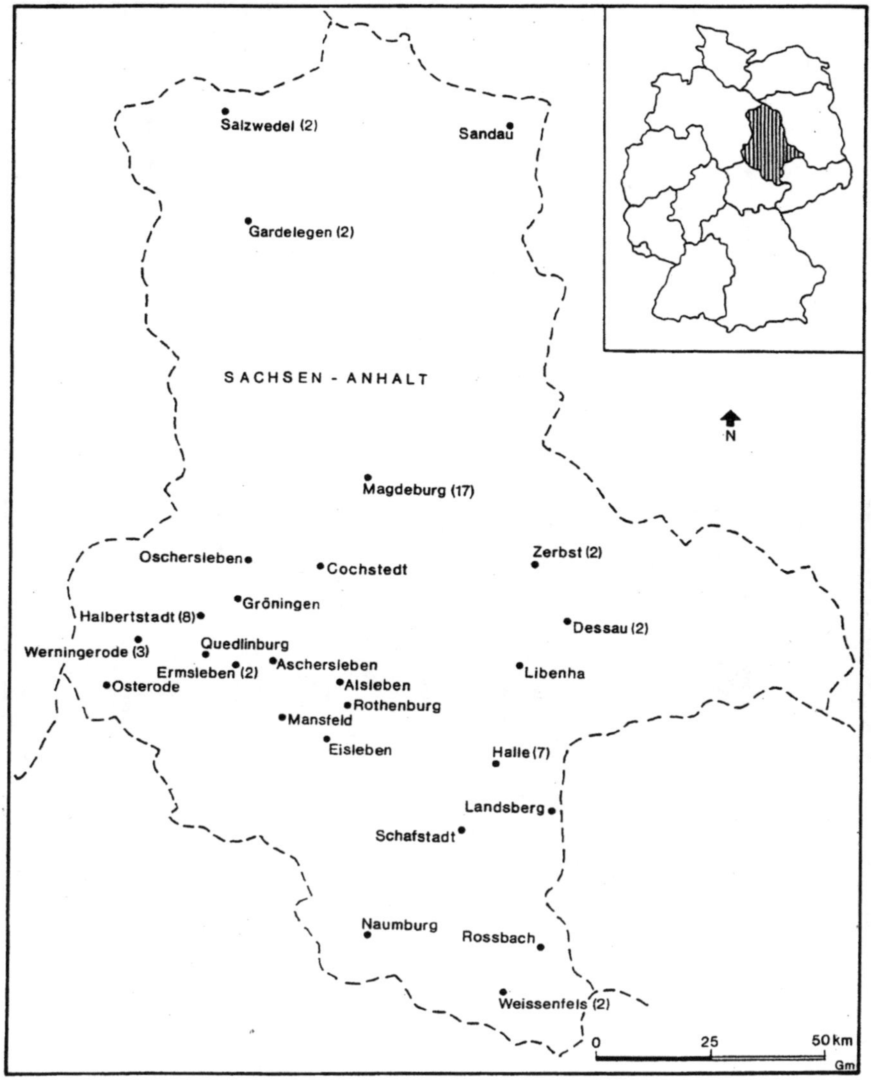

Map A2.12: Surgical recruitment from Westphalia

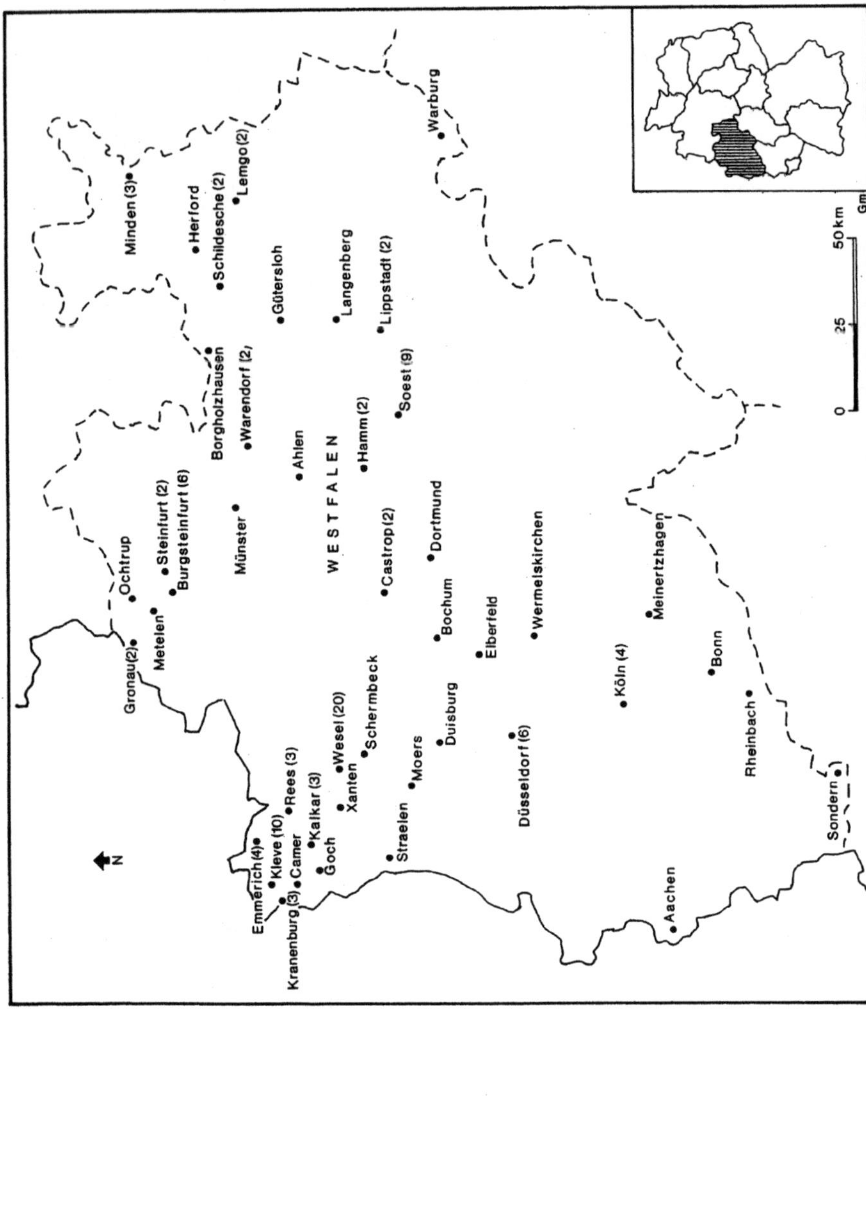

Map A2.13: Surgical recruitment from Brandenburg

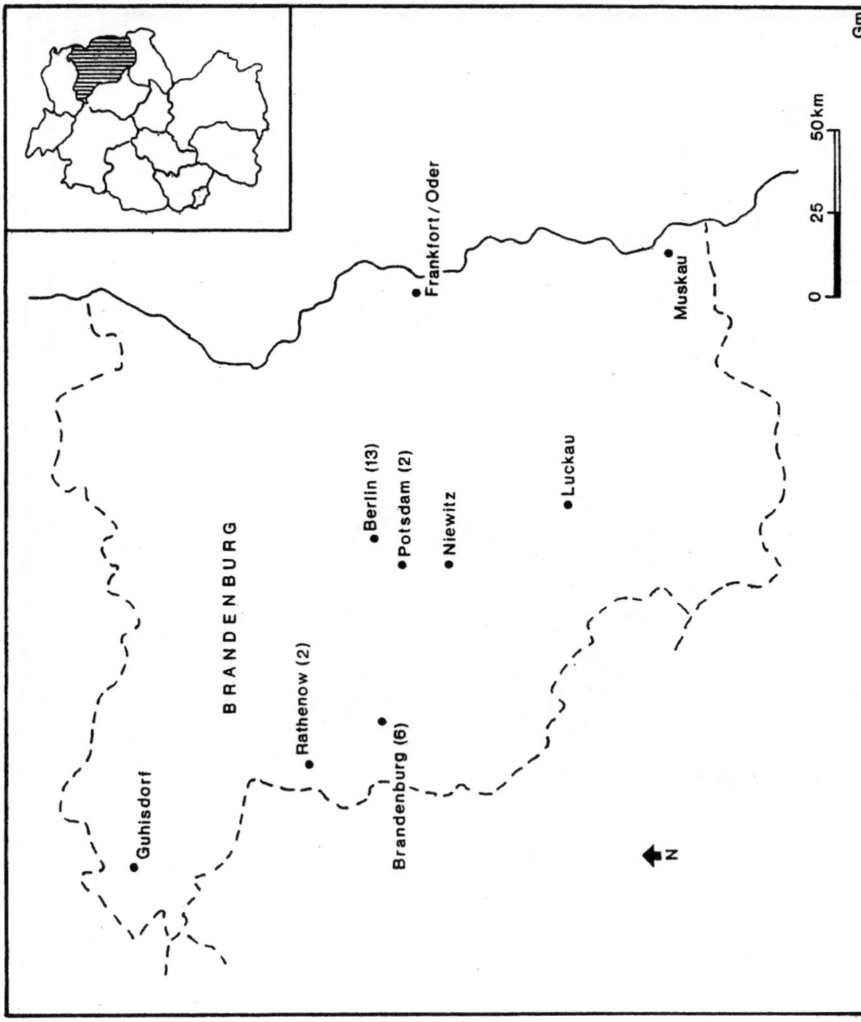

Map A2.14: Surgical recruitment from Mecklenburg-Vorpommern

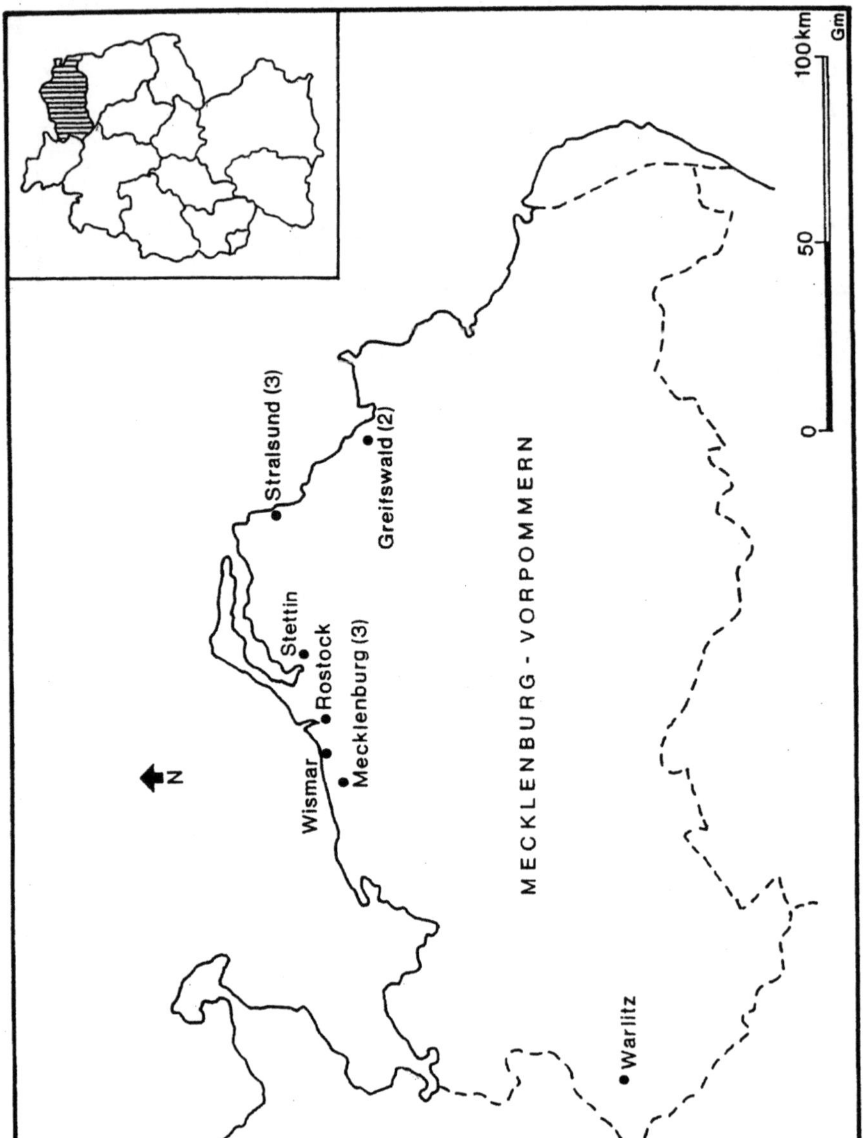

Map A2.15: Surgical recruitment from Schleswig-Holstein

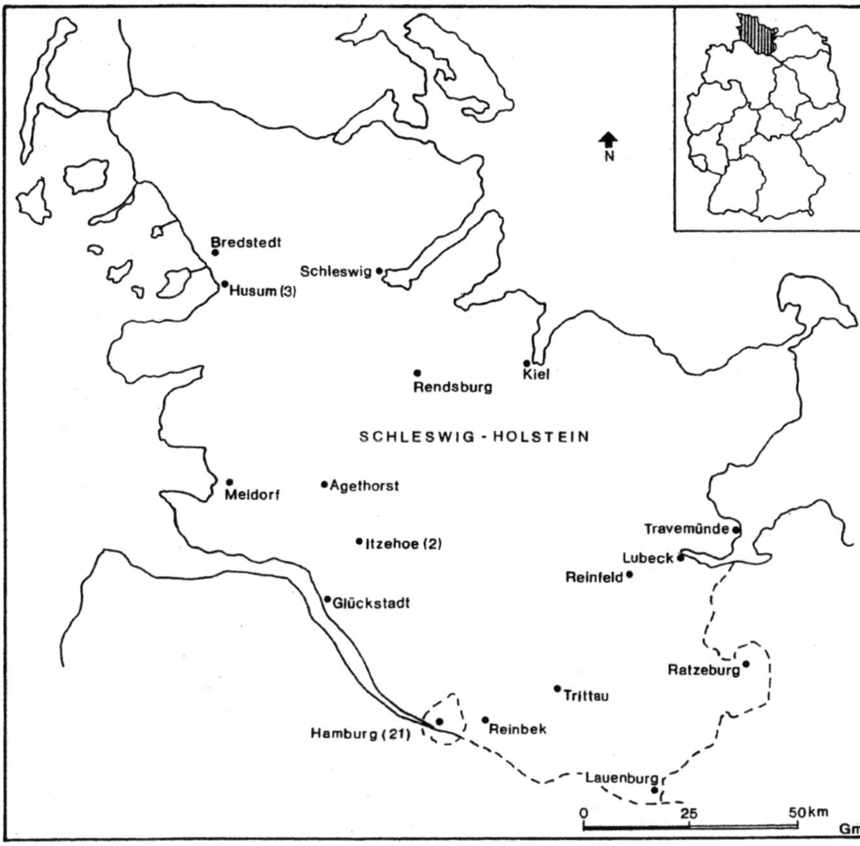

Map A2.16: Surgical recruitment from Hessen

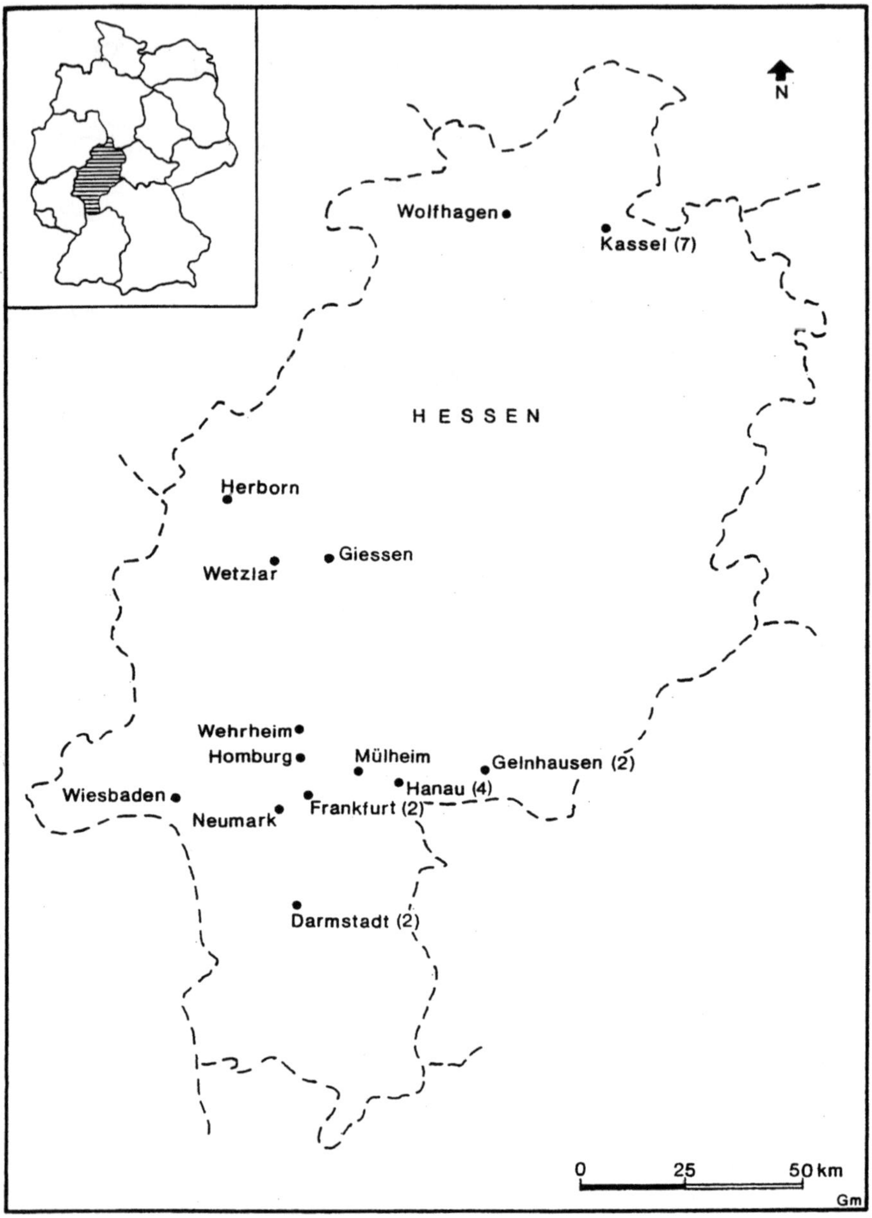

Map A2.17: Surgical recruitment from Thuringia

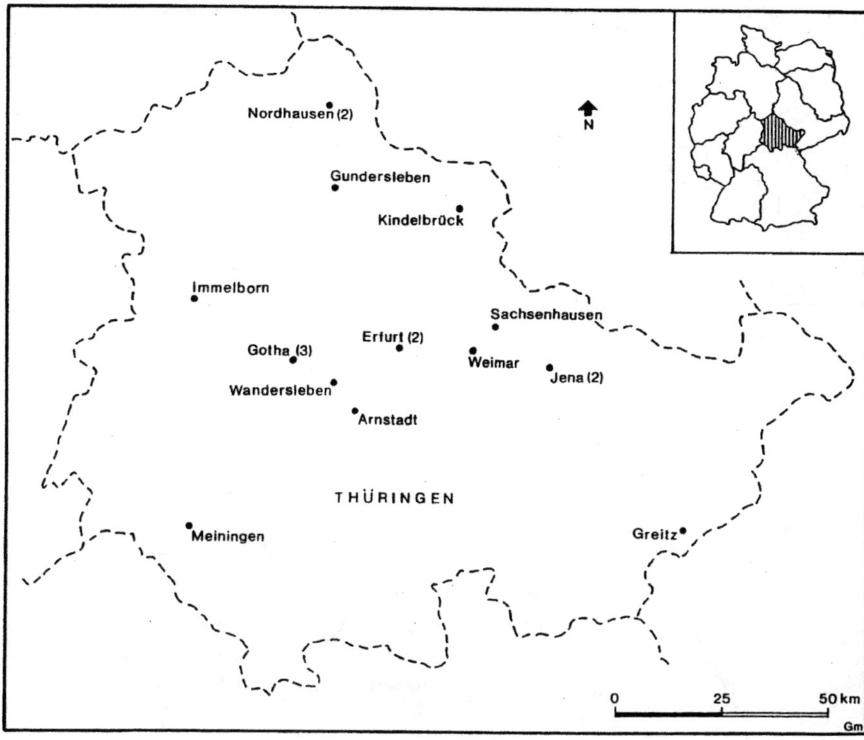

Map A2.18: Surgical recruitment from Rheinland-Pfalz

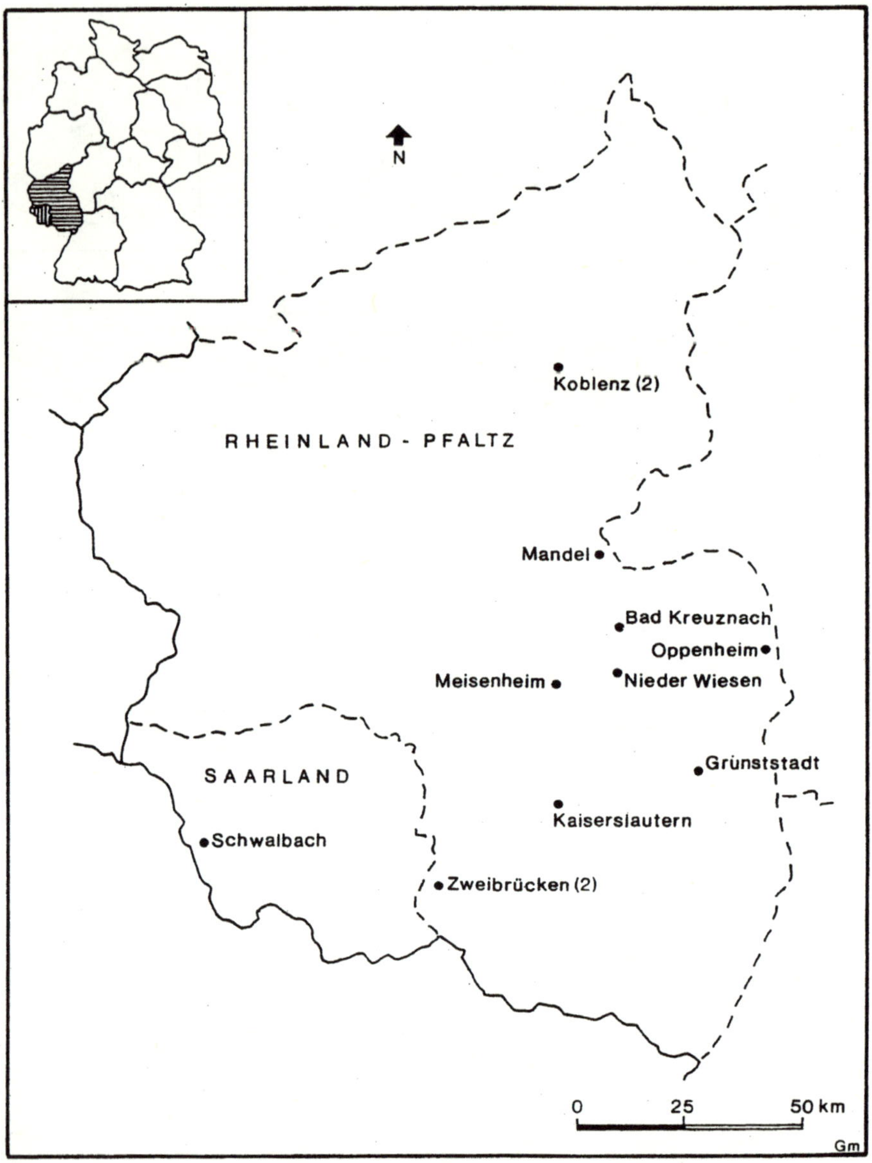

Map A2.19: Surgical recruitment from Bavaria

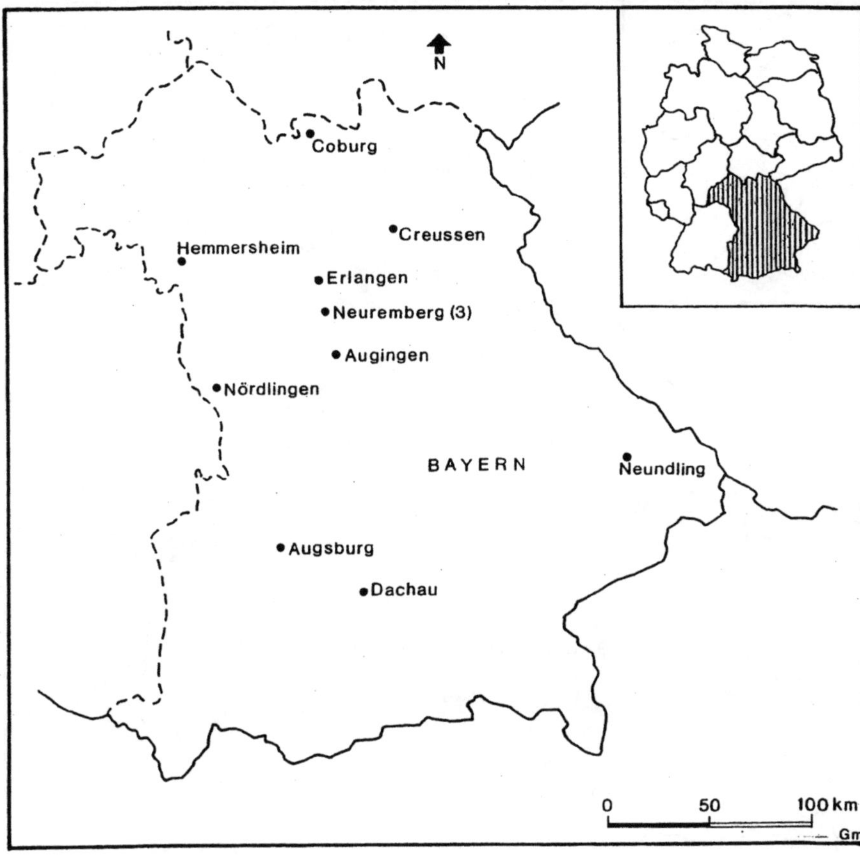

Map A2.20: Surgical recruitment from Baden-Württemberg

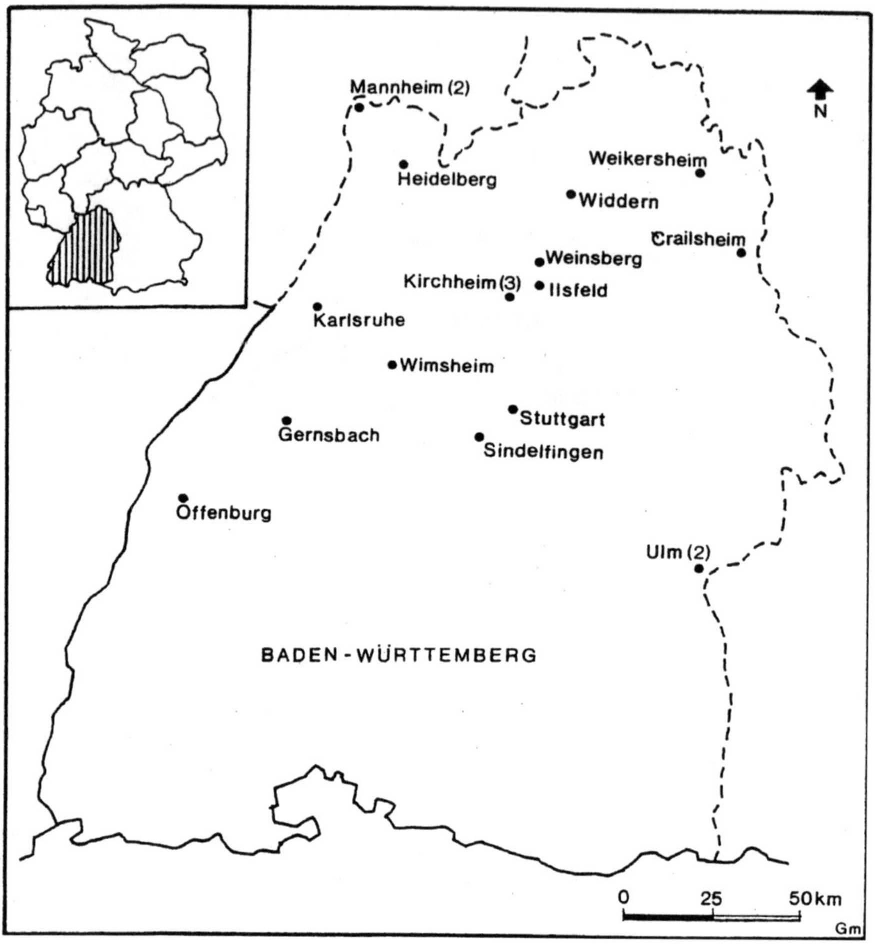

Appendix 3. Notaries used by the Company's surgeons in Batavia 1600-1800[6]

M. van Aerden (2x)
N. Bergen van der Grijp (8x)
J. van de Bergh (1x)
J.N. Bestbier (4x)
E. Blomhert (14x)
J. Bolsward (1x)
B.H. Brooks (2x)
J. de Brouwer (1x)
A. Codde (1x)
J. Rijklof Costers (2x)
J. Greving (5x)
N. Crul (8x)
A. Deldijn ((7x)
A. Dinter (7x)
D. Dispontijn (6x)
P. Dobberlaar (3x)
A. Domburg (6x)
D. van Es (10x)
G.G. Franchimont (3x)
J. Freeman (3x)
J.P. Fremi (5x)
G.F. Fuijttingh (3x)
G. van Gierssen (4x)
J.L. Gousset (4x)
C. van Grootelande (1x)
M.D. van Haak (5x)
M. Hommes (1x)
A. Huijsman (3x)
J.M. de Jonge (3x)
C. Jongbloet (1x)
P.J. Bert (1x)
Cl. de With (2x)
J. Levier (13x)
N. Maas (2x)
P. Maidens
J. Meichman (1x) F. Michault (6x)
F. Michault (6x), C. van Outers
P. van Leeuwen (4x)
P.W. Lammens (2x)
P. Uldering (1x)
Th. Van Rhee (1x)
D. Reguleth (19x)
J. Reijssens (1x)
F. Robbé (4x)
L. Rolff (12x)
S.L. Garnison (2x)
L.W. van Schellebeek (3x)
H. Scheltus (16x)
C. Schoute (10x)
J. Seullijn (7x)
A. Smoelnaar (1x)
C. Veenendaal (5x)
F. Verboom (3x)
A.C. Verspeijck(6x)
A. Veth (1x)
J. van Visvliet (8x)
J. van der Voort (8x)
W. Huijsen (1x)
W. Wargaren (7x)
C. Wetgen (1x)
A. Wickelhuijsen (3x)
C. van der Wijngaart (1x)
R.J. Wiltens (2x)
A.J. Zalle (15x)

Appendix 4. Ship's surgeons who died on board and whose collection of books is listed

Name	*Rank*	*Date of death*	*Books*	*Source*
Abbing, J.	First surgeon	16/5/1723	Two Bibles	VOC 5794
Winter, J. de	First surgeon	28/10/1742	Some books	VOC 12.993
Veltjes, G.	First surgeon	22/11/1743	Some books	VOC 14.435
Mester, W.A.	First Surgeon	24/1/1745	11 medical books	VOC 6170
Bello, W.	First surgeon	22/7/1745	Some books	VOC 6173
Roelofsz, J.	First surgeon	17/1/1748	Some old books and a New Testament	VOC 6219
Sorgen, C. van	First surgeon	7/4/1754	11 surgical books	VOC 13.071
Hulst, H. van der	First surgeon	14/11/1755	Several books	VOC 14.773
Verzeijl, J.	First surgeon	9/3/1756	Bible	VOC 14.775
Weemeijer, H.	First surgeon	29/11/1764	Two black books	VOC 14.475
Ulman, M.	First surgeon	21/12/1764	58 books	VOC 6447
Elikman, L.	First surgeon	25/1/1766	Some books	VOC 6464
Brauns, C.	First surgeon	20/6/1769	Two books	VOC 6524
Stilzer, J.W.	First surgeon	31/10/1770	German books	VOC 14.489
Cate, B. ten	First surgeon	23/8/1773	Some books	VOC 14.496
Meijer, J.F. (MD)	First surgeon	24/9/1782	Six books	VOC 14.510
Neiman, J.	First surgeon	20/4/1786	Spiritual books	VOC 14.514
Jager, Christoph	Hospitalier	19/2/1789	Various	VOC 14.813
Kemp, H. van der	Surgeon's mate	6/11/1719	Some books	VOC 14.139
Piscator, H.	Surgeon's mate	21/1/1740	Some books	VOC 6096

Curvemaker, J.	Surgeon's mate	17/1/1752	Some books	VOC 14.764
Gouwenaar, Jan	Surgeon's mate	16/8/1752	Surgical	VOC 14.766
Name	*Rank*	*Date of death*	*Books*	*Source*
Hink, P.E.	Surgeon's mate	8/3/1755	Some books	VOC 6296
Dake, Jan	Surgeon's mate	29/11/1758	14 books	VOC 14.466
Belkol, W.	Surgeon's mate	24/3/1759	40 books	VOC 6378
Willemsvaart, J.	Surgeon's mate	15/1/1766	Some books	VOC 6464
Maas, F.	Surgeon's mate	26/2/1769	Four books	VOC 6507
Roger, Isaak	Surgeon's mate	31/10/1770	Some books	VOC 6540
Scharl, B.	Surgeon's mate	25/12/1770	Several books	VOC 6536
Keijser, Jan	Surgeon's mate	14/9/1782	35 books	VOC 14.510

Mellingen, J. van	Third surgeon	07/04/1721	Some books	VOC 5767
Bovet, J.	Third surgeon	6/3/1722	Surgical books	VOC 5891
Twent, S.H.	Third surgeon	20/6/1734	Some old books	VOC 5590
Vernerius, J.	Third surgeon	1/4/1738	Some books	VOC 6086
Walmeester, S.	Third Surgeon	11/10/1752	Bible	VOC 14.866
Josse, Pieter	Third surgeon	21/9/1762	Some books	VOC 6401
Boom, Claas	Third surgeon	14.4.1763	15 books	VOC 14.787
Sande, P. van de	Third surgeon	13/7/1763	Some books	VOC 6424
Sion, J.G.	Third surgeon	15/1/1766	Five books	VOC 6464
Weijers, M.	Third surgeon	27/11/1768	Surgical books	VOC 14.486
Worms, W.	Third surgeon	3/1/1771	Several old books	VOC 6536
Swart, H.	Third surgeon	4/3/1774	Some old books	VOC 6592
Anspach, J.C.	Third surgeon	21/2/1779	Some books	VOC 6672

Appendix 5. Ship's surgeons who died on board and were in the possession of instruments

Name	*Rank*	*Date of death*	*Instruments*	*Source*
J. Abbing	First surgeon	16/5/1723	1 long box with surgical instrument; 50 needles	VOC 5794
W. Belkol	First surgeon	24/7/1729	Some surgical instruments; 4 lancets; 1 silver cylinder for lancets; and 4 lancets	VOC 6378
J. de Winter	First surgeon	28/10/1742	Some instruments	VOC 12.993
W.A. Mester	First surgeon	24/1/1745	1 box with instruments	VOC 6170
B. Enema	First surgeon	9/2/1745	1 chest with surgical instruments; some medicines	VOC 14.746
R. Fokking	First surgeon	5/1/1747	3 chests with instruments; 3 cylinders with instruments	VOC 14.438
J. Roelofsz	First surgeon	17/1/1748	1 cylinder with small instruments; 1 silver catheter; 12 pair of tweezers (*prince en princetten*)	VOC 6219
J.F. Muller	First surgeon	12/9/1750	Small box with weights	VOC 6257
C. van Sorgen	First surgeon	7/4/1754	Box with instruments: 1 knife for the trepan; 1 syringe; 1 silver *signatorium*, 1 silver *lenghsigklaer (?);* 1 iron needle; 2 pieces of steel; 1 pair of iron forceps for molars; 1 pair of iron forceps; 2 pairs of scissors; 2 pairs of forceps; 2 scrapers; 1 dental instrument; 1 saw; 1 small saw; 1 curved saw; 1 knife, 2 ball-scoops, 3 gauges (*brandijzertjes*).	VOC 13.071
Jan Verzijl	First surgeon	9/3/1756	1 box of instruments	VOC 14.475

Name	*Rank*	*Date of death*	*Instruments*	*Source*
H.D. Weemeijer	First surgeon	29/11/1764	1 box with surgical instruments; 4 lancets; 1 iron syringe; 2 silver gauges (*sondeerijzers*); 1 box with surgical instruments; 2 lancets; 1 *hultor-lenticularis* (spectacles?); 1 key belonging to the trepan; 3 crowns; 1 perforative; 1 depressor; 2 *elevatoriums*; 2 bone-rasps; 1 small chisel; 1 trocard; 1 trepan; 1 saw; 1 syringe	VOC 14.475
M. Ulman	First surgeon	21/12/1764	1 small bag with surgical instruments; 1 silver spatula; 1 silver catheter; 1 small cylinder with 13 lancets; 1 small cylinder with 12 surgical instruments; many medicines (Sal. Sedlicense; Berlin Blue; Cortex Peruvian; white vitriol; Resina Jalappa (root of jalap from which one could make powder of Jalap); Spanish green; Spanish flies; salsaparilla; Oculi cancrie; Fol. Sennae)	VOC 6447
L. Elikman	First surgeon	25/1/1766	1 small cylinder with 6 silver lancets; 1 bag filled with five instruments of steel; 1 tourniquet; one small box with instruments; 2 small black cylinders with 7 lancets; 6 pair of pincers; 2 silver instruments.	VOC 6464

Name	*Rank*	*Date of death*	*Instruments*	*Source*
C. Brauns	First surgeon	20/6/1769	1 wooden chest with 4 gauges (*sondeer ijzers)*; 4 ball scoops; 1 curved pair of forceps; 1 surgical knife; 1 curved knife; 1 straight pair of forceps; 1 trepan with 2 forceps; 1 pair of curved scissors; 1 lancet; 1 probe; 1 pair of silver forceps; 1 cylinder with six lancets; 1 pair of forceps; 3 irons for trepaning; 1 small saw; 1 saw with 2 blades; 1 syringe; 1 curved ball scoop, 1 silver catheter, 1 pair of forceps, 1 pair of straight scissors; 2 spatula; 1 silver spatula; 2 spatula; 2 lancets; 1 tourniquet; 1 dental screw.	VOC 6524
J.W. Stilzer	First surgeon	31/10/1770	1 box with 4 lancets; 1 syringe of tin for clistering; 1 box with surgical instruments; 1 cylinder with iron syringes; 1 box with pieces of iron; 6 pieces of iron	VOC 14.489
E. Lambert	First surgeon	29/1/1771	Some surgical instruments	VOC 6350
B. ten Cate	First surgeon	23/8/1773	1 small bag with surgical instruments	VOC 14.496
J.F. Meijer	First surgeon	24/9/1782	Chest of instruments with 5 lancets and 3 silver instruments; 3 scissors, small box with 27 surgical instruments.	VOC 14.510
J. Neiman	First surgeon	20/4/1786	Lancets	VOC 14.514
Chr.G. Jager	Hospitalier	19/2/1789	1 box with some surgical instruments (sold for five guilders); 1 medical chest; one operating table	VOC 14.813

Name	*Rank*	*Date of death*	*Instruments*	*Source*
W. Meijer	Surgeon's mate	1/11/1719	1 cylinder with instruments	VOC 5742
H. van der Kemp	Surgeon's mate	6/11/1719	Box with surgical instruments	VOC 14.139
J. Gouwenaar	Surgeon's mate	16/8/1752	1 cylinder with 4 lancets; 1 cylinder for ointments; some instruments; 1 cylinder with instruments	VOC 14.766
P.E. Hink	Surgeon's mate	8/3/1755	Some surgical instruments	VOC 6296
J. van Willemsvaart	Surgeon's mate	15/1/1766	Some surgical instruments; 1 scissor; 1 silver spatula	VOC 6464
V. Maas	Surgeon's mate	26/2/1769	1 small bag with instruments	VOC 6507
B. Scharl	Surgeon's mate	25/12/1770	1 box with instruments	VOC 6536
J. van Melligem	Third surgeon	7/4/1721	1 cylinder with surgical instruments	VOC 5767
J. Bovet	Third surgeon	6/3/1722	1 cylinder with instruments; several surgical instruments	VOC 5891
S.H. Twent	Third surgeon	20/6/1734	4 lancets; 1 syringe; 1 cylinder for instruments; 1 pelican (dental forceps)	VOC 5990
H.H. Henke	Third surgeon	27/3/1741	Cylinder with instruments	VOC 6066
N. Lameij	Third surgeon	10/7/1745	1 pair of dental forceps; 2 lancets	VOC 14.433
Chr. Nasbij	Third surgeon	13/1/1751	Some instruments	VOC 6552
P. Josse	Third surgeon	21/9/1762	1 small box with instruments	VOC 6401
C. Boom	Third surgeon	14.4.1763	Three surgical instruments	VOC 14.787
P. van der Sande	Third surgeon	13/7/1763	1 small box with instruments; 1 box with ointments	VOC 6424

Name	*Rank*	*Date of death*	*Instruments*	*Source*
J.G. Sion	Third surgeon	15/1/1766	Some surgical instruments	VOC 6464
M. Weijers	Third surgeon	27/11/1768	Some instruments	VOC 14.486
W. Worms	Third surgeon	3/1/1771	1 small bag with instruments	VOC 6536
H. Swart	Third surgeon	4/3/1774	1 box with instruments	VOC 6592
J.C. Anspach	Third surgeon	21/2/1779	Some surgical instruments	VOC 6672
J. Spies	Third surgeon	28/4/1720	3 lancets	VOC 5738

Archives and bibliography

Arsip Nasional, Jakarta (*National Archives Indonesia, Jakarta*):
- J.A. van der Chijs, Inventaris van 's Lands-Archief
  Resolutie Hospitalen 1766-1768;
  Testamenten;

Westfries Archief (*Westfrisian Archive, Hoorn*),
- Gerechterlijk Archief Hoorn: Keuren en Ordonnantiën
- Doop-, Trouw-, en Begraafregisters Hoorn van 1581 tot en met 1811 (*Registers of births, deaths and marriages 1581-1811*)
- Chirurgijnsarchief Hoorn (*Surgeons' Guild Hoorn*)
- Doop, Trouw en Begraafregisters Enkhuizen (*Registers of births, deaths and marriages Enkhuizen*)
- Handtvesten, privilegien, willekeuren ende ordonnantien der stadt Enckhuysen (Enckhuysen, Egbert van den Hoof, 1667)

Nationaal Archief, Den Haag (*National Archives the Netherlands, The Hague*)
- De Archieven van de Verenigde Oostindische Compagnie, 1602-1811 (*Archives of the Dutch East India Company, 1602-1811*)
- Archief Radermacher (*Archives of the Radermacher family*)

Gemeente Archief, Amsterdam (*Municipal Archives, Amsterdam*)
- Doop-, Trouw- en Begraafregisters (*Registers of births, deaths and marriages*)
- Chirurgijnsgilde (*Surgeons' Guild*)
- Brouwerscollege (*Brewers' Association*)

Rijksmuseum Scheepvaartmuseum Amsterdam (*Maritime Museum, Amsterdam*)
- A.0451(39) nr.0014

Kennemerlandarchief (*Municipal Archives Haarlem 'Kennemerland'*)
- Collectie Doop-, Trouw- en Begraafregisters (*Registers of births, deaths and marriages*)
- Chirurgijnsgilde archief (*Surgeons' Guild Archives*)

Gemeentearchief Delft (*Municipal Archives Delft*)

- Collectie Doop-, Trouw- en Begraafregisters circa 1367-1811 (*Registers of births, deaths and marriages*). These registers have been consulted online on: www.archief.delft.nl.

Gemeentearchief Rotterdam (*Municipal Archives Rotterdam*)

- Collectie Doop-, Trouw- en Begraafregisters (*Registers of births, deaths and marriages*) These registers have been consulted online on: www.gemeente archief.rotterdam.nl
- Chirurgijnsgildearchief (*Surgeons' Guild archives*)

Gemeentearchief Arnhem (*Municipality Archives Arnhem*)

- Collectie Doop-, Trouw- en Begraafregisters (*Registers of births, deaths and marriages*)

Gemeentearchief Utrecht (*Municipality Archives Utrecht*)

- Collectie Doop-, Trouw- en Begraafregisters (*Registers of births, deaths and marriages*)

Public Records Office, Kew, London

- Records of the High Court of Admiralty and colonial Vice-Admiral courts

The genealogical database of The Church of Jesus Christ of Latter-day Saints (the Mormons, Salt Lake City) (http://www.familysearch.org/)

Several municipal archives have 'linked' their primary sources (registers of births, deaths, and marriages) to the genealogical database of Gensdata (S)ISIS, which can be found on http://www.gensdata.nl/sisis. Other primary sources may be found on : http://geneaknowhow.net/digi/bronnen.html

Bibliography

Grell, O.P., and A. Cunningham, *Health Care and Poor Relief in Protestant Europe 1500-1700* (London, 1997).

Acda, G.M.W., *Voor en achter de mast. Het leven van de zeeman in de zeventiende en achttiende eeuw* (Bussum, 1976).

Actes du Xième Colloque Franco-Allemand d'Histoire de la Médecine Navale et d'Outre-Mer (Paris, 1987), no. IX.

Actes du Xième Colloque Franco-Allemand d'Histoire de la Médecine Navale et d'Outre-Mer (Hambourg, 1988), no. XII.

Aerts, R. and L. Hoogkamp, *De Gelderse Pallas. Gymnasium Illustre. Gelderse Universiteit. Rijksathenaeum te Harderwijk 1600-1800* (Barneveld, 1986).

Alsop, J.D., 'Sea-surgeons, Health and England's Maritime Expansion: The West African Trade 1553-1660', *The Mariner's Mirror*, 76 (1990) 3, 215-221.

Alsop, J.D., 'Sickness in the British Mediterranean fleet: The Tiger's Journal of 1706', *War & Society*, 11 (October 1993) 2, 57-76.

Anderson, Ph., *The English in Western India; being the early history of the factory at Surat, of Bombay, and the subordinate factories on the Western coast* (London, 1854).

Annema, J.T., 'Het erfrecht in Friesland', *Jaarboek van het Centraal Bureau voor Genealogie*, 55 (2001).

Arnold, D. (ed.) *Warm Climates and Western Medicine: The emergence of tropical medicine 1500-1900* (Amsterdam, 1996).

Asaert, G. et al, *Maritieme Geschiedenis der Nederlanden* (Bussum, 1976-1978), 4 vols..

Aymard, M. (ed.), *Dutch Capitalism and World Capitalism* (Cambridge University Press, 1982)

Bala, P., *Imperialism and Medicine in Bengal. A Social-Historical Perspective* (New Delhi, 1991).

Ballintijn, G., *Rumphius, de blinde ziener van Ambon* (Wormerveer, **s.a.**).

Barend-van Haeften, M., *Oost-Indië Gespiegeld. Nicolaas de Graaf, een schrijvend chirurgijn in dienst van de VOC* (Zutphen, 1992).

Barge, J.A.J., 'Het geneeskundig onderwijs aan de Leidse universiteit in de 18e eeuw', *Nederlands Tijdschrijft van Geneeskunde*, 78, I (1934) 1, 47-69.

Basham, A.L., *The Wonder that was India* (New York, 1959).

Baumann, E.D., *Uit drie eeuwen Nederlandse geneeskunde* (Amsterdam, 1952).

Beers, J.K. and C. Bakker, *Westfriezen naar de Oost. De kamers der VOC te Hoorn en Enkhuizen en hun recruteringsgebied 1700-1800* (Schagen, 1990).

Bethlehem, J., and A.C. Meijer (eds.), *VOC en Cultuur. Wetenschappelijke en culturele relaties tussen Europa en Azië ten tijde van de Verenigde Oostindische Compagnie* (Amsterdam, 1993).

Beukers, H., and A.M. Luyendijk-Elshout et al (eds.), *Red-Hair Medicine. Dutch-Japanese Medical Relations*, Nieuwe Nederlandse Bijdragen tot de Geschiedenis der Geneeskunde en der Natuurwetenschappen 36 (Amsterdam, 1991).

Bik, J.G.W.F., *Vijf eeuwen medisch leven in een Hollandse stad* (Assen, 1955).

Blake, N.F. (ed.), *The Canterbury Tales by Geoffrey Chaucer* (London, 1980).

Blussé, J.L et al (eds), *De Dagregisters van het kasteel Zeelandia, Taiwan 1629-1662*, 4 vols. (The Hague, 1986-2000).

Blussé, J.L., *Strange Company: Chinese Settlers, mestizo women and the Dutch in VOC Batavia* (Leiden, 1986).

Blussé, L., *Bitters bruid. Een koloniaal huwelijksdrama in de Gouden Eeuw* (Amsterdam, 1997).

Blussé, L., 'Doctor at Sea: Chou Mei-yeh's voyage to the West (1710-1711)', in De

Poorter, E. (ed.), *As the Twig is bent ... Essays in honour of Frits Vos* (Amsterdam, 1990), 7-30.

Boekenoogen, G.J., 'Namen en wapens van Leidsche Chirurgijns', *Leids Jaarboekje* (Leiden, 1929), 79-101.

Bonke, H., *De zeven reizen van de Jonge Lieve. Biografie van een VOC-schip, 1760-1761* (Nijmegen, 1999).

Bontekoe, C., *Alle de philosophische, medicinische, chymische werken* (Amsterdam, 1698).

Bontekoe, Willem IJsbrantsz, *Journaal ofte gedenkwaardige beschrijvinge, wegens de wonderbaerlijke Oost-Indische reijze, van Willem Ysebrants Bontekoe van Hoorn, begrijpende veel wonderlijke ende gevaarlijke zaaken, hem op dezelve reijse wedervaren: Begonnen den 18. december 1618 ende voleijnd den 16. november 1625* (Hoorn, 1646).

Bontius, J., *De Medicina Indorum* (Leiden, 1642).

Boockmann, H. et al, *Mitten in Europa. Deutsche Geschichte* (Berlin, 1984).

Boog Watson, W.N., 'The plague on HMS "Theseus", Jaffa 1799', *Journal of the Royal Naval Medical Service,*. 56 (1970), 260-264.

Boog Watson, W.N., 'Thomas Robertson, Naval Surgeon, 1793-1828', *Bulletin of the History of Medicine* 46 (1972), 131-149.

Boomgaard, P, R. Sciortino, and I. Smyth (eds.), *Health care in Java. Past en present* (Leiden, 1996).

Boomgaard, P., 'Smallpox, vaccination, and the Pax Neerlandica Indonesia, 1550-1930', *Bijdragen tot de Taal-, Land- en Volkenkunde (Journal of the Humanities and Social Sciences of Southeast Asia and Oceania)* 159, 2003, 4: 590-617.

Boon, P., *Bouwers van de zee: zeevarenden van het Westfriese platteland, c. 1680-1720* (Leiden, 1996).

Boucher, M., 'The Cape Passage: Some observations on health hazards about Dutch East Indiamen outward-bound', *Historia, Amptelijke orgaan van die Historiese Genootschap van Suid-Afrika*, 26 (1981), 1, 24-36.

Boxer, C.R., 'The Carreira da India, 1650-1750', *Mariners Mirror* 46 (1960) 1-10.

Boxer, C.R., 'The Dutch East-Indiamen: Their sailors, their navigators, and life on board, 1602-1795', *Mariner's Mirror*, 49 (1963), 81-104.

Boxer, C.R., *The Dutch Seaborne Empire 1600-1800* (London, 1973).

Boxer, C.R., *The Portuguese Seaborne Empire 1418-1825* (London, 1969).

Brans, P.H., 'Beiträge zur Geschichte der Schiffspharmazie in den Niederlanden und in Niederländische Indien', *Veröffentlichungen des Internationale Geschichte des Pharmazie N.F.*, 13 (1958), 59-71.

Brans, P.H., 'De geneesmiddelenvoorziening bij de admiraliteiten en bij de Oost-Indische Compagnie', *Pharmaceutisch Weekblad* 98 (1963), 596-608.

Brans, P.H., 'Overzicht van de geschiedenis der pharmacie in Nederlands Oost-Indië', *Pharmaceutisch Weekblad* 47/48 (1951), 841-880.

Breedveld, P.H. and J.L.M. Hendrix, *Het Journaal van de scheepschirurgijn J.W. Daman (1735-1783). Gezondheid en ziekte aan boord van een Oostindiëvaarder* (Nijmegen, 1987), Scripta Tironum 12.

Breuker, Ph.H., and A. Janse, *Negen eeuwen Friesland-Holland. Geschiedenis van een haat-liefde verhouding* (Leeuwarden, 1997).

Broeze, F.J.A, Bruijn, J.R., and F.S. Gaastra (eds.), *Maritieme Geschiedenis der Nederlanden* III (Bussum, 1977).

Brouwer Ancher, A.J.M., 'Oude ordonnantiën betreffende genees-, heel-, en verloskundigen, apothekers, kwakzalvers enz.', *Nederlands Tijdschrift voor Geneeskunde* 25 (1899), 1173-1197.

Bruford, W.H., *Germany in the eighteenth century. The social background of the literary revival* (Cambridge, 1959).

Bruijn, I.D.R. and G.W. Bruijn, 'An eighteenth century medical hearing and the first observation of Tropical Phagedaena', *Medical History* 35 (1991) 3, 295-307.

Bruijn, I.D.R., 'The Health Care Organization of the Dutch East India Company at Home', *Social History of Medicine* 7 (1994) 3, 359-382.

Bruijn, J.R. and F.S. Gaastra (eds.), *Ships, Sailors and Spices, East India Companies and their Shipping in the Sixteenth, Seventeenth and Eighteenth Centuries* (Amsterdam, 1993), NEHA Series III.

Bruijn, J.R. and J. Lucassen, *Op de Schepen der Oost-Indische Compagnie: vijf artikelen van J. de Hullu* (Groningen, 1980).

Bruijn, J.R., 'Commandanten van Oost-Indiëvaarders in de achttiende eeuw', *Tijdschrift voor Zeegeschiedenis* 20 (2001) 1, 4-14.

Bruijn, J.R., 'De personeelsbehoefte van de VOC overzee en aan boord, bezien in Aziatisch en Nederlands perspectief', *Bijdragen en Mededelingen voor de Geschiedenis der Nederlanden* XCI (1976), 218-248.

Bruijn, J.R., 'Dutch Men-of-War. Those on board c. 1700-1750', *Acta Historiae Neerlandicae; Studies on the History of the Netherlands* (The Hague, 1974), 88-119.

Bruijn, J.R., and E.S. van Eck van Heslinga, *Muiterij, oproer en berechting op de schepen van de VOC* (Haarlem, 1980).

Bruijn, J.R., Gaastra, F.S., and I. Schöffer (eds.), *Dutch-Asiatic Shipping in the Seventeenth and Eighteenth Centuries,* Rijks Geschiedkundige Publicatiën, Grote Serie 165 (The Hague, 1987), vol. I Introductory volume.

Bruijn, J.R., Gaastra, F.S., and I. Schöffer (eds.), *Dutch-Asiatic Shipping in the Seventeenth and Eighteenth Centuries,* Rijks Geschiedkundige Publicatiën, Grote Serie 166 (The Hague, 1979), vol. II Outward-bound voyages from the Netherlands to Asia and the Cape (1595-1794).

Bruijn, J.R., Gaastra, F.S., and I. Schöffer (eds.), *Dutch-Asiatic Shipping in the Seventeenth and Eighteenth Centuries,* Rijks Geschiedkundige Publicatiën,

Grote Serie 167 (The Hague, 1979), vol. III Homeward-bound voyages from Asia and the Cape to the Netherlands (1597-1795).

Bruijn, J.R., *The Dutch Navy of the Seventeenth and Eighteenth Centuries* (Colombia, 1993).

Burema, L., *De voeding in Nederland van de middeleeuwen tot de twintigste eeuw* (Assen, 1953).

Burrows, E.H., *A History of Medicine in South Africa up to the End of the Nineteenth Century* (Cape Town/Amsterdam, 1958).

Carré, A, and J. Siré, 'Hygiène navale et fièvre des vaisseaux au XVIIIe siècle. Une épidémie mal connue: celle de l'escadre de M. de Leclue en 1783', *Revue des corps de santé* 5 (1964), 3, 305-323.

Carré, A., 'Suffren: Aspects médicaux de la campagne des Indes', *Revue de l'Histoire des Armées* 154 (1984), 112-117.

Carrubba, R.W., 'The Latin document confirming the date and institution of Wilhem ten Rhyne's M.D.', *Gesnerus* 3 / 4 (1982) 39, 473-477.

Cates, G.L., 'The voyage: a study of medical hazards on the first immigrant ships to Georgia', *Journal of the Medical Association of Georgia*, 68 (Sept 1969), 831-834.

Chaloner, E.J., Flora, H.S., and R.J. Ham, 'Amputations at the London Hospital 1852-1857', *Journal of the Royal Society of Medicine*, 94 (August 2001), 409-412.

Chaucer, G., *Canterbury Tales* (London, 1928).

Chaudhuri, K.N., *The English East India Company* (London, 1965).

Clendening, Logan (ed.), *Source Book of Medical History.* Compiled with Notes by Logan Clendening (Mineola, New York, 1960).

Coclanis, P., 'Military mortality in Tropical Asia: British troops in Tenasserim, 1827-36', *Journal of Southeast Asian Studies* 30 (1999) 1, 22-37.

Conrad, L.E., et al, *The Western Medical Tradition: 800 BC to AD 1800* (Cambridge, 1996).

Cook, H.J., *The Decline of the Old Medical Regime in Stuart London* (Ithaca, NY, 1986).

Cook, H.J., *Trials of an Ordinary Doctor: Joannes Groenevelt in Seventeenth-Century London* (London, 1994).

Crawford, D.G., *A History of the Indian Medical Service 1600-1913*, 2 vols. (London, 1914).

Crosby, A.W., *Ecological Imperialism. The Biological Expansion of Europe, 900-1900* (Cambridge, 1986).

Curtin, P.D., *Death by Migration: Europe's Encounter with the Tropical World in the Nineteenth Century* (Cambridge, 1989).

Curtin, P.D., *The World & the West: The European Challenge and the Overseas Response in the Age of Empire* (Cambridge, 2000).

Dalat, J., 'Un chirurgien de mer à la fin du XVIIIe siècle', *Revue d'Histoire de la Pharmacie* XXX, 259 (1983), 275-281.

Dalrymple, W., *White Mughals: Love and Betrayal in Eighteenth-Century India* (London, 2003).
De Blécourt, A.S., and H.F.W.D. Fischer, *Kort begrip van het oud-vaderlands burgerlijk recht* (Groningen, 1950).
De Gorter, J., *Nieuwe Gezuiverde Heelkonst* (Leiden, 1746).
De Graaf, D., 'De Koninklijke Compagnie. De Pruisische Aziatische Compagnie 'von Emden nach China' (1751-1765)', *Tijdschrift voor zeegeschiedenis* 20 (2001) 143-162.
De Graaff, H.J., 'Nederlandsch-Indische Historiografie', *Koloniaal Tijdschrift* 29 (1940) 548-569.
De Jong, J.J., *Met goed fatsoen: de elite in een Hollandse stad (Gouda 1700-1780)* (Amsterdam, 1986)
De Moor, J.A., and P.G.E.I.J. van der Velde (eds.), *De werken van Jacob Haafner*, 3 vols. (Zutphen, 1992-1997).
De Moulin, D. (ed.), *s-Rijkskweekschool voor Militaire Geneeskundigen te Utrecht (1822-1865). Verslag van een symposium gehouden te Nijmegen op 26 september 1987*, Nieuwe Nederlandse Bijdragen tot de Geschiedenis der Geneeskunde en der Natuurwetenschappen 26.
De Moulin, D., *A History of Surgery with Emphasis on the Netherlands* (Dordrecht, 1988).
De Ridder, J., 'Van aderlatingen en amputaties. Chirurgijns, barbiers en *doctores medicinae* op Walcheren', *De Wete*, 30 (2001) 1, 21-27.
De Vries, J., and A. van der Woude, *The First Modern Economy: Success, Failure, and Perseverance of the Dutch Economy, 1500-1815* (Cambridge, 1997).
De Vries, J., *De economische achteruitgang der Republiek in de achttiende eeuw* (Leiden, 1968).
De Wet, G.C. (ed.), *Resolusies van die Politieke Raad, V: 1716-1719* (Kaapstad, 1964).
Dekkers, O. (ed.), *Een Bunschoter VOC-chirurgijn. 'Dagelijkse aantekeningen; van de reis naar Oost-Indië in 1654 door Gijsbert Heeck (1619-1669)* (Bunschoten, 2001).
Dessert, Daniel, *La Royale. Vaisseaux et marins du Roi-Soleil* (s.l., 1996).
Diederiks, H.A., et al, *Van agrarische samenleving naar verzorgingsstaat* (Groningen, 1994).
Diffie, B.W. and G.D. Winius, *Foundations of the Portuguese Empire, 1415-1580*, I (Minneapolis, 1978).
Dillo, I.G., *De nadagen van de Verenigde Oostindische Compagnie, 1783-1795. Schepen en Zeevarenden* (Amsterdam, 1992).
Dolmans, M.Th.R.M., 'Militaire hospitalen in het Romeinse rijk', *Geschiedenis der Geneeskunde* I (1983), 19-26.
Dorland's Pocket Medical Dictionary (Philadelphia, 1982).

Dorren, G., *Eenheid en verscheidenheid. De burgers van Haarlem in de Gouden Eeuw* (Amsterdam, 2001).
Doulan, P., 'The Dutch in Japan', *History Today*, vol. 50 (4) (2000), 36-42.
Duffin, J., *History of Medicine: A Scandalously Short Introduction* (London, 2001).
Dulieu, L., 'Pierre Chirac et les maladies des équipages des vaisseaux', *Revue de l'Histoire des Sciences* 37 (1984), 65-70.
Earles, M.P., 'A case of mass poisoning with mercury vapour on board H.M.S. "Triumph" at Cadiz, 1810', *Medical History* 8 (1964), 281-286.
Eijck, J.A.M., *De gezondheidszorg te Breda voor 1700* (Nijmegen, 1990), Scripta Tironum 22.
Eloy, J., 'Relations de voyages de Charles-Ghislain Wilmet, chirurgien major à la Compagnie maritime des Indes Néerlandaises', in manuscript form, offered to the *Annuaire d'Histoires Regionales et Locales, Le Vieux Châtelet* (1984).
Ernst, W., and B. Harris, *Race, Science and Medicine, 1700-1960* (London, 1999).
Faber, J.A., *Drie eeuwen Friesland. Economische en sociale ontwikkelingen van 1500 tot 1800* (Wageningen, 1972), 2 vols., AAG Bijdragen 17
Faber, J.A., et al, 'Population changes and economic developments in the Netherlands, a historical survey', *AAG Bijdragen* 12 (Wageningen, 1965), 47-114.
Fabre, A., 'Les traditions de la médicine de l'avant', *Médicine et Armées* 8 (1980), 781-786.
Fischer, K.D., 'Arzneikisten. Die Schiffsapotheke im Wandel der Zeiten', *Jahrbuch der Schifffahrt* 1978.
Foster, W. (ed.), *The English Factories in India 1618-1669* (London, 1906-1927), 13 vols.
French, R., *Medicine before Science: The Business of Medicine from the Middle Ages to the Enlightenment* (Cambridge, 2003).
Frijhoff, W., and M. Spies, *1650 Bevochten Eendracht* (The Hague, 1999).
Gaastra, F.S., *Bewind en beleid bij de VOC 1672-1702* (Zutphen, 1989).
Gaastra, F.S., *De Geschiedenis van de VOC* (Haarlem, 1982).
Gabriel, R.A. and Karen S. Metz, *A History of Military Medicine* (Westport, 1992).
Garrison, F.H., *An Introduction to the History of Medicine* (Philadelphia and London, 1929).
Gawronski, J.H.G. (ed.) *Hollandia Compendium. A Contribution to the History, Archaeology, Classification and Lexicography of a 150 ft Dutch East Indiaman (1747-1750)* (Amsterdam, 1992).
Gawronski, J.H.G. (ed.), *Jaarrapport Stichting VOC-schip* (Amsterdam, 1986).
Gawronski, J.H.G., *De Hollandia en de Amsterdam: twee schepen en een bedrijf. Organisatie en materiële cultuur van de VOC in Amsterdam in de jaren 1740-1750* (Amsterdam, 1993), unpublished dissertation.
Gehlen, A.F., *Notariële akten uit de 17^e en 18^e eeuw: handleiding voor gebruikers* (Zutphen, 1986).

Gemert, Lia van (ed.), *Joh.v an Beverwijck. De schat der gezondheid* (Amsterdam, 1992).
Gessel, M. van, and A. Kieskamp (eds.), *Ongeluckig, of droevigh verhaal van 't schip de Gouden Buys 1695. Een Enkhuizer VOC-schip strandt bij zuidelijk Afrika* (Amsterdam, 1995).
Gijsberti Hodenpijl, A.K.A., 'De ziekten aan boord van de schepen van de Oost-Indische compagnie in de eerste helft van de achttiende eeuw', *Nederlandsch Tijdschrift voor Geneeskunde* 62 (1918) IB.
Gijsberti Hodenpijl, A.K.A., 'Het gebruik van inlandsche geneesmiddelen in den compagniestijd', *Nederlands Tijdschrift voor Geneeskunde* 66 (1922) II, 1651-1654.
Gijsberti Hodenpijl, A.KA., 'De scheurbuik (scorbut) op 's-Compagnies schepen uit het vaderland komende in het jaar 1730', *Nederlandsch Tijdschrift voor Geneeskunde* 66 (1922) I, 496-501.
Gijswijt-Hofstra, M. (ed.), *Op zoek naar genezing. Medische geschiedenis van Nederland vanaf de zestiende eeuw* (Amsterdam, 1995).
Godinho, V.M., 'The Portuguese and the Carreira da India' 1497-1810', in Bruijn, J.R. and F.S. Gaastra (eds.), *Ships, Sailors and Spices. East India Companies and their Shipping. The Sixteenth, Seventeenth and Eighteenth Centuries* (Amsterdam, 1993).
Gordon, E.C., 'Scurvy and Anson's voyage round the world: 1740-44. An Analysis of the Royal Navy's Worst Outbreak', *American Neptune* 44 (1984), 155-166.
Gosse, Ph., 'Sea surgeons', *Edinburgh Review or Critical Journal* 484 (April 1923), vol. 237, 319-330.
Granshaw, L. and R. Porter (eds.), *The Hospital in History* (London 1989).
Grell, O.P., and A. Cunningham (eds.), *Health Care and Poor Relief in Protestant Europe 1500-1700* (London, 1997).
Grooss, K.S., *Cornelis Solingen. Een zeventiende eeuwse chirurgijn en zijn instrumenten* (Leiden, 1990).
Groustra, F.N., and J.R. Bruijn, 'Een kentering in de gezondheid aan boord. Bataafse vloten naar Oost- en West-Indië, 1802', *Tijdschrift voor Zeegeschiedenis* 14 (1995) 1, 25-50.
Grubb, F., 'Morbidity and mortality on the North Atlantic passage: Eighteenth-century German immigration', *Journal of Interdisciplinary History* 17 (1987) 3, 565-585.
Gulik, T.M. van, 'The role of the Dutch in the introduction of Western surgery in feudal Japan', *Netherlands Journal of Surgery* 37 (1985) 6, 161-166.
Haan, F. de, *Uit de nadagen van de 'Loffelijke compagnie'. Een keuze uit de geschriften samengesteld door Rob Nieuwenhuys* (Amsterdam, 1984).
Hacquebord, L., *Smeerenburg. Het verblijf van Nederlandse walvisvaarders op de westkust van Spitsbergen in de zeventiende eeuw.* (Groningen, 1984).

Haggard, H.W., *Devils, Drugs & Doctors: The Story of the Science of Healing from Medicine-Man to Doctor* (New York, 1953).
Hallema, A., 'Iets over de organisatie van den geneeskundigen dienst en de inrichting der zoogenaamde medische politie ten plattelande gedurende de 18de eeuw', *Nederlands Tijdschrift voor Geneeskunde* 85 (1941) 3, 36, 3608-3615.
Haneveld, G.T., 'De Scheepsartsen van Columbus', *Arts & Auto*, 58, 1118-1119.
Haneveld, G.T., 'Medische aspecten van de slag bij Doggersbank', *Tijdschrift voor de Geschiedenis van Geneeskunde, Natuurwetenschappen, Wiskunde en Techniek* 5 (1982) 2, 78-88.
Hanna, W.A., *Indonesian Banda. Colonialism and Its Aftermath in the Nutmeg Islands* (s.l., s.a.).
Hart, S., *Schrift en Getal: een keuze uit de demografische-, economische- en sociaal-historische studiën op grond van Amsterdamse en Zaanse archivalia, 1600-1800* (Dordrecht, 1976).
Haudrère, Ph., 'Les flottes des Compagnies des Indes 1600-1857', *V Journées franco-brittanniques d'histoire de la marine. III Journées d'histoire maritime et d'archéologie navale* (Vincennes, 1996).
Haver-Droeze, J.J., 'De geneeskundige dienst bij de Nederlandsch-Oost-Indische Compagnie', *Nederlandsch Tijdschrift voor Geneeskunde* 65 (1921) 1, 2535-2560.
Heine, H., 'Das Sklavenschiff', *Sämtliche Werke* (Stuttgart, s.a.), II, (264).
Heine, H., 'Geständnisse, Memoiren und kleinere autobiographische Schriften bearbeitet von G. Heinemann' XV, *Historisch-kritische Gesamtausgabe der Werke* (Hamburg, 1982).
Heine, H., *Sämtliche Werke, in zwölf Bänden* VII (Leipzig, s.a.).
Hellinga, G., 'De Amsterdamsche gasthuizen beoordeeld door vreemdelingen I', *Nederlands Tijdschrift voor Geneeskunde* 76 (1932) II, 23, 2800-2817.
Hellinga, G., 'De Amsterdamsche gasthuizen, beoordeeld door vreemdelingen II', *Nederlands Tijdschrift voor Geneeskunde* 77 (1933) II, 1410-1424.
Hellinga, G., 'De Gasthuischirurgijns en de algemeene wijkvergadering. Episode uit de geschiedenis van het Amsterdamsche St. Pietersgasthuis in het eerste jaar der Bataafsche vrijheid', *Nederlands Tijdschrift voor Geneeskunde* 71 (1927) II, 23, 2370-2372.
Hellinga, G., 'De geschiedenis der geneeskundige armverzorging, buiten de gasthuizen te Amsterdam I', *Nederlands Tijdschrift voor Geneeskunde* 76 (1932) III, 4219-4235.
Hellinga, G., 'De geschiedenis der geneeskundige armverzorging, buiten de gasthuizen te Amsterdam II', *Nederlands Tijdschrift voor Geneeskunde* 77 (1933) I, 528-543.
Hellinga, G., 'Een en ander over de overeenkomsten aangegaan gedurende het tijdvak 1651-1699 tusschen regenten van het Amsterdamsche St. Pieters Gasten Pesthuis en cureerders', *Nederlands Tijdschrift voor Geneeskunde* 73 (1929) II, 36, 4141-4146.

Hellinga, G., 'Een en ander over de positie der 17de en 18de eeuwsche gasthuis-chirurgijns in Amsterdam', *Nederlands Tijdschrift voor Geneeskunde* 70 (1926) II, 30-41.

Hellinga, G., 'Een en ander over het aandeel van het Amsterdamsche St. Pietersgasthuis in vroeger tijden "logheeren, cureeren ende accommodeeren" van zieke en gewonde soldaten en matrozen', *Nederlands Tijdschrift voor Geneeskunde* 73 (1929) I, 1720-1731.

Hellinga, G., 'Een en ander over van oudsher ingeslopen misbruiken bij het opnemen van zieken in de Amsterdamsche gasthuizen, en de daartegen genomen maatregelen', *Nederlands Tijdschrift voor Geneeskunde* 68 (1924) II, 2230-2239.

Hellinga, G., 'Een en ander uit de geschiedenis der Amsterdamsche gasthuizen. Het Sint Pieters-Gasthuis en Pesthuis', *Nederlands Tijdschrift voor Geneeskunde* 67 (1923) I, 43-47.

Hellinga, G., 'Geschiedenis der geneeskundige armenverzorging buiten de gasthuizen te Amsterdam', *Nederlands Tijdschrift voor Geneeskunde* 77 (1933) I, 5, 528-543.

Hellinga, G., 'Het Amsterdamsche Dol- of Krankzinnigenhuis', *Nederlands Tijdschrift voor Geneeskunde* 76 (1932) II, 14, 1603-1620.

Heringa, J., et al, *Geschiedenis van Drenthe* (Meppel, 1985).

Hernández-Sáenz, L.M., 'Seamen, Surgeons and empire: Spanish naval medical reform and Mexican medicine in the late colonial period', *The Northern Mariner*, X, 1 (2000), 21-36.

Holland, B.K., 'Treatments for bubonic plague: reports from seventeenth century British epidemics', *Journal of the Royal Society of Medicine* 93 (2000), 322-324.

Horstmanshof, H.F.J., 'Galenus: produktief schrijver en scherpzinnig hofarts', *Leidraad* (April 1992), 13-14.

Houben, G.M.M., 'Medicinale gewichten', *Arts en Wereld* (1975), 59-69.

Houtzager, H.L. et al, *Delft en de Oost-Indische Compagnie* (Amsterdam, 1987).

Houtzager, H.L., and M.J. van Lieburg (eds.), *De Stichting Historia Medicinae 1967-1987* (Amsterdam, 1987).

Hovy, L. *Ceylonees Plakkaatboek. Plakkaten en andere wetten uitgevaardigd door het Nederlandse bestuur op Ceylon, 1638-1796* (Hilversum, 1991), 2 vols..

Howard, M.R., 'Red jackets and red noses: alcohol and the British Napoleonic soldier', *Journal of the Royal Society of Medicine* 93 (2000), 38-41.

Huard, P., 'La médecine navale Française aux XVIIe et XVIIIe siècles', *La Semaine des hôpitaux de Paris* 37 (20.23.1961), 3624-3626.

Huisman, F.G., *Stadsbesef en Stadsbelang. Gezondheidszorg en medisch beroep in Groningen, 1500-1730* (Amsterdam, 1992).

Huisman, T., *De vier gedaanten van de arts* (Leiden, Museum Boerhaave, s.a.).

Huizenga, E., *Tussen autoriteit en empirie. De Middelnederlandse chirurgieën in de veertiende en vijftiende eeuw en hun maatschappelijke context* (Hilversum, 2003).

Huizenga, E., *Tussen autoriteit en empirie. De Middelnederlandse chirurgieën in de veertiende en vijftiende eeuw en hun maatschappelijke context* (Hilversum, 2003).
Imhof, A.E., 'The hospital in the eighteenth century: for whom?', *Journal of Social History* 10 (1977), 4, 448-470.
Israel, J. I., *The Dutch Republic: Its Rise, Greatness, and Fall 1477-1806* (New York, 1995).
Israel, J.I., *Dutch Primacy in World Trade, 1585-1740* (Oxford, 1989).
Israel, J.I., *Nederland als centrum van de wereldhandel 1585-1740* (Franeker, 1991).
Jacobs, E.M., *Koopman in Azië. De handel van de Verenigde Oost-Indische Compagnie tijdens de achttiende eeuw* (Zutphen, 2000).
Jacobs, J., *Een zegenrijk gewest. Nieuw-Nederland in de zeventiende eeuw* (Amsterdam, 1999).
Jansen, H.P.H., *Middeleeuwse Geschiedenis der Nederlanden* (Utrecht, 1972).
Jensen, J.N.J., 'Van een Duitschen barbier op Hollandsche schepen in de 18^e^ eeuw', *Het Nederlandsche Zeewezen*, 22 (1916), 324-356.
Jetter, D., *Geschiedenis van de geneeskunde* (Zwolle, 1992).
Jobse-Van Putten, J., *Eenvoudig maar voedzaam. Cultuurgeschiedenis van de dagelijkse maaltijd in Nederland* (Nijmegen, 1995).
Johnson, S., *The Oxford Authors* (Oxford, 1984).
Jones, E., *Wives, whores, and concubines: Early modern Dutch marriage law and the transmission of family wealth in Asia* (Berkeley, 2000).
Jonkman, J., 'Collegium Medico-Pharmaceuticum te Enkhuizen in 1786', *Pharmaceutisch Weekblad*, 22 (1913), 641-646.
Kaiser, W., 'Der Marinearzt Louis Rouppe und sein Beitrag zur Medicina Nautica', *Janus* 61 (1974), 1-14.
Keay, J., *The Honourable Company; A History of the English East India Company* (London, 1991).
Keevil, J.J., Lloyd, Chr., and J.L.S. Coulter, *Medicine and the Navy 1200-1900*, 4 vols. (Edinburgh, 1957-1963).
Kerkhof, A.H.M., 'Over de geneeskundige verzorging in het Staatse leger', *Geschiedenis der Geneeskunde*, 5 (1998), 3, 143-148.
Kerkhof, A.H.M., *Over de geneeskundige verzorging in het Staatse leger* (Nijmegen, 1976).
Ketting, H., *De Amsterdamse chirurgijns: van ambacht naar professie, 1750-1798* (Amsterdam, 1988), unpublished masters thesis.
Ketting, H., *Leven, werk en rebellie aan boord van Oost-Indiëvaarders (1595-1650)* (Amsterdam, 2003).
Kipling, R., *Traffics and Discoveries* (London, 1904).
Kleiweg de Zwaan, J.P., 'Denkbeelden der inlanders van onzen Indischen archipel omtrent het ontstaan van ziekten', *Onze Koloniën*, series 10, no. 3 (Baarn, 1914).

Knotter, A., and J.L. van Zanden, 'Immigratie en arbeidsmarkt in Amsterdam in de zeventiende eeuw', *Tijdschrift voor Sociale Geschiedenis* 13 (1987) 4, 403-431.

Kolff, G., 'Realia register op de generale resolutien van het kasteel Batavia 1632-1805', *Uitgegeven door het Bataviaasch Genootschap van Kunsten en Wetenschappen*, 3 vols. (The Hague, 1882-1885).

Koninkx, C., 'L'alimentation et la pathologie des déficiences alimentaires dans la navigation au long cours au XVIIIe siècle', *Revue d'Histoire Moderne et Contemporaine* 30 (1983), 109-138.

Koninkx, C., 'Voeding op zee in de achttiende eeuw. Een kwantitatief en vergelijkend onderzoek', *Marine Academie Mededelingen* XXV (1978-1979), 3-23.

Koninkx, C., 'Ziekten op Zee. Pathologie van de Ziekten in de Grote Vaart in de Achttiende Eeuw', *Marine Academie Mededelingen* XXVI (1980-1981-1982), 33-54.

Koninkx, C., *Het eerste en tweede octrooi van de Zweeds Oost-Indische Compagnie (1731-1766)* (Brussel, 1975).

Koninkx, C., *The First and Second Charters of the Swedish East India Company (1731-1766)* (Kortrijk, 1980).

Kooijmans, L., *Onder regenten: de elite in een Hollandse stad. Hoorn 1700-1780* (Amsterdam, 1985).

Kool-Blokland, J.L., *De zorg gewogen. Zeven eeuwen godshuizen in Middelburg* (Middelburg, 1990).

Larsen, O., *Schiff und Seuche 1795-1799* (Oslo, 1968).

Lasagna, Louis, 'The Sea Disease', *The Sciences* (1980), 30-33.

Lattimore, M.I., 'Early naval medical libraries, personal and corporate', *Journal of the Royal Naval Medical Service.* 69 (1983), 156-160.

Lauw, G.M., *De Dokter Djawaschool* (Nijmegen, 1987), Scripta Trionum 9-10.

Lequin, F., *Het personeel van de VOC in Azië in de achttiende eeuw, meer in het bijzonder in de vestiging Bengalen* (Leiden, 1982).

Leuftink, A.E. *Chirurgijns Zee-Compas. De medische verzorging aan boord van Nederlandse zeeschepen gedurende de Gouden Eeuw* (Delft, 1963).

Leuftink, A.E., *De geneeskunde bij 's Lands oorlogsvloot in de 17e eeuw* (Assen, 1953).

Leuftink, A.E., *Harde heelmeesters. Zeelieden en hun dokters in de 18e eeuw* (Zutphen 1991).

Lindeboom, G.A., 'Medisch-wetenschappelijke betrekkingen tussen Noord- en Zuid-Nederland in vroeger dagen (15e-17e eeuw)', extrait du *Scalpel*, 21 (1958), 3-7.

Lindeman, R. et al (eds.), *Reisverslagen van Noord-Nederlanders uit de zestiende tot begin negentiende eeuw. Een chronologische lijst* (Rotterdam, 1994).

Lindemann, M., *Health & Society in Eighteenth Century Germany* (Baltimore, 1996).

Lindemann, M., *Medicine and Society in Early Modern Europe* (Cambridge, 1999).

Lloyd, Chr. (ed.), *The Health of Seamen. Selections from the works of Dr. James Lind, Sir Gilbert Blane and Dr. Thomas Trotter* (London, 1965).

Lloyd, Chr., 'The British Seaman 1200-1800', *Publications of the Navy Records Society*, vol. CVII (London, 1965).

Loudon, I.S.L., 'Leg ulcers in the eighteenth and early nineteenth centuries. II. Treatment', *Journal of the Royal College of General Practitioners* (1982), 301-309.

Lucassen, J., *Migrant Labour in Europe, 1600-1900* (London, 1987).

Lucassen, J., *Naar de kusten van de Noordzee. Trekarbeid in Europees Perspektief, 1600-1900* (Utrecht, 1984).

Lyons, A.S., and R.J. Petrucelli, *Medicine. An Illustrated History* (New York, 1987).

Major, R.H., *Classic Descriptions of Disease* (Illinois, 1939).

Massée, Cl., *Les chirurgiens navigants originaires des dioceses de Bordeaux et Bazas dans les écoles Saint-Côme entre 1752 et 1791* (s.l., s.a.)

McFee, W., *The Law of the Sea* (London, s.a.)

McNeil, W.H., *Plagues and Peoples* (New York, 1998).

Meilink-Roelofsz, M.A.P. et al, *De VOC in Azië* (Bussum, 1976).

Meilink-Roelofsz, M.A.P., et al, *Dutch authors on Asian History* (Dordrecht, 1988).

Merklein, Johann Jakob, *Reise nach Ostasien 1644-1653* (Windsheim, 1985).

Meulenbeld, G.J., and Dominik Wujastyk (eds.), *Studies on Indian Medical History: papers presented at the international workshop on the study of Indian medicine held at the Wellcome Institute for the History of Medicine* (Groningen, 1987).

Michel, W., *Von Leipzig nach Japan. Der Chirurg und Handelsmann Caspar Schamberger (1623-1706)* (Munich, 1999).

Mijnhardt, W.W. (ed), *Kantelend Geschiedbeeld. Nederlandse historiografie sinds 1945* (Utrecht, 1983).

Molière, J.B., *Le Malade Imaginaire* (Paris, 2002).

Mooij, A., *De Polslag van de stad. 350 jaar academische geneeskunde in Amsterdam* (Amsterdam 1999).

Moree, P., 'Predikanten en ziekentroosters aan boord van Rotterdamse Oost-Indiëvaarders', in: Van der Heijden, M., and P. van de Laar (eds.), *Rotterdammers en de VOC. Handelscompagnie, stad en burgers (1600-1800)* (Amsterdam, 2002), 161-180.

Nanninga-Uiterdijk, J., 'De geneeskunstbeoefenaren te Kampen I', *Bijdragen tot de Geschiedenis van Overijssel* 4 (1877), 26-60.

Napjus, J.W., 'De geneeskundige faculteit van de hoogeschool en Rijksathenaeum te Franeker 1585-1843', *Nederlands Tijdschrift voor Geneeskunde* 71 (1927) II, 1003-1027.

Nash, G., 'Naval Uniform', *Mariners Mirror* 41 (1956), 99.
Naval Chronicle 37 (1817).
Neuburger, M., *Geschichte der Medizin*, 2 Bände (Stuttgart, 1906).
O'Brian, P., *Master & Commander* (London, 1996).
Oberschelp, R., *Niedersachsen 1760-1820. Wirtschaft, Gesellschaft, Kultur in Land Hanover und Nachbargebieten* (Hildesheim, 1982), 2 vols., Veröffentlichungen der historischen Kommission für Niedersachsen und Bremen. XXXV Quellen und Untersuchungen zur allgemeiner Geschichte Niedersachsens in der Neuzeit, Band 4, I, and II.
Owen, D.D.R., *Eleanor of Aquitaine. Queen and Legen* (Oxford, 1993).
Owen, N.G. (ed.), *Death and Disease in Southeast Asia: Explorations in Social, Medical and Demographic History* (Oxford, 1987).
Pabbruwe, H.J., *Dr. Robertus Padtbrugge (Parijs 1637-Amersfoort 1703) Dienaar van de Verenigde Oost-Indische Compagnie, en zijn familie* (Kloosterzande, s.a.).
Page Moch, L., *Moving Europeans: Migration in Western Europe since 1650* (Bloomington, 1992).
Palmer, R., and J. Colton, *A History of the Modern World* (New York, 1978).
Paranavitana, K.D., 'Medical establishment in Sri Lanka during the Dutch period (1640-1796)', *The Journal of the Royal Asiatic Society of Sri Lanka* XXXIII (A.S. 1988/89), 103-110.
Patterson, T.J.S., 'The medical practice of the East India Company', *Society for the Social History of Medicine Bulletin* 26 (Oxford, 1980), 40-44.
Patterson, T.J.S., 'The relationship of Indian and European practitioners of medicine from the sixteenth century', in *Studies on Indian Medical History*, Meulenbeld, G.J. and D. Wuyastyk (eds.), (Groningen, 1987).
Pearson, M.N., *The New Cambridge History of India. I: The Portuguese in India* (Cambridge, 1987).
Pearson, N.N., 'The thin end of the wedge. Medical relativities as a paradigm of early modern Indian-European relations', *Modern Asian Sudies* 29, 1 (1995), 141-170.
Peeters, F.A.H. (ed.), *Bataviaasche Apotheek (1746)* (Tilburg, 1981).
Peters, M., and F. André de la Porte, *In steen geschreven. Leven en sterven van VOC-dienaren op de kust van Coromandel in India* (Amsterdam, 2002).
Philibert, H., 'L 'oeuvre scientifique outre-mer des pharmaciens de la marine et des colonies au XIXe siècle', *Medicine Tropicale*, vol. 30 (1970), 5: 587-597.
Pop, G.F., *De Geneeskunde bij het Nederlandsche Zeewezen (Geschiedkundige Nasporingen)* (Batavia, 1922).
Porter, R., *Blood and Guts: A Short History of Medicine* (London, 2003).
Porter, R., *Disease, Medicine and Society in England, 1550-1860* (London, 1993).
Postma, J.M., *The Dutch in the Atlantic Slave Trade, 1600-1815* (Cambridge, 1990).
Powell, I.L., 'Early Ship Surgeons', *Mariner's Mirror*, IX (1923) 3: 11-15.

Prakken, J.R., 'Van schouw-, schurft- en pokmeesters tot huidartsen', *Nederlands Tijdschrift voor Geneeskunde* 120 (1976) 20, 886-891.
Price, C.H., 'Medicine and Pharmacy at the Cape of Good Hope, 1652-1807', *Medical History*, 6 (1962), 169-176.
Priester, L., 'De behandeling van slaven door de slavenhandelaren van de Middelburgsche Commercie Compagnie', *Zeeuws Tijdschrift* 39 (1989) 1, 5-20.
Raben, R. and H. Spijkerman (ed.), *The Archives of the Dutch East India Company (1602-1795)* (The Hague, 1992).
Raben, R., *Batavia and Colombo: The Ethnic and Spatial Order of Two Colonial Cities 1600-1800* (Leiden, 1996).
Reinders Folmer-Van Prooijen, C., *Van goederenhandel naar slavenhandel. De Middelburgsche Commercie Compagnie 1720-1755*, Werken Uitgegeven door het Koninklijk Zeeuwsch Genootschap der Wetenschappen X (Middelburg, 2000).
Reynes, P., and Ch. Courtois-Marchal, 'Le chirurgien dentiste et la marine au XVIIIe siècle', *Actualités Odonto-Stomatologiques* 153 (1986), vol. 40, 155-168.
Ribbius, P., 'Medici en medische toestanden te Arnhem door alle tijden', *Nederlands Tijdschrift voor Geneeskunde* 71 (1927), II, 623-648.
Riley, J.C., 'Mortality on long-distance voyages in the eighteenth century', *Journal of Economic History* XLI (1981) 3, 651-656.
Ringoir, D.J., *Plattelandschirurgijns in de zeventiende en achttiende eeuw. De rekeningboeken van de 18e eeuwse Durgerdamse chirurgijn Anthonij Egberts* (Bunnik 1977).
Riordan, H.D., *Medical Mavericks*, Vol. II (Wichita, KS, 1989).
Risse, G., *Mending Bodies, Saving Souls: A History of Hospitals* (Oxford, 1999).
Robinson, G., 'Admiralty and Naval Affairs, May 1660-March 1764', *Mariners Mirror* 36 (1950) 2-17.
Robinson, V., *The Story of Medicine* (New York, 1944).
Rodger, N.A.M., *The Safeguard of the Sea: A Naval History of Britain, Vol. I: 660-1649* (London, 1997).
Rodger, N.A.M., *The Wooden World: An Anatomy of the Georgian Navy* (London, 1986).
Roelofs, G., *Die Medizinische Versorgung auf Walfangschiffen des Grönlandhandels unter Berücksichtiging der Chirurgenprotokolle*, (Bräist/Bredstedt, 1997), Studien und Materialien veröffentlicht im Nordfriisk Institut 29.
Roessingh, 'Het Veluwse inwonertal, 1526-1947', *A.A.G. Bijdragen* 11, 79-150, (Wageningen, 1964), 79-150.
Romieux, Y., 'Médicaments et médications à bord des vaisseux de la Compagnie francaise des Indes', *Les flottes des Compagnies des Indes 1600-1857*, Ph. Haudrère (ed.), (Vincennes, 1996).
Rooms, 'Medische dienst verbonden aan de troepen van de Spaans-Habsburgse

monarchie in de Zuidelijke Nederlanden (1567-1700)', *Geschiedenis der Geneeskunde*, 5, (1998) 3, 136-142.
Roos, D., *Zeeuwen en de VOC* (Middelburg, 1987).
Rutten, A.M.G., *Apothekers en Chirurgijns. Gezondheidszorg op de Benedenwindse Eilanden van de Nederlandse Antillen in de Negentiende Eeuw* (Maastricht, 1989).
Ruttten [sic], A.M.G., *Dutch Transatlantic Medicine Trade in the Eighteenth Century under the Cover of the West India Company* (Rotterdam, 2000).
Sarton, G., 'Rumphius, Plinius Indicus'(1628-1702)', *Mediz.hist.J.* (Hildesheim) 2 (1967), 167-174.
Schadewaldt, H., 'Zur Geschichte der Schiffshygiene in medizinischer Sicht', *Die Medizinische Welt* 20 (1966) 17, 1136-1142.
Schadewalt, H., 'Die Seewasserdestillation on Bord der Segelschiffe', *Aus dem Institut für Geschichte der Medizin an der Medizinischen Akademie,* 21 (Düsseldorf, 1963), 289-294.
Schadewalt, H., 'Die Wasserversorgung an Bord. Eine medizinhistorische Studie', *Gesnerus* 20 (1963), 47-88.
Schadewalt, H., 'Geschichte der Schiffschirurgie. Die Entwicklung bis zur Mitte des 19. Jahrhunderts'. *Münchner Medizinische Wochenschrift* 34 (1967), 1732-1742.
Schama, S., *The Embarrassment of Riches: An Interpretation of Dutch Culture in the Golden Age* (London, 1987).
Schaling, L., *Frikius of Storm in een glas water. Opmerkingelijke lotgevallen van een zeventiende-eeuwse reisjournaalschrijver* (Unpublished masters thesis, Amsterdam, 1992).
Schirren, C., 'Medizinische Versorgung auf Walfangschiffen im 18. Jahrhundert an hand eines Chirurgen-Protokolls des Schiffes "Conferenceraad Pretorius"', *Nordfriesisches Jahrbuch*, 29 (Braïst/Bredtstedt NF, 1993), 313-318.
Schoorl, H., and J.T. Bremer, *Varensgasten en ander volk. Vier eeuwen bedrijvigheid aan de kusten van Hollands Noorden* (Schoorl, 1987).
Schoute, D., 'Gezondheid en ziekte aan boord der Compagnie's Oost-Indiëvaarders', *Overdruk uit de Provinciale Zeeuwsche en Middelburgsche Courant van 26.02.1936 – 03.03.1936.*
Schoute, D., 'Scheepschirurgijns-journaal van een slavenschip der Middelburgsche Commercie Compagnie', *Nederlandsch Tijdschrift voor Geneeskunde* 92 (1948) IV, 45, 3645-3662.
Schoute, D., *De geneeskunde in den dienst der Oost-Indische Compagnie in Nederlandsch-Indië* (Amsterdam, 1929).
Schoute, D., *De levensloop van een ziekenhuis. Geschiedenis van het Gasthuis te Middelburg* (Middelburg, 1916).
Schoute, D., *Occidental Therapeutics in the Netherlands East Indies during the Centuries of Netherlands Settlements (1600-1900),* (Batavia, 1937).

Schoute, D., *Schets van het Middelburgsche Chirurgijns-gilde* (s.n., 1913).

Schutte, G.J., *Een Hollandse dorpssamenleving in de late achttiende eeuw: de banne Graft 1770-1810* (Franeker, 1989).

Sciortino, R.M.E., *Care-takers of Cure: A Study of Health Centre Nurses in Rural Central Java* (Amsterdam [s.n.], 1992).

Shakespeare, W., *The complete works of William Shakespeare* (London, 1923).

Sheridan, R.B., 'The Guinea Surgeons on the Middle Passage: the provision of medical services in the English slave trade.' *The International Journal of African Historical Studies* 14 (1981) 4, 601-25.

Shryock, R.H., *The Development of Modern Medicine: An Interpretation of the Social and Scientific Factors Involved* (Wisconsin, 1962).

Sicking, L., *Zeemacht en Onmacht. Maritieme politiek in de Nederlanden 1488-1558* (Amsterdam, 1998).

Sigmond, J.P., and L.H. Zuiderbaan, *Nederlanders ontdekken Australië* (Bussum, 1976).

Slenders, J.A.M., *Het Theatrum Anatomicum in de Noordelijke Nederlanden, 1555-1800* (Nijmegen, 1989), Scripta Tironum 17/18.

Slicher van Bath, B.H., 'The economic situation in the Dutch Republic during the seventeenth century', in: M. Aymard (ed), *Dutch Capitalism and World Capitalism* (Cambridge, 1982).

Slicher van Bath, B.H., *Een samenleving onder spanning: geschiedenis van het platteland in Overijssel* (Utrecht, 1977).

Stapel, F.W. (ed.), 'Pieter van Dam's Beschrijvinge van de Oostindische Compagnie', *Rijksgeschiedkundige Publicatiën* (The Hague, 1943) Grote Serie, 87.

Steege, J. van der, *Geneeskundige Berichten* (Batavia, 1779).

Stuart, K., *Defiled Trades and Social Outcasts. Honor and Ritual Pollution in Early Modern Germany* (Cambridge, 1999).

Sturdy, St. (ed.), *Medicine, Health and the Public Sphere in Britain, 1600-2000* (London, 2002).

Subba Reddy, D.V., 'An Indo-British medical classic of XVIII century. Charles Curtis on diseases of India in the fleet and in the naval hospital at Madras in 1782 and 1783', *Bulletin of the Indian Institue of the History of Medicine* 4 (1974), 193-206.

Subba Reddy, D.V., 'Charles Curtis on diseases of India in the fleet and in the naval hospital at Madras in 1782 and 1783', *Bulletin of the Indian Institute of the History of Medicine* 5(1974), 193-206.

Summerville, T., 'Letters of a surgeon's mate in the age of Smollett', *Scottish Medical Journal*, 1963, 8, 318-322.

Sutherland Shaw, J.J.S., 'The hospital ship 1608-1740', *Mariner's Mirror* 22 (1936), 422-426.

Swaving, C., 'Batavia's sanitaire geschiedenis onder het bestuur van de Oost-In-

dische maatschappij', *Nederlandsch Tijdschrift voor Geneeskunde* 14 (1878) II, 1-210.
Tavernier, J.B., *Historie van 't beleit der Hollanders in Asia* (1682).
Taylor, J. Gelman, *The Social World of Batavia: European and Eurasian in Dutch Asia* (Madison, WI, 1983).
Temkin, O., 'The role of surgery in the rise of modern medical thought', *Bulletin of the History of Medicine*, voume XXV (1951), 248-259.
Ten Doesschate, A., 'Geneeskunde in Oud-Zwolle', *Verslagen en Mededelingen uitgegeven door de Vereeniging tot beoefening Overijssels regt en geschiedenis*, 1e reeks, 45 (1928), 21e stuk, 1-89.
The Oxford Classical Dictionary (Oxford, 1996).
The Short Oxford History of English Literature (Oxford, 1994).
Thomas, D.P., 'Sailors, scurvy and science', *Journal of the Royal Society of Medicine* 90 (1997) 50-54.
Tickner, F.J. and V.C. Medvei, 'Scurvy and the health of European crews in the Indian Ocean in the seventeenth century', *Medical History* 2 (1958), 36-46.
Travers, Twiss (ed.), *The Black Book of the Admiralty*. Appendix – Part III (London, 1965, reprint), Rerum Britannicarum Medii Aevi Scriptores (Rolls Series) 55.
Turner, E.H., 'Naval medical service, 1793-1815', *Mariner's Mirror* 46 (1960) 1, 119-133.
Ultee, M. (ed), *Adapting to Conditions. War and Society in the Eighteenth Century* (Alabama, 1986).
Ultzheimer, Andreas, *Beschreibung etlicher Reisen 1596-1610* (Tübingen, 1971).
Uragoda, C.G., and L.D. Paranavitana, 'The seventeenth-century Dutch hospital in Colombo', *Medical History* 29 (1985), 182-192.
Valentin, M. and P-M Niaussat, 'Le rôle fondamental d'Amédée Lefèvre, médecin de la Marine (1798-1869), en médecine du travail et en histoire de la médecine', *Histoire des Sciences Medicales* 13 (1979), 407-417.
Van Andel, M.A., 'Geneeskunde en hygiëne op de slavenschepen in den compagnietijd', *Nederlands Tijdschrift voor Geneeskunde* 75 (1731) I, 6, 614-637.
Van Andel, M.A., 'Vrije uitoefening der geneeskunde in de 17de eeuw', *Nederlands Tijdschrift voor Geneeskunde* 58 (1914) I, 1907-1914.
Van Andel, M.A., *Chirurgijns, Vrije Meesters, Beunhazen en Kwakzalvers. De chirurgijnsgilden en de practijk der heelkunde (1400-1800)* (Amsterdam, 1946).
Van de Bijl, W.F.Th, 'Uit de geschiedenis der chirurgijnsgilden in Zeeland', *Nederlands Tijdschrift voor Geneeskunde* 77 (1933) II, 18, 2046-2064.
Van der AA, A.J., *Aardrijkskundig Woordenboek der Nederlanden*, 13 vols. (Gorinchem, 1839-1854).
Van der Boom, J.H., 'Genealogisch onderzoek in de archieven van de Verenigde Oostindische Compagnie in het Algemeen Rijksarchief te 's Gravenhage', *De Indische Navorscher*, Orgaan van de Indische Genealogische Vereniging, 10 (1997) 1, 15-40.

Van der Brug, P.H., *Malaria en malaise: de VOC in Batavia in de achttiende eeuw* (Amsterdam, 1994).
Van der Chijs, J.A., *Nederlandsch-Indisch Plakaatboek, 1602-1811*, I-XVII (Batavia/ The Hague, 1885-1900).
Van der Hoeven, J., 'Een en ander over de examens bij de chirurgijnsgilden en over het "vroedkundig examen"', *Nederlands Tijdschrift voor Geneeskunde* 81 (1937) III, 3142-3147.
Van der Hoeven, J., 'Het chirurgijnsgilde te Deventer', *Nederlands Tijdschrift voor Geneeskunde* 78 (1934) II, 1547-1559.
Van der Hoeven, M., 'Na de slag. Het veldhospitaal van Hendrik Verschuring en realisme in zeventiende eeuwse oorlogskunst', *Armamentaria* 29 (1994) 35-42.
Van der Korst, J.R.., *Een dokter van formaat. Gerad van Swieten, lijfarts van Keizerin Maria Theresia* (Amsterdam, 2003).
Van der Meij-de Leur, A.P.M., *Van olie en wijn. Geschiedenis van verpleegkunde, geneeskunde en sociale zorg* (Amsterdam, 1981).
Van der Weijde, A.J., 'Collegium Medicum Ultrajectinum', *Nederlands Tijdschrift voor Geneeskunde* 68 (1924) III, 655-666.
Van der Weijde, A.J., 'Eed voor den heelmeester in 1811', *Nederlands Tijdschrift voor Geneeskunde* 68 (1924) II, 1258.
Van der Weijde, A.J., 'Iets over steensnijden en steensnijders', *Nederlands Tijdschrift voor Geneeskunde* 68 (1924) II, 655-666.
Van der Weijde, A.J., 'Toezicht op de uitoefening der geneeskunde in 1817', *Nederlands Tijdschrift voor Geneeskunde* 67 (1923) II, 902-905.
Van der Woude, A.M., *Het Noorderkwartier. Een regionaal historisch onderzoek in de demografische en economische geschiedenis van westelijk Nederland van de late middeleeuwen tot het begin van de negentiende eeuw* (Wageningen, 1972), 3 vols..
Van Deursen, A.Th., *Een dorp in de polder: Graft in de zeventiende eeuw* (Amsterdam, 1994).
Van Dorssen, J.M.H., 'De lepra in Nederlandsch Oost-Indië tijdens de 17e en 18e eeuw', *Geneeskundig Tijdschrift voor Nederlandsch-Indië* 37 (1897), 255-324.
Van Dorssen, J.M.H., 'Willem ten Rhijne, *Geneeskundig Tijdschrift voor Nederlandsch-Indië*, 55 (1911), 134-228.
Van Eeghen, I.H., *De Gilden. Theorie en Praktijk* (Bussum, 1965).
Van Eijck van Heslinga, E.S., *Van Compagnie naar koopvaardij. De scheepvaartverbinding van de Bataafsche Republiek met de koloniën in Azië 1795-1806* (Amsterdam, 1988).
Van Gelder, R., *Het Oost-Indisch avontuur. Duitsers in dienst van de VOC (1600-1800)* (Nijmegen, 1997).
Van Gelder, R., *Naporra's Omweg: Het Leven van een VOC-matroos (1731-1793)* (Amsterdam, 2003).

Van Leur, J.C., *Indonesian Trade and Society: Essays in Asian Social and Economic History*, Selected Studies on Indonesia by Dutch Scholars, I (The Hague, 1955).

Van Lieburg, M.J., 'De genees- en heelkunde in de Noordelijke Nederlanden, gezien vanuit de stedelijke en chirurgijnsgildeordonnanties van de 16e eeuw', *Tijdschrift voor de Geschiedenis der Geneeskunde, Natuurwetenschappen, Wiskunde en Techniek* 6 (1983) 4, 169-184.

Van Lieburg, M.J., 'De geneeskundige verzorging van zieke en gewonde soldaten en matrozen te Rotterdam gedurende de 17e eeuw', *Nederlands Militair Geneeskundig Tijdschrift* 30 (1977), 33-45.

Van Loon, L., 'Het Rotterdamsche chirurgijnsgilde "S. Cosmas et Damianus" van 1467 – 1798, I', *Nederlands Tijdschrift voor Geneeskunde* 83 (1939) II, 1485-1492.

Van Loon, L., 'Het Rotterdamsche chirurgijnsgilde "S. Cosmas et Damianus" van 1467 – 1798 II', *Nederlands Tijdschrift voor Geneeskunde* 83 (1939) III, 3911-3919.

Van Petersen, J.W., *Van Zoete Wijn en Bittere Medicijn. Zes eeuwen gezondheidszorg in de Liemers en Doesburg* (Zutphen, 1989).

Van Piskijkers en Heelmeesters. Genezen in de Gouden Eeuw (Leiden, Museum Boerhaave, s.a.).

Van Rooij, H.H., and J. Gawronski, *VOC-schip Amsterdam: gebleeven op de kust van Sussex tussen Hastings en Beachyhead gestrand* (Haarlem, 1989).

Van Royen, P.C. van, Bruijn, J.R., and J. Lucassen, *"Those Emblems of Hell"? European sailors and the maritime labour market, 1570-1870* (New Foundland, 1997).

Van Royen, P.C. van, *Zeevarenden op de koopvaardijvloot omstreeks 1700* (Amsterdam, 1987).

Van Till, M., 'Social care in eighteenth century Batavia. The poorhouse, 1725-1750', *Itinerario* XIX (1995) 1, 18-31.

Van Vliet, A.P., *Vissers & kapers: de zeevisserij vanuit het Maasmondgebied en de Duinkerker kapers (ca. 1580-1648)* (The Hague, 1994).

Van Zanden, J.L., and A. van Riel, *Nederland 1780-1914. Staat, instituties en economische ontwikkeling* (Amsterdam, 2000).

Veirac, J. and B. Hussum, 'Antwoord over de rotkoorts op de Oost-Indische schepen', *Verhandelingen uitgegeven door het Zeeuwsch Genootschap der Wetenschappen* VI (Middelburg, 1769-1792), 3-225.

Veldman, J.E., 'Chirurgie van de roodharige barbaren; Hollandse medici in Japan, 1600-1870', *Nederlands Tijdschrift voor Geneeskunde* 145 (2001) 52, 2542-2547.

Voegen van Engelen, J., 'De Surinaamsche artz 1786-1788', *Publications of the Foundation for Scientific Research in Surinam and the Netherlands Antilles* 109 (1981) no. 4.

Völker, 'Die Gebruder Schaarschmid. Zum 200. Todestag von August Schaarschmid (1720-1791)', *Zeitschrift gesammte Inn. med.* 47 (1992), 168-176.
Von Römer, L.S.A.M., *Historical Sketches. An introduction to the Fourth Congress of the Far Eastern Association of Tropical Medicine* (Batavia, 1921) .
Wagenaar, L.J., 'Het eiland Ontrust bij Batavia als onderdeel van het VOC-scheepsbedrijf in de 17de en 18de eeuw', *Antiek* 25 (1990) 2, 65-80.
Wagenaar, L.J., *Galle, VOC-vestiging in Ceylon. Beschrijving van een koloniale samenleving aan de vooravond van de Singalese opstand tegen het Nederlands gezag, 1760* (Amsterdam, 1994).
Warnsinck, J.C.M. (ed.), *De Reisen van Nicolaus de Graaff gedaan naar alle gewesten des werelds. Beginnende 1639 tot 1687 incluis*, Werken uitgegeven door de Linschoten-Vereeniging, XXXIII (The Hague, 1930).
Watt, J., 'Medical perspectives of some voyages of discovery', *TransMedSoclondon* 95 (1978/1979), 61-91.
Watt, J., 'Nutrition in adverse environments; forgotten lessons of maritime nutrition', *Human Nutrition* 36A (1982), 35-45.
Watt, J., 'Some forgotten contributions of naval surgeons', *Journal of the Royal Society of Medicine* 78 (1985), 753-762.
Watt, J., 'Surgeons of the Mary Rose', *Mariner's Mirror* 69 (1983) I, 3-18.
Watt, J., 'The burns of seafarers under oars, sail and steam', *Injury: the British Journal of Accident Surgery*, Vol. 12, 1, 69-81.
Watts, Sh., *Epidemics and History: Disease, power and Imperialism* (London, 1977).
Wendte, J.F., 'De Hoornse stadsarts Dr. Pilgrom Hermansz Hulleman en zijn voor- en nageslacht', *Gens Nostra*, 55 (2000), 3, 115-122.
Wijnands, D.O., 'De relaties van de Zweedse botanicus/naturalist Carl Petter Thunberg (1743-1828) met Nederlandse genootschappen', *Teylers Magazine* 28 (1990), 11-26.
Winton, R., 'Food and fitness at sea', *The Medical Journal of Australia*, 2 (1980), 411-412.
Wilson, R., *Pious Traders in Medicine: A German Pharmaceutical network in Eighteenth-Centruy North America* (State College, PA, 2000).
Wittop Koning, D.A., *De oude apotheek* (Delft, 1966).
Wright, D.S., 'The history and development of the medical services of H.M. dockyard, Chatham, 1625-1966', *Journal of the Royal Naval Medical Service*, 54 (1968), 25-68.
Wrigley, E.A. (ed.), *Identifying People in the Past* (London, 1973).
Wunderlich, C.A., *Geschichte der Medicin* (Suttgart, 1859).
Zorn, E., 'Schiffärtsmedizin im Wandel der Zeiten', *Medizinische Klinik* 69 (1974), 529-534.

Zuckerman, A., 'Scurvy and the ventilaton of ships in the Royal Navy; Samuel Suttons contribution', *Eighteenth Century Studies* 10 (1976/7), 222-234.
Zwitzer, H.L., *'De militie van den staat'. Het leger van de Republiek der Verenigde Nederlanden* (Amsterdam, 1991).

Notes

Notes to Introduction

1 O'Brian, P., *Master & Commander* (London, 1996), 38.
2 Translation by the author. Bontekoe, W.IJ., *Journael ofte Gedenckwaerdige beschrijvinghe van de Oost-Indische reijse van – Begrijpende veel wonderlijcke en gevaerlijcke saecken hem daer in wedervaren; begonnende den 18 December 1618 en vol-eind den 16 November 1625* (Hoorn, 1646).
3 ...*verregaande onbekwaamheid en van een uiterst geringe intelligentie*. Roos, D., *Zeeuwen en de VOC*, (Middelburg, 1987), 127. Translation by the author.
4 Translation by the author. Voegen van Engelen, J., *De Surinaamsche Artz 1786-1788* (Facsimili, Utrecht, 1982), 84. *In ons Vaderland, daar de Heelkunde op den veragtelijksten voet is, en eeniglijk in onze voornaame steden door eenige bekwame handartzen voor een volstrekt verval bewaard wordt, beginnen onze ScheepsDoctoren hun onderwijs met baardscheren, daarna komt'er Pleisters smeeren en Aderlaaten bij; de Patroon stopt zijnen leerling vervolgens een kort Begrip van Ontleed en Heelkunde in de Hand; een gelukkig geheugen en eenige geradbraakte Latijnsche Kunstwoorden volmaakten de zaak. Een jammerlijk Examen volgt, eenige Guldens worden betaald, en zie daar mijn Aesculaap voorzien van een zeebrief waarbij hem geoorloofd wordt de zeebouwende Onderdaanen van den Staat door alle de vier Werelddelen te medicamenteeren tot 'er geenezing of de Dood na volgt.*
5 De Moor, J.A., and P.G.E.I.J. van der Velde (eds.), *De werken van Jacob Haafner*, III (Zutphen, 1997), 281-282.
6 De Moor, and Van der Velde (eds), *De werken van Jacob Haafner*, I (Zutphen, 1992), 104. Translation by the author.
7 Grell, O.P., and A. Cunningham, *Health Care and Poor Relief in Protestant Europe 1500-1700* (London, 1997), 1.
8 Brans, P.H., 'Beiträge zur Geschichte der Schiffspharmazie in den Niederlanden und in Niederländische Indien', *Veröffentlichungen des Internationale Geschichte des Pharmazie N.F.*, 13 (1958), 61.
9 Broeze, F.J.A., Bruijn, J.R., and F.S. Gaastra (eds.), *Maritieme Geschiedenis der Nederlanden* (Bussum, 1977), III, 177.
10 Bruford, W.H., *Germany in the Eighteenth Century: The Social Background of the Literary Revival* (Cambridge, 1959), 258.
11 Ibid., 258.
12 Stuart, K., *Defiled Trades and Social Outcasts: Honor and Ritual Pollution in Early Modern Germany* (Cambridge, 1999).
13 Except from J.R. Bruijn's article on Dutch VOC masters (*schippers*) (Bruijn, J.R., 'Commandanten van Oost-Indiëvaarders in de achttiende eeuw', *Tijdschrift voor Zeegeschiedenis* 20 (2001) 1, 4-14), Perry Moree's 'Predikanten en ziekentroosters aan boord van Rotterdamse Oost-Indiëvaarders', and Van Gelder's thesis on some 40 German soldiers in the service of the VOC (Van Gelder, R., *Het Oost-Indisch avontuur. Duitsers in dienst van de VOC (1600-1800)* (Nijmegen, 1997), not much has been written about other professional groups of employees of the Dutch East India Company.
14 Lindemann, M., *Medicine and Society in Early Modern Europe* (Cambridge, 1999), 141-147.
15 To name the most significant: Brug, P.H. van der, *Malaria en malaise: de VOC in Batavia in de achttiende eeuw* (Amsterdam, 1994); Dorssen, J.M.H. van, 'De lepra in Nederlandsch

Oost-Indië tijdens de 17e en 18e eeuw', *Geneeskundig Tijdschrift voor Nederlandsch-Indië*, 37 (1897), 255-324; Dorssen, J.M.H. van, 'Willem ten Rhijne, *Geneeskundig Tijdschrift voor Nederlandsch-Indië*, 51 (1911), 134-228; Gijsberti Hodenpijl, A.K.A., 'De ziekten aan boord van de schepen van de Oost-Indische compagnie in de eerste helft van de achttiende eeuw', *Nederlandsch Tijdschrift voor Geneeskunde* 62 (1918); Gijsberti Hodenpijl, A.K.A., 'De scheurbuik (scorbut) op 's-Compagnies schepen uit het vaderland komende in het jaar 1730', *Nederlandsch Tijdschrift voor Geneeskunde*, 66 (1922) I, 496-501; Haver-Droeze, J.J., 'De geneeskundige dienst bij de Nederlandsch-Oost-Indische Compagnie', *Nederlandsch Tijdschrift voor Geneeskunde* 65 (1921), I, 2535-2560; Bruijn, J.R. and J. Lucassen, *Op de Schepen der Oost-Indische Compagnie: vijf artikelen van J. de Hullu* (Groningen, 1980); Koninkx, C., 'Ziekten op Zee. Pathologie van de Ziekten in de Grote Vaart in de Achttiende Eeuw', *Marine Academie Mededelingen* XXVI (1980-1981-1982), 34-48; Leuftink, A.E., *Harde Heelmeesters. Zeelieden en hun dokters in de 18e eeuw* (Zutphen 1991), 37; Pop, G.F., *De Geneeskunde bij het Nederlandsche Zeewezen (Geschiedkundige Nasporingen)* (Batavia, 1922); Von Roemer, L.S.A.M., *Historical Sketches. An Introduction to the fourth Congress of the Far Eastern Association of Tropical Medicine* (Batavia, 1921); Schoute, D., *De geneeskunde in den dienst der Oost-Indische Compagnie in Nederlandsch-Indie* (Amsterdam, 1929); Swaving, C., 'Batavia's sanitaire geschiedenis onder het bestuur van de Oost-Indische maatschappij', *Nederlandsch Tijdschrift voor Geneeskunde* II (1878) 14, 1-210.

Notes to Chapter 1

1 Chaucer, G., *Canterbury Tales* (London, 1928), 160.
Esculapius or Asclepios; in Homer's *Iliad*, he is a hero, the 'blameless physician', a god of healing.
Deyscordes is Pedanius Dioscorides (*circa* 41-68), a military physician who studied and recorded the medical uses of plants and wrote what is probably the first thorough systematic *materia medica*, which became the basis for all subsequent studies and writings on pharmacology, including *materia medica*.
Rufus is Rufus of Ephesus (*circa* 110-180) who made significant anatomical observations. He described, *inter alia* the correct course of the optic nerves, and was a highly respected physician.
Ypocras is Hippocrates (460-377 BC) who attributed all diseases to an imbalance of body fluids.
Haly is Haly Abbas (930-994) or Ali ibn al-'Abbas al-Majusi, whose major work was *Liber Regius*; the *Liber Regius* was translated into Latin in the eleventh century by Constantinus Africanus who published it as his own work, entitled *Libri Pantechni*. It belonged to the typical mediaeval medical literature and was very popular in Europe.
Galyen is Galen (Galienus) of Pergamon (131-201) who elaborated Hippocrates's system of humoral pathology into a science called Galenism.
Serapion and Damascien (Damascenus) are ambiguous: the former may have been Greek or Arab, the latter a Muslim or Christian, depending upon the particular identification. (Blake, N.F. (ed.), *The Canterbury Tales by Geoffrey Chaucer* (London, 1980), 49). During the Ptolemaic times, Serapis was a local Egyptian deity who rivalled Asclepios among the populace of Egypt as a god of healing.
Razis is Abu Bakr Muhammad ibn Zakarija ar-Razi, or Rhazes (*circa* 850-923) who exerted great influence on the medicine and surgery of the West. His *opus magnum* was *al-Hawi*, known in Europe as *Liber Continens* or *Liber medicinalis ad Almansorum*, a compilation of Greek, Indian, and Arabic sources, translated into Latin in the second half of the thirteenth century.
Avycen is Avicenna (980-1037) or Abu 'ali al-Husayn ibn 'Abd Allah ibn Sina, a Persian whose *Canon Medicina* is one of the most influential medical books ever written.
Averrois must be Averroës (1126-1198) a physician-philosopher of Cordoba.
Damascien, see Serapion above.

Constantyn, or rather Constantinus Africanus (*circa* 1080-1087) was crucial to the introduction of the ideas of Hippocrates and Galen at the University of Salerno. He maintained a continuity with the ancient world. He travelled for four decades in Syria, India, Egypt, and Ethiopia, accumulating medical manuscripts, which he studied and translated.

The prominent medical Arabs were closely associated with the rise of the medical school at Montpellier which was founded circa 738. Prominent pupils were, *inter alia*, Gilbertus Anglicus (in Chaucer's text, Gilbertyn) and Bernard de Gordon (here, Bernard), the leading representatives of Anglo-Norman medicine.

Gatesden: Chaucer refers to John Gaddesden (?1280-1361), who was an instructor in Merton College, Oxford, and later a court physician to Edward II. (Chaucer, G., *Canterbury Tales* (London, 1928), 132). Gaddesden is the author of *Rosa Anglica Practica Medicinae.*

2 Shakespeare, W., T*he Complete Works of William Shakespeare: Henry IV, act.* 1, *scene* II (London, 1923), 498.

3 Molière, *Le Malade Imaginaire* (Paris, 2002): Troisième Intermède, 88-89.

4 French, R., *Medicine before Science: The Business of Medicine from the Middle Ages to the Enlightenment* (Cambridge, 2003), 121.

5 Imhof, A.E., 'The hospital in the eighteenth century: for whom?', *Journal of Social History* 10 (1977) 4, 448. This stands contrary to Huizenga's view who states that during the fourteenth century the idea about health and disease changed: health became perceived as (more) positive than in earlier times as a result of which (municipal) measures were taken to guarantee the health of as many people as possible. Huizenga does not substantiate this opinion. Huizenga, E., *Tussen autoriteit en empirie. De Middelnederlandse chirurgieën in de veertiende en vijftiende eeuw en hun maatschappelijke context* (Hilversum, 2003) 86.

6 Imhof, 'The hospital in the eighteenth century', 451.

7 Granshaw, L., and R. Porter (eds.), *The Hospital in History* (London, 1989), 21.

8 Imhof, 'The hospital in the eighteenth century', 449.

9 Lindemann, M., *Medicine and Society in Early Modern Europe* (Cambridge, 1999), 139.

10 Garrison, F.H., *An Introduction to the History of Medicine* (Philadelphia and London, 1929), 93-94.

11 Conrad, L.E., et al, *The Western Medical Tradition: 800 BC to AD 1800* (Cambridge, 1996), 80.

12 De Moulin, D., *A History of Surgery with emphasis on the Netherlands* (Dordrecht, 1988), 29-30.

13 McNeil, W.H., *Plagues and Peoples* (Oxford, 1977), 236.

14 Shryock, R.H., *The Development of Modern Medicine. An Interpretation of the Social and Scientific Factors Involved* (Madison, WI, 1962), 5.

15 Huizenga, *Tussen autoriteit en empirie*, 44.

16 Temkin, O., 'The role of surgery in the rise of modern medical thought', *Bulletin of the Hisotry of Medicine*, vol. XXV, 1951, 252.

17 De Moulin, *A History of Surgery*, 44.

18 Conrad, *The Western Medical Tradition*, 162-163.

19 French, *Medicine before Science*, 120.

20 Watts, Sh., *Epidemics and History: Disease, Power and Imperialism* (London, 1977), 12.

21 Wats, *Epidemics and History*, 15.

22 Risse, G., *Mending Bodies, Saving Souls: A History of* Hospitals (Oxford, 1999), 201.

23 Grell, O.P., and A. Cunningham, *Health Care and Poor Relief in Protestant Europe 1500-1700* (London, 1997).

24 Grell and Cunningham, *Health Care and Poor Relief*, 51; Risse, *Mending Bodies*, 216.

25 Grell and Cunningham, *Health Care and Poor Relief*, 5, 51.

26 Conrad, *The Western Medical Tradition*, 293.

27 De Moulin, *A History of Surgery*, 66-67.

28 Cook, H.J., *The Decline of the Old Medical Regime in Stuart London* (Ithaca, 1986), 46.

29 Cook, *The Decline of the Old Medical Regime*, 28.

30 Keevil, J.J., *Medicine and the Navy 1200-1900* I, (London, 1957), 127.
31 Keevil, *Medicine and the Navy* I, 137.
32 Garrison, *Introduction to the History of Medicine*, 341.
33 De Moulin, *A History of Surgery*, 54.
34 Lyons, A.S., and R.J. Petrucelli, *Medicine: An Illustrated History* (New York, 1987), 381.
35 Lindemann, *Medicine and Society in Early Modern Europe*, 217.
36 Charles-Francois Félix (1650-1703), the king's first surgeon, had successfully performed an operation for fistula-in-ano on his royal patron in 1687. De Moulin, *History of Surgery*, 106.
37 Conrad, *The Western Medical Tradition*, 437-438.
38 Larsen, O., *Schiff und Seuche 1795-1799* (Oslo, 1968), 27-28.
39 Hernández-Sáenz, L.M., 'Seamen, surgeons and empire: Spanish naval medical reform and Mexican medicine in the late colonial period', *The Northern Mariner* X, 1 (2000), 22-28. Conrad, *The Western Medical Tradition*, 231.
40 Garrison, *Introduction to the History of Medicine*, 218-219.
41 Conrad, *The Western Medical Tradition*, 311-315.
42 Franciscus de le Boë Sylvius, physician, physiologist, anatomist and chemist who is also considered to be the founder of the seventeenth century iatrochemical school of medicine, which held that all phenomena of life and disease are based on chemical action.
43 Lindemann, *Medicine and Society in Early Modern Europe*, 75-77.
44 French, *Medicine before Science*, 187.
45 Barge, J.A.J., 'Het geneeskundig onderwijs aan de Leidsche universiteit in de achttiende eeuw', *Nederlands Tijdschrift voor Geneeskunde* 78, I, (1934), 1, 50-54.
46 Conrad, *The Western Medical Tradition*, 384-384.
47 Cook, H.J., *Trials of an Ordinary Doctor. Joannes Groenevelt in Seventeenth-Century London* (London, 1994), 56, 69, 82, 102.
48 Aerts, R., and L. Hoogkamp, *De Gelderse Pallas. Gymnasium Illustre. Gelderse Universiteit. Rijksathenaeum te Harderwijk 1600-1800* (Barneveld, 1986), 50. By the age of nineteen De Gorter became a master-surgeon, and three years later he graduated at Leiden.
49 Van Deursen, A.Th., *Een dorp in de polder. Graft in de zeventiende eeuw* (Amsterdam, 1994) 112-113.
50 Cook, *The Decline of the Old Medical Regime*, 28.
51 Schoute, D., *Schets van het Middelburgsche chirurgijns-gilde* (s.n., 1913), 43.
52 Mooij, A., *De Polslag van de stad. 350 jaar academische geneeskunde in Amsterdam*, (Amsterdam, 1999), 37.
53 Cook, *Trials of an Ordinary Doctor*, 81.
54 Brouwer Ancher, A.J.M., 'Oude ordonnantiën betreffende genees-, heel-, en verloskundigen, apothekers, kwakzalvers enz.', *Nederlands Tijdschrift voor Geneeskunde* 25 (1899), 1174.
55 Van Andel, M.A., 'Vrije uitoefening der geneeskunde in de 17de eeuw', *Nederlands Tijdschrift voor Geneeskunde* 58 (1914) I, 1908-1910.
56 Mooij, *De Polslag van de stad*, 47.
57 Van Petersen, J.W., *Van Zoete Wijn en Bittere Medicijn. Zes eeuwen gezondheidszorg in de Liemers en Doesburg* (Zutphen, 1989), 75.
58 Keevil, *Medicine and the Navy* I, 127.
59 Bik, J.G.W.F., *Vijf eeuwen medisch leven in een Hollandse stad* (Assen, 1955), 9.
60 De Moulin, *A History of Surgery*, 66.
61 Van Petersen, *Van Zoete Wijn en Bittere Medicijn*, 74.
62 Huisman, F.G., *Stadsbesef en stadsbelang. Gezondheidszorg en medisch beroep in Groningen, 1500-1730* (Amsterdam, 1992), 172-173.
63 Ketting, H., *De Amsterdamse chirurgijns: van ambacht naar professie.1750-1798*, unpublished thesis (Amsterdam, 1988), 28
64 Mooij, *De polslag van de stad*, 80-82.
65 Van Eeghen, I.H., *De Gilden. Theorie en Praktijk* (Bussum, 1965), 73.
66 Van Lieburg, M.J., 'De Genees- en Heelkunde in de Noordleijke Nederlanden, gezien

vanuit de stedelijke en chirurgijnsgilde-ordonnantiën van de zestiende eeuw', *Tijdschrift voor de Geschiedenis der Geneeskunde, Natuurwetenschappen, Wiskunde en Techniek* 6(19183) 4, 179.

67 Van Eeghen, *De Gilden.*, 73; Brouwer Ancher, 'Oude ordonnantiën', 1183-1184.

68 Ribbius, P., 'Medici en medische toestanden te Arnhem door alle tijden', *Nederlands Tijdschrift voor Geneeskunde* 71 (1927), II, 635.

69 Schoute, *Schets van het Middelburgsche Chirurgijns-gilde*, 36-38.

70 Loudon, I.S.L., 'Leg ulcers in the eighteenth and early nineteenth centuries. II. Treatment', *Journal of the Royal College of General Practitioners*, 1982, 301.

71 Brouwer Ancher, 'Oude ordonnantiën', 1185.

72 De Moulin, *A History of Surgery*, 69.

73 'innerlijcke en uitterlijcke accidenten van het menschen lichaem beneefens desselfs bandagie'.

74 Dorren, G., *Eenheid en verscheidenheid. De burgers van Haarlem in de Gouden Eeuw* (Amsterdam, 2001), 103.

75 Temkin, O., 'The role of surgery in the rise of modern medical thought', *Bulletin of the Hisotry of Medicine*, 252.

76 Watt, J., 'Surgeons of the Mary Rose', *Mariners Mirror* 69 (1983), 7.

77 De Moulin, *A History of Surgery*, 86.

78 Ibid., 90.

79 Jan van Beverwijck, M.D., studied medicine in Leiden, after which his *peregrinatio academica* took him to France, Italy, and Switzerland. He became the City-Physician and *praelector anatomiae* of Dordrecht. He wrote several treatises, *inter alia*, *De calculo renum et visicae* published in 1638 and *Heelkonste* ('Surgery') of 1645. These also appear in his collected works of 1651. He was one of the first on the European continent to recognise the accuracy of Harvey's theory of the circulation of blood.

80 Ambroise Paré, barber surgeon. Modern French surgery entered Holland towards the end of the sixteenth century by way of the collected works of Paré (*Oeuvres Complêtes*) which were published in Dutch in 1592. Made a master surgeon in 1554 by King Henry II, he published his magnificent treatise *l'Anatomie universelle du corps humain* ('A Universal Surgery') in 1561.

81 The author Gabelhoven has not been identified.

82 Wilhelm Fabricius Hildanus. *Observationum & curationum chirurgicarum centuriae (I-V) nunc primum simul in unum opus congestae, ac in duo volumina distributae. Quorum prius continet centuria I. II. & III.* He is considered by some to be the 'father of surgery in Germany'. The comments of Hildanus are probably the comments on Hildanus which were published in Rotterdam in 1656. Hildanus was an authority on kidney stones.

83 Paulus Barbette was a physician who emigrated from Alsace and obtained his doctorate at Leiden. He established himself in Amsterdam and became a close friend of Francois de le Boë Sylvius. He published a compendium of surgery: *Chirurgie nae de hedendaeghse practijk beschreven*, followed by a treatise on surgical anatomy in 1659 (*Anatomica Practica*). Furthermore, he wrote a book on medicine, *Praxis Barbettiana*, and an account of the plague that struck Amsterdam in 1655.

84 Nicolaas Zas was the first *lector anatomicus* of Rotterdam, especially concerned with the instructing of surgeons. The book mentioned here is *Den dauw der dieren ende welle des waters*, which was published in Rotterdam, 1660.

85 Louis de Bils, or Louys de Bils, or Ludovicus de Bilsius. Anatomist. In 1659 he published *Kopije van zekere ample acte van Jr. Louijs de Bils rakende de wetenschap van de oprechte anatomije des menselijken lichaams* in Rotterdam. He was the first to discover a practical way to conserve dead bodies for anatomical purposes. He also proposed establishing an anatomy theatre and anatomical collection in Rotterdam. His *opera omni* would include *Aan alle ware liefhebbers der anatomie* (Rotterdam, 1659); *Anatomische beschrijvinge van een wanschepsel, geboren op de Elderschans buijten Aerdenburg* (Middelburg, 1659); *Epistolica dissertatio: qua verus hepatis circa chylum, & partier ductus chiliferi hactenus dicti usus,*

docetur (Rotterdam, 1659); *Omnibus verae anatomes studiosis* (Rotterdam, 1660); *Specimina anatomica* (Rotterdam, 1661); and *Responsio ad admonitiones d.i. Johannis ab Horne* (Rotterdam, 1661).

86 The Amsterdam *Pharmacopeia Amstelredamensis* of 1636.

87 Carolus Battus (*circa* 1540-1617) translated many medical works, notably by French surgeons, particularly the *Opera Omni* of Ambroisius Paré. Battus was a physician in Dordrecht.

88 This author has not been found.

89 Not identified.

90 The works of Paracelsus.

91 Van Loon, L., 'Het Rotterdamsche chirurgijnsgilde "S. Cosmas et Damianus" van 1467 – 1798', II, *Nederlands Tijdschrift voor Geneeskunde* 83 (1939) III, 3911-3919, page 3911.

92 Rembertus Dodonaeus (1517-1585).

93 *Item een boeck waer in op verscheijde manieren getoont wert het fabrijck des menelijcke lichaems*: Schoute, D., *Schets van het Middelburgsche Chirurgijnsgilde* (s.n., 1913), 34.

94 Cornelis van Solingen, a (sea-)surgeon as well as physician. Published *Manuele Operatien der Chirurgie* in 1684, which became a book used by surgeon-apprentices until far into the eighteenth century. The text of the *Manuele Operatien* is based on Van Solingen's many experiences as a ship's surgeon.

95 De Moulin, *A History of Surgery*, 136.

96 *Alhoewel de Geneesheer de voorrang heeft in het verslag geven daarom heeft hij geen meerder geloofwaardigheid in het oordeelen. Want het verslag moet afgenomen worden uit de kundigheid en wetenschap in de Ontleedkunde en dierlijke huishouding, maar niet uit den voorrang; weshalven men een kundig Heelmeester meer geloof heeft te geven dan aan een onkundig Geneesheer*. De Gorter, J., *Nieuwe Gezuiverde Heelkonst*, § 1205.

97 Jansen, H.P.H., *Middeleeuwse geschiedenis der Nederlanden* (Utrecht, 1972), 184.

98 Ten Doesschate, A., 'Geneeskunde in Oud-Zwolle', *Verslagen en Mededelingen uitgegeven door de Vereeniging tot beoefening Overijssels regt en geschiedenis*, 1st vol., 45 (1928), 21, 9.

99 Ribbius, P., 'Medici en medische toestanden te Arnhem door alle tijden', *Nederlands Tijdschrift voor Geneeskunde* 71 (1927), II, 625, 627.

100 Van Loon, 'Het Rotterdamsche chirurgijnsgilde', 1486.

101 Nanninga-Uiterdijk, J., 'De geneeskunstbeoefenaren te Kampen I', *Bijdragen tot de Geschiedenis van Overijssel* 4 (1877), 27.

102 Bik, *Vijf eeuwen medisch leven in een Hollandse stad*, 15.

103 Hellinga, G., 'De geschiedenis der geneeskundige armverzorging, buiten de gasthuizen te Amsterdam', I, *Nederlands Tijdschrift voor Geneeskunde* 77 (1933), 4221.

104 Lindemann, *Medicine and Society*, 167-168.

105 Hellinga, G., 'De geschiedenis der geneeskundige armverzorging, buiten de gasthuizen te Amsterdam', II, *Nederlands Tijdschrift voor Geneeskunde* 77 (1933), 531.

106 Hart, S., *Geschrift en Getal. Een keuze uit de demografische, economische- en sociaal-historische studieën op grond van Amsterdamse en Zaanse archivalia, 1600-1800* (Dordrecht 1976), 119.

107 Schoute, D., *De levensloop van een ziekenhuis. Geschiedenis van het Gasthuis te Middelburg* (Middelburg, 1916), 44.

108 Ibid., 49, 61.

109 Sciortino, R.M.E., *Care-takers of Cure: a Study of Health Centre Nurses in Rural Central Java* (Amsterdam, 1992), 21.

110 Mooij, *De polslag van de stad*, 53.

111 Ibid., 50.

112 Ibid., 53.

113 Ketting, *De Amsterdamse chirurgijns*, 20.

114 Wendte, J.F., 'De Hoornse stadarts dr. Pilgrom Hermansz Hulleman en zijn voor- en nageslacht', *Gens Nostra*, 55 (2000), 3, 116-117.

115 Van Gelder, R., *Het Oost-Indisch avontuur. Duitsers in dienst van de VOC (1600-1800)*, (Nijmegen, 1997), 70.

116 Hallema, A., 'Iets over de organisatie van den geneeskundigen dienst en de inrichting der zoogenaamde medische politie ten plattelande gedurende de 18de eeuw', *Nederlands Tijdschrift voor Geneeskunde* 85, (1941) 3, 36, 3610.
117 Ringoir, D.J., *Plattelandschirurgijns in de zeventiende en achttiende eeuw. De rekeningboeken van de 18e eeuwse Durgerdamse chirurgijn Anthonij Egberts* (Bunnik, 1977), 16.
118 Van der Hoeven, M., 'Na de slag. Het veldhospitaal van Hendrik Verschuring en realisme in zeventiende eeuwse oorlogskunst', *Armamentaria* 29 (1994) 35-42, 37.
119 Kerkhof, A.H.M., *Over de geneeskundige verzorging in het Staatse leger* (Nijmegen, 1976), 49-56.
120 Van der Hoeven, 'Na de slag', 37.
121 Kerkhof, 'Over de geneeskundige verzorging', 143-148.
122 Ten Doesschate, 'Geneeskunde in Oud-Zwolle', 49.
123 De Moulin, *A History of Surgery*, 42.

Notes to Chapter 2

1 Some traces of maritime medicine are found in Antiquity. In the *Corpus Hippocraticum*, tetanus is mentioned, as the master of a cargo boat suffered from it (Schadewaldt, H., 'Geschichte der Schiffschirurgie. Die Entwicklung bis zur mitte des 19. Jahrhunderts', *Münchener Medizinischer Wochenschrift* 34 (1967) 1732-1742). Sometimes, among the crews of classical Greek and Roman fleets, it appears a ship's physician is listed, mostly to care for wounded sailors injured in naval engagements (Zorn, E., *Schiffärtzmedizin im Wandel der Zeiten*, 529). According to the German medical historian H. Schadewalt, the *Lex Didia* stipulated that the *Duumviri Navales* had to take care of health and hygiene on board (Schadewalt, H., 'Geschichte der Schiffschirurgie. Die Entwicklung bis zur mitte des 19. Jahrhunderts'. *Münchener Medizinischer Wochenschrift* 34/1967, 1732-1742, p. 1735). According to the Oxford Classical Dictionary, the *Duumviri Navales* were two officers, established by a tribunician *Lex Decia* in 311 BC, with the primary function of coastal defence. Each of them commanded ten warships (The Oxford Classical Dictionary, Oxford University Press 1996, 499). As voyages in those days were necessarily short (the ships were mainly rowed because sailing techniques were still rather simple), the coastline was hugged. Fighting tactics were relatively primitive, maritime medical care, if present, must have been rather limited in scope.
The Rhodian Sea law, or *Lex Rhodia*, was based on maritime customary law originating in ancient Rhodes. However, the origins of the Lex Rhodia, the foundation of modern maritime jurisprudence, are, in the words of the early-twentieth-century historian William McFee, "lost in the cataclysms which overwhelmed the Mediterranean world after the collapse of the Roman Empire" (McFee, W., *The Law of the Sea* (London, n.d.)). The regulations not only concentrated on the liability for the cost of lost or damaged cargo, but the third part contains three short chapters that deal with fighting sailors:
(chapter v) If sailors set to fighting, let them fight with words and let no man strike another. If a man A strikes B on the head and opens it or injures him in some other way, let A pay B his doctor's fees and expenses and his wages for the whole time he is away from work taken care of himself.
(chapter vi) Sailors are fighting, and A strikes B with a stone or a log. B returns the blow; he did it from necessity. Even if A dies, if it is proved that he gave the first blow, whether with a stone, log, or axe, B, who struck and killed him, is to go harmless. A suffered what he wished to inflict.
(chapter vii) One of the captains, merchants or sailors, strikes a man with his fist and blinds him, or gives him a kick and happens to cause a hernia. The assailant is to pay the doctor's bill and for the eye, twelve gold pieces, for the hernia, ten. If the man dies, his assailant can be tried for murder. (W. McFee, *The Law of the Sea* (London, n.d.) Appendix I, The Rhodian Law, 276-285).

The chapters emphasise that one is liable for the doctor's fees as a result of the injuries incurred. In a primitive way, the sailor of Antiquity was protected against the odd troublemaker on board. More, apparently, was not needed.

2 McFee, W., *The Law of the Sea* (London, n.d.), 38-40.

3 Ibid., Appendix I, The Rhodian Law, 276-285, and Appendix II, The Law of Oleron, 285-292.

4 The nineteenth-century historian Walter Ashburner, editor and critic of the Rhodian Law, noted that by the end of the sixteenth century there were almost as many codes as ports, basically identical, all founded on the Rhodian Codex, but with many diverse clauses. The circumstances with which the codes dealt did not change materially from the time of its original composition until the time when it ceased to be copied. The American legal expert R.D. Benedict believes that the Rhodian Law was a myth and is lacking in all historical factuality, save one sentence. According to Benedict, the myth is based on a fifteenth-century document called "Fragments Pertaining to Nautical Affairs Which Are Commonly Called the Nautical Law of the Rhodians". The Dutchman Cornelius van Bijnkershoek (1673-1743), jurist and inventor of what is known as the "three-mile limit" (based on the thesis that sovereignty over the sea, or territorial waters, extended as far as a cannon could shoot), called this document "the fabrication of some hungry little Greek".

5 Twiss, T. (ed.), *The Black Book of Admiralty*, III, (London 1965), 189.

6 Keevill, J.J., *Medicine and the Navy 1200-1900* (four vols.) I (1200-1649), (London, 1957) I, 10.

7 Zorn, E., 'Schiffärtzmedizin im Wandel der Zeiten', *Medizinische Klinik* 69 (1974), 530.

8 Keevill, *Medicine and the Navy 1200-1900* I, 85-85. According to J. Duffin, the first quarantine can be traced to the town of Ragusa (now Dubrovnik) in 1377. J. Duffin, *History of Medicine: A Scandalously Short Introduction* (Toronto, 2001), 142.

9 Keevil, *Medicine and the Navy 1200-1900* I , 20.

10 Ibid., 25.

11 Rodger, N.A.M., *The Safeguard of the Sea: A Naval History of Britain*. vol. I (London 1997), 306.

12 Keevill, *Medicine and the Navy 1200-1900* I, 57.

13 Keay, J., *The Honourable Company: A History of the English East India Company* (London, 1983), 6.

14 Diseases introduced by the Spanish was one of the causes of the disintegration of the Inca Empire.

15 Crosby A.W., *Ecological Imperialism: The Biological Expansion of Europe, 900-1900* (Cambridge, 1986), 199.

16 Sheridan, R.B., 'The Guinea Surgeons on the Middle Passage: the provision of medical services in the English slave trade', *The International Journal of African Historical Studies* 14 (1981) 4, 602.

17 Crosby, *Ecological Imperialism*, 135.

18 Schoute, D., *De geneeskunde in den dienst der Oost-Indische Compagnie in Nederlandsch-Indië* (Amsterdam 1929), 152.

19 Arnold, D. (ed), *Warm Climates & Western Medicine: The Emergence of Tropical Medicine 1500-1900* (Amsterdam, 1996), 31.

20 Ibid., 22-23.

21 Pearson, M.N., *The New Cambridge History of India I: The Portuguese In India* (Cambridge, 1987), 93.

22 Subba Reddy, D.V., 'An Indo-British medical classic of XVIII century. Charles Curtis on diseases of India in the fleet and in the naval hospital at Madras in 1782 and 1783', *Bulletin of the Indian Institute of the History of Medicine* 4 (1974), 194.

23 Boxer, C.R., *The Portuguese Seaborne Empire 1418-1825* (London, 1969), 131.

24 Diffie, B.W., and G.D. Winius, *Foundations of the Portuguese Empire, 1415-1580*, (University Minnesota, 1978), 178.

25 These diseases were caused by the lack of vitamins which were, however, not identified until the twentieth century.

26 Bruijn, J.R., and F.S. Gaastra (eds.), *Ships, Sailors and Spices, East India Companies and Their Shipping in the Sixteenth, Seventeenth and Eighteenth Centuries* (Amsterdam, 1993), 45.
27 Bruijn and Gaastra (eds.), *Ships, Sailors and Spices*, 46.
28 Boxer, C.R., 'The Carreira Da India, 1650-1750', *Mariners Mirror* 46 (1960) 1-10.
29 Dalrymple, W., *White Mughals. Love and Betrayal in Eighteenth-Century India* (London, 2003), 12. Dalrymple states this from J.B. Tavernier, *Travels in India* (Translated by W. Ball, ed. W. Crooke), 2 vols., Oxford, 1925.
30 Dalrymple, W., *White Mughals*, 6.
31 Meulenbeld, G.J., and Dominik Wujastyk (eds.), *Studies on Indian Medical History: Papers Presented at the International Workshop on the Study of Indian Medicine held at the Wellcome Institute for the History of Medicine* (Groningen, 1987), 121.
32 Foster, W. (ed.), *The English Factories in India 1618-1669* (London, 1906-27), 13 vols., Vol. vol.
33 Hernández-Sáenz, L.M., 'Seamen, surgeons and empire: Spanish naval medical reform and Mexican medicine in the late colonial period', *The Northern Mariner* X (2000) 1, 22-28. Conrad, L.I et al, *The Western Medical Tradition. 800 BC to AD 1800* (Cambridge, 1996), 231.
34 Watt, J., 'Some forgotten contributions of naval surgeons', *Journal of the Royal Society of Medicine* 78 (1985) 753. Also, with Henry VIII, bigger warships were built in which more men were packed for ever-increasing periods. As a result, epidemics on board became commonplace (Keevil, *Medicine and the Navy 1200-1900* I, 60-61).
35 Watt, J., 'Surgeons of the Mary Rose. The practice of surgery in Tudor England', *Mariners Mirror* 69 (1983) 6.
36 Keevil, *Medicine and the Navy 1200-1900 I (1200-1649)*, 142.
37 In 1588, during the Dutch Revolt, Philip II of Spain sent an Armada to invade England along with a Spanish army from Flanders. England's defeat of this fleet constituted the first naval battle to be fought entirely with heavy guns. Philip II employed 85 surgeons as well as several physicians on the 141 ships with crews totalling circa 30,000 men. Apart from the fact that the defeat of the Armada prevented England from being invaded and the Dutch Republic from becoming extinct, while dealing a heavy blow to the prestige of the greatest European power of the epoch, the Armada battle has enduring historical significance as the first major naval gun battle under sail and as the moment from which, for over two-and-a-half centuries, the heavily armed sailing warship dominated the seas.
38 Rodger, *The Safeguard of the Sea* I, 306.
39 Watt, J., 'Surgeons of the Mary Rose', 3.
40 Patterson, T.J.S., 'The medical practice of the East India Company', *Society for the Social History of Medicine Bulletin*, 2 (1980), 41.
41 Meulenbeld, and Wujastyk (eds), *Studies on Indian Medical History*, 123.
42 Keevil, *Medicine and the Navy 1200-1900* I, 110/111.
43 Patterson, 'The medicial practice of the East India Company', 40.
44 A foreign brother being an apprentice who, at the end of his seven-year term of service was admitted to the Company without examination and usually received his licence from the diocesan bishop of the country district where he intended to practise. Keevil, *Medicine and the Navy 1200-1900* I, 140.
45 Ibid., 140.
46 Ibid., 141.
47 Boog Watson, W.N., 'Thomas Robertson, Naval Surgeon, 1793-1828', *Bulletin of the History of Medicine*, 46 (1972), 134.
48 Keevill, *Medicine and the Navy 1200-1900* I, 202/3.
49 Ibid., 203.
50 Broeze, F.J.A., Bruijn, J.R. , and F.S. Gaastra (eds), *Maritieme Geschiedenis der Nederlanden* III (Bussum, 1977), 147.
51 Van Vliet, A.P., *Vissers & Kapers. De zeevisserij vanuit het Maasmondgebied en de Duinkerker kapers (ca. 1580-1648)* (The Hague, 1994), 46.

52 Ibid., 39.
53 Ibid., 162.
54 Broeze, Bruijn, and Gaastra (eds), *Maritieme Geschiedenis der Nederlanden* III, 177; Roelofs, G., *Die Medizinische Versorgung auf Walfangschiffen des Grönlandhandels unter Berücksichtigung der Chirurgenprotocolle* (Bredstedt, 1997), 8.
55 Roelofs, *Die Medizinische Versorgung auf Walfangschiffen*, 9.
56 Leuftink, *De geneeskunde bij 's Lands oorlogsvloot* (Assen, 1953), 15.
57 Sicking, L., *Zeemacht en Onmacht. Maritieme politiek in de Nederlanden. 1488-1558* (Amsterdam, 1998), 204. A hospital ship is a vessel equipped primarily to receive sick and wounded sailors, to provide them with interim treatement and to convey them to hospitals or lodgings on land.
58 Leuftink, *De geneeskunde bij 's Lands oorlogsvloot*, 16.
59 Ibid., 37.
60 Bruijn, J.R., *The Dutch Navy of the Seventeenth and Eighteenth Centuries* (CIT???, 1993), 138.
61 Jan Huijghen van Linschoten spent six years (1583 1589) in Goa, in the Portuguese service. He served pretty much as a 'commercial spy'. There he quietly compiled a dossier on the eastern sea routes, which he smuggled back to the Netherlands. Published in Holland in 1595/6 and translated into English in 1598, Van Linschoten's works were crucial to the early Dutch and English trade expeditions to India and the East Indies.
62 The Dutch ship's surgeon, in the employ of the Habsburg/Dutch Admiralty earned fifteen guilders a month in 1550. Sicking, *Zeemacht en Onmacht*, 202.
63 A Company captain earned between 65 and 80 Dutch guilders whereas a sailor earned between 9 to 11 Dutch guilders a month. A third surgeon earned between 14 and 18 guilders; a surgeon's mate between 22 and 30 guilders and a senior surgeon between 34 and 60 Dutch guilders.
64 Bruijn, I.D.R., 'The health care organization of the Dutch East India Company at home', *The Social History of Medicine* 7 (1994) 3, 366.
65 Bruijn, 'The health care organization of the Dutch East India Company', 368.
66 Westfries Archief (Westfrisian archives or WA): Archive Hoorn, inventory no. 1815(a).
67 See, for instance, Brans, P.H., 'De geneesmiddelvoorziening bij de admiraliteiten en bij de Oost-Indische Compagnie', *Pharmaceutisch Weekblad* 98 (1963), 596-608, page 599.
68 WA, Archive Hoorn. This ordinance is one of the ca. 250 documents which unfortunately have been lost. There still exists a printed form of the ordinance in the archive in Hoorn. See also, Leuftink, A.E., *Geneeskunde bij 's Lands Oorlogsvloot* (Assen, 1953), 35.
69 Leuftink, *De geneeskunde bij 's Lands oorlogsvloot*, 34.
70 Ibid., 34.
71 Gemeentearchief Amsterdam (Municipality Archives of Amsterdam) or GAA, Inventory 366 (Surgeon's Guild): Miseroy 255 folio 2616; Gastman 251 folio 613; and Sluijs nr. 255 folio 359.
72 GAA, inventory 366, no. 251.
73 National Archives (NA), VOC 110: 04-09-1686 and NA, VOC 110: 08-10-1687.
74 Koninkx, C., *Het eerste en tweede octrooi van de Zweedse Oost-Indische Compagnie (1731-1766)* (Brussel, 1975), 284.
75 Israel, J., *The Dutch Republic: Its Rise, Greatness and Fall 1477-1806* (New York, 1995), 307.
76 '*Ordonnantie van 't Collegie der Doctoren ende Chirurgijns anno 1636 den 7 December*' in: *Handtvesten, privilegien, willekeuren ende ordonnantien der stadt Enckhuysen* (Enckhuysen, Egbert van den Hoof, 1667), 264-269.
77 NA, VOC 234: 05-12-1652.
78 Schoute, *De geneeskunde in den dienst der Oost-Indische Compagnie in Nederlandsch-Indië*, 17.
79 Nationaal Archief (NA, National Archives, The Hague), VOC 241: 17.07.1681
80 Leuftink, *Harde Heelmeesters. Zeelieden en hun dokters in de 18e eeuw* (Zutphen 1991), 31.
81 Ibid., 35.
82 Van Andel, M.A., *Chirurgijns, Vrije Meesters, Beunhazen en Kwakzalvers. De chirurgijnsgilden en de practijk der heelkunde 1400-1800* (Amsterdam, 1946), 109-110.

83 De Ridder, J., 'Van Aderlaten en Amputaties', *De Wete* 30 (2001) 1, 25.
84 Ibid., 25.
85 NA, VOC 126: 28-09-1751.
86 De Wet, G.C., *Resolusies van die Politieke Raad.* V*: 1716-1719*: 26-9-1719.
87 "… wijl mijn maat d'ondermeester overleeden is, en den ander oppermeester doot kranck leijt en is het groot getal van onse siecken soodanigh aangenomen hebbe als ick kan bijbrengen dat het mijn onmogelijck is daer van in het particulier journaal te houden …", NA, VOC 5082.
88 Eloy, J., 'Rélations de Voyages de Charles-Ghislain Wilmet. Chirurgien major à la Cie Maritime des Indes Neêrlandaises', *Annuaire d'Histoires Régionales et Locales 'Le Vieux Châtelet'*, (1984), 115-134, p. 122. Charles Ghislain Wilmet wrote several letters about his voyages as ship's surgeon to his family in Belgium. His letters were brought back to the Republic to be posted there by returning 'friends'. Born in the village Gembloux near Namur on 28 October, 1757, Wilmet travelled to Rotterdam at the beginning of 1779 to lodge with a 'friend' Master-Surgeon Van Putten who had his shop and home in the Breestraat. Wilmet wrote to his aunt and uncle on 11 March 1779 that he had been to the Chamber of Rotterdam to present his letters and certificates. The authorities were quite interested in him as a prospective employee and they told him that he would be tested on his surgical knowledge in order to determine his rank (first surgeon, first surgeon's mate or third surgeon). Passing his exam with honours, he subsequently sailed (probably) on the *Willem Frederik* (a vessel with a crew of more than 300 men) as first a ship's surgeon. In 1782, he was employed by the merchant fleet; in 1784, on the whaling fleet and at the Admirality of Rotterdam, and in 1785 and in 1790 again, by the Company's. Clearly, he must have, at least, enjoyed his work as a ship's surgeon. Though Wilmet did not write much about his work, he does describe small parcels to be delivered to friends. Charles Ghislain Wilmet continued working as a first ship's surgeon until his demise in Asia in 1791.
89 Ketting, H., *Leven, werk en rebellie aan boord van Oost-Indiëvaarders (1595-1650)* (Amsterdam, 2003), 85.
90 Warnsinck, J.C.M. (ed.), *De Reisen van Nicolaus de Graaff gedaan naar alle gewesten des werelds. Beginnende 1639 tot 1687 incluis*, Werken Linschoten-Vereeniging, XXXIII (The Hague, 1930), Oost-Indische Spiegel, 58-63.
91 According to G.F. Pop, the middle cabin on starboard was allocated to the senior surgeon, and as such, this surgeon was a 'member' of the captain's cabin. The surgeon's mate slept in a self-made cabin of canvas in the *kerk* or *voorcajuit* (the foremost cabin), and the third surgeon slept in the gunner's cabin. G.F. Pop, *De geneeskunde bij het Nederlandsche zeewezen (Geschiedkundige Nasporingen)* (Batavia, 1922), 251.
92 Leuftink, *Harde Heelmeesters*, 39.
93 Burrows, E.H., *A History of Medicine in South Africa up to the End of the Nineteenth Century* (Cape Town & Amsterdam 1958), 23. Van der Chijs, J.A., *Nederlandsch-Indisch Plakaatboek, 1602-1811*, II (The Hague 1886), 08.03.1658: article 40: The promise is that the injured and ill will be treated and cured by the surgeons; article 66: all surgeons and surgeon's mates should be at the service of the ill and injured, except those who suffer from venereal disease; article 67: the patient's quarter-mates should help the patient; article 68: the crew should clean the ship regularly; and article 69: the ship's company should use only designated areas as a toilet. The article letter of 02.03.1634 mentions that if a sailor lost an arm or leg, the Company would pay a certain sum by way of compensation; all surgeons had to be in the service of the vessel's company for which the surgeons only received their wages and no other compensation; the surgeons are allowed to be paid extra for the treatment of venereal diseases and injuries that result from incidents outside the service; moreover, quarter-mates should support their patients and clean the vessel each morning (translated and summarised by the author).
94 NA, VOC 111: 10-12-1695.
95 Ketting, *Leven, werk en rebellie*, 128.

96 No whet-stones needed for the sharpening of knives were ever mentioned. P. Sterk, former Dutch Navy barber, and currently hairdresser in Amsterdam as well as an amateur-historian of the history of barbers, confirmed that a 'shaving knife' or razor for personal use has to be sharpened at least once a week. If used professionally, as in a barber's shop, at least once a day. I refer to chapter 7 for the particulars of those lists of possessions.

97 NA, VOC 14.826.

98 Van Rooij, H.J., and J. Gawronski, *VOC-schip Amsterdam: gebleeven – op de kust van Sussex tussen Hastings en Beachyhead gestrand* (Haarlem, 1989), 58: it also had a dependance on the wharf.

99 Van der Chijs, J.A. (ed), *Nederlandsch-Indisch Plakaatboek* IV *1709-1743* (Batavia/'s-Gravenhage 1887), 447-448.

100 Van Rooij, and Gawronski, *VOC-schip Amsterdam*, 64-66.

101 For instance, Sir Gilbert Blane (1749-1834) suggested the following ingredients for the medical chests of the English Navy (which suggestions were adopted) at the end of the eighteenth century. Blane's medicines do not differ much from those of the VOC's medical chests (Lloyd, Chr., *Medicine and the Navy 1200-1900* III*: 1714-1815* (London, 1961), 54).

Sir Gilbert Blane's proposed medical chest

Peruvian bark	Calomel	Emitic tarta	Ipeccacuanha
Opium	Purging salts	Senna leaves	Aloes
Ammoniacum	Balsam of Copaiva	Cantharides	Capsicum
Traumatic Balsam	Camphor	Castor	Chamomile flowers or Hops
Cinnamon	Prepared Chalk or Oyster shells	Conserve of Roses	Cordial Confection
Cordial Confection	Cathartic extract	Extract of Hemlock	Extract of Logwood
Gentian	Dried Squills	Golden Sulphur of Antimony	Flower of Sulphur
Cream of Tartar	Vinegar	White Vitriol	Wormwood
Flowers of Zinc	Ginger	Gum Arabic	Gum Guiacum
Powder of Jalap	Laudanum	Linseed	Magnesia
Manna Whole Mustard Seed	Myrrh	Crude Mercury	Corrosive Sublimate
Nitre	Oil of Almonds	Castor oil	Linseed oil
Essential oil of Mint	Jamaica pepper	Blistering plaster	Quassia
Salt of Harshorn	Salt of Steel	Salt of Wormwood	Castile Soap
Sarsaparilla	Serpentary	Spermaceti	Rectified spirit of wine
Weak spirit of Vitriol	Spirit of Mindererus	Spirit of Turpentine	

102 Kool-Blokland, J.L., *De Zorg Gewogen. Zeven Eeuwen Godshuizen in Middelburg* (Middelburg, 1990), 433-437.

103 NA, VOC 154: 19-02-1682. Renate Wilson's *Pious Traders in Medicine* (2000) made it clear how much the charitable works of the Halle Pietists depended on income from

their medical trade (in medical substances). Although it does seem a very natural extra business activity for ship's surgeons to engage in as medicines were valuable in comparison with their weight and bulk, I have not found any evidence of systematic trade in these substances (see chapter 6).

104 Romieux, Y., 'Médicaments et médications à bord des vaisseux de la Compagnie francaise des Indes', in: Haudrères, Ph. (ed), *Les flottes des Compagnies des Indes 1600-1857* (Vincennes, 1996), 120.

105 NA, VOC 253: 02-06-1681.

106 Breedveld, P.H., and J.L.M. Hendrikx, *Het journaal van de scheepschirurgijn J.W. Daman (1735-1783). Gezondheid en ziekten aan boord van een oostindiëvaarder*, Scripta Tironum 12 (Nijmegen, 1987).

107 See chapter 1.

108 Warnsinck, J.C.M. (ed.), *De Reisen van Nicolaus de Graaff gedaan naar alle gewesten des werelds. Beginnende 1639 tot 1687 incluis*, Werken uitgegeven door de Linschoten-Vereeniging, XXXIII (The Hague, 1930) 140.

109 NA, VOC 11.356.

110 Dekkers, O. (ed), *Een Bunschoter VOC chirurgijn. 'Dagelijkse aantekeningen' van de reis naar Oost-Indië in 1654 door Gijsbert Heeck (1619-1669)* (Bunschoten, 2001), 86.

111 Lloyd, *Medicine and the Navy 1200-1900.* III*: 1714-1815*, 64.

112 NA, VOC 147: 22-08-1630.

113 NA, VOC 104: 11-10-1656.

114 Gawronski, J. (ed.), *Hollandia Compendium. A Contribution to the History, Archaeology, Classification and Lexicography of a 150 ft Dutch East Indiaman (1747-1750)* (Amsterdam, 1992), 231-242.

115 NA, VOC 14.411.

116 NA, VOC 12.893.

117 NA, VOC 13.240.

118 NA, VOC 13.136.

119 Burrows states that for the period 1730 to 1749 130 ship's surgeon's logs were found in the archives of the Cape. See: Burrows, *A history of medicine in South Africa*, 25.

120 Boon, P., *Bouwers van de zee: zeevarenden van het Westfriese platteland, c. 1680-1720* (Leiden, 1996), 129,130.

121 Boxer, C.R., *The Dutch Seaborne Empire 1600-1800* (London, 1973), 92.

122 Van Gelder, R., *'Naporra's Omweg: Het Leven van een VOC-matroos (1731-1793)* (Amsterdam, 2003), 129.

123 Bruijn, J.R.,'De personeelsbehoefte van de VOC overzee en aan boord, bezien in Aziatisch en Nederlands perspectief', *Bijdragen en Mededelingen van de Geschiedenis der Nederlanden* XCI (1976), 222; Boxer, *The Dutch Seaborne Empire*, 51; and Van der Woude, A.M., *Het Noorderkwartier: een regionaal historisch onderzoek in de demografische en economische geschiedenis van westelijk Nederland van de late Middeleeuwen tot het begin van de negentiende eeuw*, AAG Bijdragen 16 (Wageningen, 1972) II, 366-367.

124 Bruijn, *The Dutch Navy of the Seventeenth and Eighteenth Centuries*, 195.

125 Bruijn, 'The Health Care Organization of the Dutch East India Company', 366.

126 Bruijn, et al. (eds.), *Dutch Asiatic Shipping* I, 159.

127 Bruijn, J.R., and J. Lucassen (eds.) *Op de schepen der Oost-Indische Compagnie. Vijf artikelen van J. de Hullu* (Groningen, 1980), 120.

128 NA, VOC 11.356.

129 Bruijn, 'De personeelsbehoefte van de VOC', 223. These high mortality rates were, in all probability, the result of typhus epidemics on board, see further under *Fevers and Typhus* of this chapter.

130 Bruijn, et al. (eds.), *Dutch Asiatic Shipping* I, 163.

131 Koninkx, C., 'Ziekten op Zee. Pathologie van de Ziekten in de Grote Vaart in de Achttiende Eeuw'. *Marine Academie Mededelingen* XXVI (1980-1981-1982).

132 Bruijn, et al. (eds.), *Dutch Asiatic Shipping* I, 162.

133 Koninkx, 'Ziekten op Zee', 41.

134 Bruijn, et al. (eds.), *Dutch Asiatic Shipping*, I, 160; and Schoute, D., 'Gezondheid en ziekte aan boord der Compagnie's Oost-Indiëvaarders', *Overdruk uit de Provinciale Zeeuwsche en Middelburgsche Courant van 26.02.1936 – 03.03.1936.*
135 Lloyd, *Medicine and the Navy 1200-1900*. III*: 1714-1815*, 293.
136 Gordon, E.C., 'Scurvy and Anson's voyage round the world: 1740-44. An analysis of the Royal Navy's worst outbreak.', *American Neptune* 44 (1984), 155-166, 155.
137 Lloyd, Chr. (ed.), *The Health of Seamen: Selections from the works of Dr. James Lind, Sir Gilbert Blane and Dr. Thomas Trotter* (London 1965), 20-21.
138 Bruijn, and Gaastra (eds.), *Ships, Sailors and Spices*, 81.
139 Dalat, J., 'Un chirurgien de mer à la fin du XVIIIe siècle', *Revue d'Histoire de la Pharmacie* XXX, 259 (1983) 275.
140 Bruijn, and Gaastra (eds.), *Ships, Sailors and Spices*, 92.
141 Koninckx, 'Ziekten op Zee', 34-35.
142 Bruijn, and Gaastra (eds.), *Ships, Sailors and Spices*, 134.
143 Koninckx, *The First and Second Charters of the Swedish East India Company, 1731-1766* (Kortrijk, 1980), 347-349.
144 Koninckx, C., 'L'alimentation et la pathologie des déficiences alimentaires dans la navigation au long cours au XVIIIe siècle', *Revue d'Histoire Moderne et Contemporaine* (1983), 30, 137.
145 Watt, J., 'Some forgotten contributions of naval surgeons', *Journal of the Royal Society of Medicine* 78 (1985). 757.
146 Dekkers (ed.), *Een Bunschoter VOC chirurgijn*, 86.
147 Ibid., 114.
148 Ibid., 130.
149 Bruijn et al. (eds.), *Dutch Asiatic Shipping*, I, 165/166.
150 Blussé, J.L., *Strange Company: Chinese Settlers, Mestizo Women and the Dutch in VOC Batavia* (Leiden, 1986), 30
151 Van der Brug, P.H., *Malaria en malaise : de VOC in Batavia in de achttiende eeuw* (Amsterdam, 1994). I also refer to chapter 4 under *The crisis of the eighteenth century.*
152 *The Economist*, 21 July 2001, pages 68-69: The origins of Malaria.
153 Ibid.
154 Ultee, M. (ed), *Adapting to Conditions: War and Society in the Eighteenth Century* (Alabama, 1986), 27-34.
155 Van der Brug, P.H., *Malaria en malaise*, 200.
156 Ibid., 27.
157 Ultee, *Adapting to Conditions*, 35.
158 Bruijn, and Gaastra (eds.), *Ships, Sailors and Spices*, 99.
159 Ibid., 110.
160 Ibid., 147.
161 De Graaf, D., 'De Koninklijke Compagnie. De Pruisische Aziatische Compagnie 'von Emden nach China' (1751-1765)', *Tijdschrift voor Zeegeschiedenis* 20 (2001) 143-162.
162 Meulenbeld, and Wujastyk (eds.), *Studies on Indian Medical History*, 120.
163 In 1694, medical (and surgical) experiences of both the East and West Indies were united in Bontius, J., Piso, G., and G. Markgraef, *Oost- en West-Indische warande: Vervattende aldaar de leef- en geneeskomst. Met een verhaal van de specerijen, boom- en aardgewassen, dieren etc. in oost- en West Indien voorvallende*. In which was also included *De nieuw verbeterde chirurgijns scheepkist.*
164 Schoute, *De geneeskunde in den dienst der Oost-Indische compagnie in Nederlandsch-Indië*, 120.
165 Von Roemer, L.S.A.M., *Historical Sketches. An Introduction to the Fourth Congres of the Far Eastern Association of Tropical Medicine* (Batavia, 1921), 223.
166 NA, VOC 4123, folio 1037 recto, 1043 recto.
167 NA. 1.10.69. Archief Rademacher, 91.
168 Ibid.
169 Ibid.

170 NA, VOC 4123, folio 1033 verso and 1039 recto.
171 Ibid., folio 1036 recto.
172 NA, VOC 121: 27.08.1736; VOC 12: 26.02.1739
173 NA. 1.10.69. Archief Radermacher 91.
174 Veirac, J., and B. Hussum, 'Antwoord over de rotkoorts op de Oost-Indische schepen', *Verhandelingen van het Zeeuwsch Genootschap der Wetenschappen* VI (Middelburg, 1769-1792).
175 NA, VOC 5151.

Notes to Chapter 3

1 Only occasionally was an academically trained *doctor medicinae* to be found at the medical service of the Company in Asia, as this service was thought to be more surgical in character and was not well paid compared to a practice at home. Furthermore, any physician who did hire on was soon drawn into the administrative apparatus of the Company in Asia. One example is Dr Bontius who went to Asia in 1627 and who described several tropical diseases like beri-beri, tetanus, dysentery, cholera, Indian fevers and Amboinese pocks (framboesia), as well as Asian herbs in his *De Medicina Indorum* (Leiden, 1642). He was soon promoted to *fiscaal* of the Council of the Indies (Schoute, D., *De geneeskunde in den dienst der Oost-Indische Compagnie in Nederlandsch-Indië*, (Amsterdam, 1929), 119-126). Dr Robertus Padtbrugge was another example; he obtained his doctorate at the medical faculty of Leiden University in 1663, set sail for Batavia in 1664 and in 1666 had already been appointed member of the court of justice in Ceylon. (Pabbruwe, H.J., *Dr Robertus Padtbrugge (Parijs 1637 – Amersfoort 1703), Dienaar van de Verenigde Oost-Indische Compagnie en zijn familie* (Kloosterzande, n.d.)). The physician Willem ten Rhijne who was sent to Batavia to advise the *Hoge Regering* was made a member of the same council in 1681.

2 Risse, G., *Mending Bodies, Saving Souls: A History of* Hospitals (Oxford, 1999), 216-216.

3 Ibid., 236. States would also try to increase their strength by promoting their population's health, as a part of the political and mercantilist goals of various European states.

4 The research for this chapter is mainly based on the resolutions made by the Gentlemen XVII and the Chamber Amsterdam, as those for Zeeland and the smaller chambers are either virtually non-existent or not indexed. As far as Batavia and the other overseas settlements are concerned, the research has been done in the ordinances of the Council of the Indies, which were published in Van der Chijs, J.A., *Nederlandsch-Indisch Plakaatboek, 1602-1811*, I-XVII (Batavia/The Hague, 1885-1895), in the resolutions of the Council of the Indies, which are found in the National Archives of The Hague (*Nationaal Archief, NA*), and in the *Overgekomen Brieven en Papieren*. The existing literature on the Dutch medical overseas organisation such as Schoute, D., *De geneeskunde in den dienst der Oost-Indische Compagnie in Nederlandsch-Indië* (Amsterdam, 1929) and the English translation *Occidental Therapeutics in the Netherlands East Indies during three centuries of Netherlands settlement (1600-1900)* (Batavia, 1937), Von Römer, L.S.A.M., *Historical Sketches. An introduction to the Fourth Congress of the Far Eastern Association of Tropical Medicine* (Batavia, 1921), J.N.H. van Dorssen, 'De lepra in Nederlandsch Oost-Indië tijdens de 17de en 18de eeuw', *Geneeskundig Tijdschrift voor Nederlandsch-Indië* 37 (1897) 255-324, and 'Willem ten Rhijne', *Geneeskundig Tijdschrift voor Nederlandsch-Indie* 51 (1922) 135-228, though admirable studies, are rather old fashioned and contain practically no references. The research of the past 20 years has led to many new insights, such as those of Van der Brug, P.H in *Malaria en Malaise. De VOC in Batavia in de achttiende eeuw* (Amsterdam, 1994). Leuftink, A.E., *Harde Heelmeesters. Zeelieden en hun dokters in de 18de eeuw* (Zutphen, 1991) contains a profound study of Cape Town hospitals. For those who are interested in a more detailed description of the South African medical organisation during the period of the Company, I refer to Leuftink and Burrows (Burrows, E.H., *A History of Medicine in South Africa up to the End of the Nineteenth Century* (Cape Town/Amsterdam, 1958).

5 NA, VOC 238: 24.01.1669, and VOC 247: 16.04.1708.

6 NA, VOC 238: 11.01.1669; J.J. de Jong, *Met goed fatsoen: de elite in een Hollandse stad (Gouda 1700-1780)* (Amsterdam, 1986), 379.

7 NA, VOC 227: 21.06.1612.

8 NA, VOC 235: 31.01.1658.

9 NA, VOC 241: 31.07.1678; VOC 250: 08.12.1718.

10 Bruiijn, I.D.R., 'The Health Care Organization of the Dutch East India Company at Home', *Social History of Medicine* 7 (1994) 3, 359-382.

11 NA, VOC 234: 05.12.1652; VOC 236: 30.06.1659; VOC 246: 21.01.1706.

12 Leuftink, *Harde Heelmeesters*, 47.

13 Hellinga, G., 'De geschiedenis der geneeskundige armverzorging, buiten de gasthuizen te Amsterdam', I, *Nederlands Tijdschrift voor Geneeskunde* 76 (1932) III, 4224.

14 NA, VOC 364: 03.09.1672; VOC 366: 04.09.1742.

15 Rodger, N.A.M., *The Wooden World: An Anatomy of the Georgian Navy* (London, 1986), 20: On merchant ships it was, and remains, the master who holds command (although sometimes he is called 'captain'), while in the navy, the master was simply the navigator. Because a fully educated surgeon was called 'master' or 'master-surgeon' in the Republic, I have used 'captain' for the master of a Dutch East Indiaman in order not to confuse him with a surgeon.

16 NA, VOC 280: 04.06.1772 ; 15.06.1772; 18.06.1772.

17 NA, VOC 299: 14.07.1791.

18 Böeseken, A.J., *Resolusien van die Politieke Raad*, IV (Kaapstad, 1962): 8-11-1708. Benraath, it appears, was a difficult man. Because of his quarrelsome, overbearing character, coupled with his licentious life, the Political Council judged it better to repatriate him in 1712. He duly arrived in Amsterdam in 1713, and did not enlist with the Company again.

19 This hospital ship was later captured by the English.

20 NA, VOC 280: 25.11.1771; 09.12.1771.

21 NA, VOC 280: 22.04.1772.

22 Bruijn, J.R., 'De personeelsbehoefte van de VOC overzee en aan boord, bezien in Aziatisch en Nederlands perspectief', *Bijdragen en Mededelingen betreffende de Geschiedenis der Nederlanden* XCI (1976), 222.

23 NA, VOC 111: 10.12.1695. In all probability, it was typhus that caused the highest mortality rates and not scurvy.

24 NA, VOC 124: 29.03.1745; 30.08.1745; VOC 127: 15.10.1754; VOC 128: 01.04.1755; 09.04.1755.

25 In 1783, the Company paid a full surgeon three guilders, and a surgeon's mate one guilder (1,10) for every member of the crew brought to the Cape alive. If they survived the voyage to Batavia, the premium was slightly higher, namely five guilders for a full surgeon and two guilders (2,10) for a surgeon's mate (NA, VOC 138, 19.11.1783). This turned out to be quite a costly affair, especially when these payments had to be paid out in Batavia. Consequently, the Council of the Indies requested the directors in the Republic to revert to the old practise of lump sums (NA, VOC 139: 28.04.1786; 21.03.1791). In 1791, it was decided to pay a lump sum (douceur) of 150 guilders to a chief surgeon and a 100 guilders to a surgeon's mate.

26 NA, VOC 111: 10.12.1695; VOC 122: 26.02.1739; VOC 14329: 04.09.1743; VOC 126: 28.09.1751; VOC 134: 14.03.1771; VOC 184: 02.04.1774; VOC 141: 08.12.1788; VOC 206: 04.01.1794.

27 NA, VOC 126: 28.9.1751.

28 NA, VOC 121: 27.08.1736; VOC 12: 26.02.1739.

29 Boxer, C.R., 'The Dutch East-Indiamen: their sailors, their navigators and life on board, 1602-1795', *Mariner's Mirror* 49 (1963), 81-104, 98.

30 Veirac, J., and B. Hussum, 'Antwoord over de rotkoorts op de Oost-Indische schepen', *Verhandelingen van het Zeeuwsch Genootschap der Wetenschappen* VI Middelburg (1769-1792) 3-225; see also Leuftink, *Harde Heelmeesters*, 143-6.

31 Schoute, D., *De levensloop van een ziekenhuis. Geschiedenis van het gasthuis te Middelburg* (Middelburg, 1916), 63.
32 NA, VOC 181: 10.04.1773.
33 NA, VOC 184: as an appendix to resolution 02.04.1774.
34 NA, VOC 135: 02.04.1774.
35 NA, VOC 287: 24.06.1779; 26.08.1779; 06.09.1779; VOC 288: 10.02.1780.
36 NA, VOC 138: 15.05.1784.
37 NA, VOC 181: 06.10.1772.
38 Leuftink, *Harde Heelmeesters*, 143.
39 Lines from an anonymous contributor in the *Naval Chronicle*, 1817, 37: 334.
40 Bruijn, J.R., Gaastra, F.S., and I. Schöffer (eds.), *Dutch Asiatic Shipping in the seventeenth and eighteenth centuries*, I, (The Hague 1987), 119-121.
41 Van der Chijs, J.A., *Nederlandsch-Indisch Plakaatboek, 1602-1811*, I (The Hague, 1885): 17.03.1632.
42 Raben, R., *Batavia and Colombo. The Ethnic and Spatial Order of Two Colonial Cities 1600-1800* (Leiden, 1996), 278. No proof has been found in the National Archives of The Hague, nor those of Djakarta, of the existence of a surgical guild in Batavia, Colombo, or, for that matter, the Cape of Good Hope.
43 Raben, *Batavia and Colombo*, 281.
44 Van der Chijs, *Nederlandsch-Indisch Plakaatboek, 1602-1811*, I (The Hague 1885),: 12.03.1642, Ibid.: 17.03.1632.
45 Schama, S., *The Embarrassment of Riches*, 576.
46 Granshaw, L., and R. Porter (eds.), *The* Hospital *in History* (London, 1990), 150.
47 Ibid., 172.
48 Ibid., 4.
49 Keevil, *Medicine and the Navy* II, 283.
50 Conrad, L.I. et al., *The Western Medical Tradition. 800 BC to AD 1800* (Cambridge, 1996), 231.
51 Anderson, Ph., *The English in Western India: being the early history of the Factory at Surat, of Bombay, and the subordinate factories on the Western coast* (London, 1854), 63.
52 Granshaw and Porter, *The Hospital*, 181.
53 Swaving, C., 'Batavia's sanitaire geschiedenis onder het bestuur van de Oost-Indische Maatschappij', *Nederlandsch Tijdschrift voor Geneeskunde* (1878), 8.
54 NA, VOC 1394, folio 760-762: Bericht van de prakticijns van het Hospitaal Batavia, 30.11.1683.
55 NA, VOC 147: 24.08.1626.
56 Although ship's surgeons were examined in the Republic, it could happen that *derde meesters* and *ondermeesters* were promoted long before they were professionally competent to act in this capacity; they were therefore examined and/or certified in Batavia.
57 J. Bontius, *Iac.Bontii in Indijs Archiatri De medicina Indorum* (Leiden, 1642) translated into English as *An account of the Diseases, Natural History and Medicines of the East Indies, translated from the Latin of James Bontius, Physician to the Dutch settlement at Batavia* (London, 1769).
58 Schoute, *Occidental Therapeutics*, 27.
59 In the Republic, as elsewhere, no vessel was built especially to serve as a permanent floating hospital. Instead, it was practice to outfit a particular vessel for temporary use when the need arose. Such ships were usually the least seaworthy available at the moment. Boog Watson, W.N., 'Thomas Robertson, Naval Surgeon, 1793-1828', *Bulletin of the History of Medicine* 46 (1972), 45. In the eighteenth century, the *Admiraalschip*, which was usually anchored at the roadstead, served as a hospital ship. Otherwise, this ship served as a lodging for sailors waiting for their next destination.
60 Van der Chijs, *Nederlandsch-Indisch Plakaatboek, 1602-1811*, I (The Hague, 1885), 01.11.1638.
61 Sciortino, R., *Care-takers of Cure: A Study of Health Centre Nurses in Rural Central Java* (Amsterdam, 1992), 50.

62 Realia Register op de Generale Resolutiën van het Kasteel Batavia 1632-1805. Uitgegeven door het Bataviaasch Genootschap van Kunsten en Wetenschappen, I (Leiden, 1882): 12.03.1642.
63 Employees with a higher status, usually with a merchant rank, were allowed to lodge with friends in case of illness. The word 'friend' included mere acquaintancies. It follows that only lower-ranking servants used the hospital.
64 Von Röemer, *Historical Sketches*, 165.
65 Oost-Indische Spiegel, 9, in: *Reisen van Nicolaus de Graaff. Gedaan naar alle gewesten des Werelds. Beginnende 1639 tot 1687 incluis*. Uitgegeven en toegelicht door J.C.M. Warnsinck. Werken uitgegeven door de Linschoten Vereeniging XXXIII (The Hague, 1986).
66 Van Gelder, R., *'Naporra's Omweg: Het Leven van een VOC-matroos (1731-1793)* (Amsterdam, 2003), 315.
67 Boog Watson, 'Thomas Robertson, Naval Surgeon, 1793-1828', *Bulletin of the History of Medicine* 46 (1972) 132.
68 Arsip Nasional Republik Indonesia (ANRI) 6: Resoluties Hospitalen 1766-67. Not identified: Salvation?
69 Stapel, F.W. (ed.), *Pieter van Dam's Beschrijvinge van de Oostindische Compagnie*, Rijks Geschiedkundige Publicatiën (RGP) 87 (The Hague, 1943), 209.
70 Stapel, *Pieter van Dam's Beschrijvinge*, RPG 87, 209.
71 Blussé, L., *Strange Company*, 18-19.
72 Gaastra, F., *De Geschiedenis van de VOC* (Zutphen, 1991), 71-72. Bruijn, J.R., Gaastra, F.S. and I. Schöffer (eds.), *Dutch Asiatic Shipping in the seventeenth and eighteenth centuries* (The Hague, 1987), I, 124.
73 Raben, R., et al, *The Archives of the Dutch East India Company 1602-1795* (The Hague, 1992), 27.
74 At a funeral, for instance, the cortège followed according to rank: directly after the deceased came the family members, the members of the *Hoge Regering*, possibly accompanied with governors of outer factories. Then followed friends and the councillors of Justice, the aldermen, the vicars, the members of the drainage boards, the commissioners of marriage, chief merchants and captains, merchants and ship masters, and then came the chief surgeons, after which followed a number of lower-ranked employees. See Van der Chijs, *Nederlandsch-Indisch Plakaatboek*, IV, 09.08.1718.
75 Taylor, J. Gelman, *The Social World of Batavia* (London, 1983), 4. Rank, however, did not have to be related to a specific function; a person could be a surgeon with the rank of a merchant. This clarified the issue of a person's status in the Company hierarchy and it also clarified what extra remunerations that person was entitled to, often in the form of wine or arak and rice. In pre-modern Western Europe, payment in kind was a normal practice.
76 Van der Chijs, *Nederlandsch-Indisch Plakaatboek*, V: 18.09.1744. This was to be followed some years later in the Republic. When Dr De Famars inspected the hospital ship at Den Helder in 1774, he found that the surgeons who worked there had granted themselves the designation 'practitioners' (*praktizijns*) because they treated internal diseases for which they demanded to be recognised. De Famars judgment of these 'practitioners' was very scathing. Leuftink, *Harde Heelmeesters*, 143.
77 Van der Chijs, *Nederlandsch-Indisch Plakaatboek*, VI: 29.12.1752.
78 NA, VOC 838: 02.04.1762.
79 NA, VOC 1072: folio 297.
80 The surgeons vouched for the use of instruments (by paying a sum) and had to return them in the Netherlands.
81 Van der Chijs, *Nederlandsch-Indisch Plakaatboek*, II: 24.7.1667 and 03.11.1667; Brans, P.H., 'Overzicht van de geschiedenis der pharmacie in Nederlands Oost-Indië', *Pharmaceutisch Weekblad*, 47/48 (1951): 841, 862.
82 Van der Chijs, *Nederlandsch-Indisch Plakaatboek*, V: 18.09.1744.
83 Van der Chijs, *Nederlandsch-Indisch Plakaatboek*, II: 03.11.1667.
84 NA, VOC 828.
85 Van der Chijs, *Nederlandsch-Indisch Plakaatboek*, III: 10.04.1682

86 Ibid., V: 18.09.1744
87 Peeters, F.A.H. (ed.), *Bataviaasche Apotheek* (Tilburg, 1981).
88 Van der Chijs, *Nederlandsch-Indisch Plakaatboek*, VI: 14.07.1752.
89 Stapel, *Pieter van Dam's Beschrijvinge'*, RGP 87, 209.
90 Schoute, *De geneeskunde*, 143-145.
91 Ibid., 143-145.
92 Van der Chijs, *Nederlandsch-Indisch Plakaatboek,* II: 9.1.1664.
93 NA, VOC 1266, folio 572-579; Von Roemer, *Historical Sketches*, 184.
94 Van Dorssen, J.M.H., 'Willem ten Rhijne', *Geneeskundig Tijdschrift voor Nederlandsch-Indië*, 51 (1911) 148-150.
95 Van der Chijs, *Nederlandsch-Indisch Plakaatboek*, V: 27.09.1745, and X: 27.08.1770, 25.11.1777; and Von Römer, *Historical Sketches*, 192.
96 Arsip Nasional Jakarta (ANRI), notarial archives 1757-1758.
97 Von Römer, *Historical Sketches*, 193.
98 Van der Chijs, *Nederlandsch-Indisch Plakaatboek*, II: 21.9.1648.
99 Ibid., V: 10.10.1690.
100 Realia Register op de Generale Resolutiën van het Kasteel Batavia 1632-1805. Uitgegeven door het Bataviaasch Genootschap van Kunsten en Wetenschappen, I (Leiden, 1882, two vols.): 13.09.1651.
101 Van der Chijs, *Nederlandsch-Indisch Plakaatboek*, I: 13.09.1640; II: 13.09.1651, and V: 30.07.1745.
102 600 rixdollars from the municipality and 50 rixdollars from the Chinese hospital.
103 Van der Chijs, *Nederlandsch-Indisch Plakaatboek*, V: 29.03.1750.
104 Ibid., VI: 31.05.1754, and VII: 26.06.1761 and *idem* 03.06.1757.
105 Ibid., VIII: 02.05.1769.
106 Raben, *Batavia and Colombo*, 274.
107 Van Till, M., 'Social Care in Eighteenth Century Batavia: The Poorhouse, 1725-1750', *Itinerario* XIX (1995), 1, 19.
108 Schoute, *Occidental Therapeutics*, 39.
109 Van der Chijs, *Nederlandsch-Indisch Plakaatboek*, III: 15.01.1682 and 6.2.1682.
110 Ibid., III: 19.5.1692.
111 Ibid., III:10.10.1690.
112 Van Dorssen. J.M.H., 'De lepra', *Geneeskundig Tijdschrift voor Nederlands-Indië* 37 (Batavia, 1897), 260-264.
113 Van der Chijs, *Nederlandsch-Indisch Plakaatboek,* II: 23.4.1666.
114 Ibid., II: 5.8.1667.
115 Ibid., III: 12.05.1679.
116 Ibid., III: 19.08.1681 and Van Dorssen, 'De lepra', 300.
117 Van Dorsen, 'Willem ten Rhijne', 186.
118 Van der Chijs, *Nederlandsch-Indisch Plakaatboek*, III: 12.4.1708.
119 171 patients in 1695, Van Dorssen, 'De lepra', 314.
120 Van der Chijs, *Nederlandsch-Indisch Plakaatboek*, III: 12.4.1708.
121 Van Dorssen, 'De lepra', 303.
122 Circa 1730, the Chinese comprised 20 per cent of the city's population. Between 1680 and 1740, the number of Chinese doubled, an influx called Hong Tai, while the total population actually decreased. The same can be said for the suburbs and "Ommelanden" (surrounding countryside). Blussé, *Strange Company*, 83-84.
123 Blussé, *Strange Company*, 81.
124 Raben, *Batavia and Colombo*, 201.
125 Realia Register op de Generale Resolutiën van het Casteel Batavia: 28.06.1635.
126 Van der Chijs, *Nederlandsch-Indisch Plakaatboek*, I: 13.08.1640. This was initiated by the Probate Board (*Collegie van Boedelmeesteren*) which was formed in 1640, consisting of two Europeans and two Chinese. This institution administered the legacies of Chinese citizens whose children were still minors. A comparable institution for the Dutch and Eur-

Asian population was the *Collegie van Weesmeesteren*. The administrators petitioned the Government for a piece of land on which to construct a hospital to accommodate needy Chinese, orphaned, disabled, aged, or ill.

127 Ibid., I: 28.12.1640.
128 Ibid., I: 6.2.1641 and III: 07.12.1706.
129 Ibid., I: 28.02.1667.
130 Ibid., VI: 27.08.1754.
131 Gaastra, *De geschiedenis van de VOC*, 87.
132 Paranavitana, K.D., 'Medical establishment in Sri Lanka during the Dutch Period (1640-1796),' *Journal of the Royal Asiatic Society of Sri Lanka*, 33 (AS 1988/89), 106.
133 Peters, M., and F. André de la Porte, *In steen geschreven. Leven en sterven van VOC-dienaren op de kust van Coromandel in India* (Amsterdam, 2002), 86.
134 Burrows, *A History of Medicine in South Africa*, 32. This hospital was the second European hospital in sub-Saharan Africa (the Portuguese hospital at Mozambique dates from 1507).
135 Burrows, *A History of Medicine*, 43.
136 Ibid., 54. At the smaller trading posts in Asia, the surgeons came to be called *hospitaliers*.
137 Price, C.H., 'Medicine and Pharmacy at the Cape of Good Hope, 1652-1807', *Medical History* 6 (1962), 169-176.
138 De Wet, G.D., *Resolusies van de Politieke Raad* V (1964), 12.10.1717.
139 NA, VOC 829, 10.10.1709.
140 Von Römer, *Historical Sketches*, 63.
141 K.D. Paranavitana, 'Medical Establishments in Sri Lanka during the Duth Period (1640-1796)', 103-110; and C.G. Uragoda and K.D. Paranavitana, 'The Seventeenth-Century Dutch Hospital', *Medical History* 29 (1985), 186.
142 Blussé, *Strange Company*, 16/17.
143 Van der Brug, P.H., *Malaria en Malaise. De VOC in Batavia in de achttiende eeuw* (Amsterdam, 1994).
144 Ibid., 201-202.
145 Von Römer, *Historical Sketches*, 164.
146 Van der Chijs, *Nederlandsch-Indisch Plakaatboek*, IV: 02.10.1731.
147 Ibid., IV: 02.10.1731, 17.12.1733 and 15.01.1735.
148 Ibid., IV: 07.05.1734.
149 Schoute, *De Geneeskunde*, 220.
150 Van der Chijs, *Nederlandsch-Indisch Plakaatboek*, V: 04.06.1743 and 27.8.1743.
151 Ibid., VI: 14.09.1753. This physician earned more on the condition that he cured only patients holding a higher rank than soldier or sailor!
152 Ibid., VI: 29.12.1752.
153 The exact meaning of this word is not known. In all probability it was someone who used oils and fats to produce all kinds of products, like candles. Another possibility is that the *smeerboer* boiled oil from which the ointments that were put on wounds were made.
154 ANRI, no. 6, 05.03.1766.
155 Ibid., 1766-1767.
156 Van der Chijs, *Nederlandsch-Indisch Plakaatboek*, V: 23.08.1743.
157 Ibid., VI: 01.10.1751.
158 Schoute, *Occidental Therapeutics*, 59.
159 Van der Chijs, *Nederlandsch-Indisch Plakaatboek*, V: October 1746.
160 Ibid., VI: 04.04.1752.
161 Ibid., VII: 30.06.1761
162 Ibid., VI: 16.02.1751.
163 Schoute, *Occidental Therapeutics*, 69.
164 Van der Chijs, *Nederlandsch-Indisch Plakaatboek*, V: 13.11.1744, and NA, VOC 773: 13.11.1744.
165 Ibid., V 13.11.1744.
166 Ibid., VII: 28.05.1756.
167 ANRI 6: 1766-67.

168 Schoute, *Occidental Therapeutics*, 38-39.
169 Van der Chijs, *Nederlandsch-Indisch Plakaatboek,* VII: 31.12.1757
170 Schoute, *Occidental Therapeutics*, 72-73.
171 Van der Chijs, *Nederlandsch-Indisch Plakaatboek*, X: 19.3.1773.
172 Ibid., X: 4.9.1775.
173 Ibid., X: 14.2.1777.
174 Schoute, *Occidental Therapeutics*, 80.
175 Van der Chijs, *Nederlandsch-Indisch Plakaatboek*, XI: 27.8.1779.
176 The medical reform in New Spain, revolutionary in one way, was severely hindered, especially by the lack of funding for these hospitals by the Crown. Hernández-Sáenz, L.M., 'Seamen, Surgeons and Empire: Spanish Naval Medical Reform and Mexican Medicine in the Late Colonial period', *The Northern Mariner*, X, 1 (2000), 22-28.

Notes to Chapter 4

1 Warnsinck, J.C.M. (ed.), *De Reisen van Nicolaus de Graaff gedaan naar alle gewesten des werelds. Beginnende 1639 tot 1687 incluis*, Werken uitgegeven door de Linschooten-Vereeniging, XXXIII (The Hague, 1930), 3.
2 Dekkers, O. (ed), *Een Bunschoter VOC-chirurgijn. 'Dagelijkse aantekeningen' van de reis naar Oost-Indië in 1654 door Gijsbert Heeck (1619-1669)* (Bunschoten, 2001), 16.
3 Lindemann, M., *Health & Society in Eighteenth Century Germany* (Baltimore, 1996), 122.
4 Barend-Van Haeften, M., *Oost-Indië Gespiegeld. Nicolaas de Graaff, een schrijvend chirurgijn in dienst van de VOC* (Zutphen, 1992), 17.
5 Translation by the author. Bontekoe, W.I.J., *Journael ofte Gedenckwaerdige beschrijvinghe van de Oost-Indische reijse van – Begrijpende veel wonderlijcke en gevaerlijcke saecken hem daer in wedervaren; begonnende den 18 December 1618 en vol-eind den 16 November 1625* (Hoorn, 1646).
6 Tavernier, J.B., *Historie van 't beleit der Hollanders in Asia* (1682), translation from *Les six voyages de Jean Baptiste Tavernier: qu'il fait en Turquie, en Perse, et aux Indes, pendant l'espace de quarante ans … accompagnez d'observations sur la qualité, la religion, le gouvernement, les coûtumes et le commerce de chaque païs, avec les figures, le poids et la valeur des monnoyes qui y ont cours* (Bruxelles, 1679). During the eighteenth century, numerous complaints were made by officials of the Company, who alleged that the quality of the ship's surgeons was not quite what it should have been. I also refer to Barend-Van Haeften, *Oost-Indië Gespiegeld*, 35.
7 Haver Droeze, J.J., 'De geneeskundige dienst bij de Nederlandse Oost-Indische Compagnie', *Nederlands Tijdschrift voor Geschiedenis* (1921), I, 2539.
8 Rijksmuseum "Scheepvaartmuseum Amsterdam", S446 BIII (20): *Wij hebben elendig volk, veele kinderen, swakke, off oude luijden, die nu geheel sijn afgemartelt. God beware ons als wij naar zee gaan....*
9 Van Gelder, R., *'Naporra's Omweg: Het Leven van een VOC-matroos (1731-1793)* (Amsterdam, 2003), 127, 176.
10 NA, VOC 13.987. Translated into English by the author: *Hertz viele geliebte Eltern. Ich thue ihnen zu wissen, das ich hier in das Schif, über die 2200 Hollandischen Gulden, an Kaufmanschaft habe, als an Frantz-wein, an Reinische Weine, an Bier, und Brandewein, an lange Pfeiffen, an roht Charlaacken, an super fein Blau-Laacken, und an einige Kleinigkeiten mehr. Ich wünsche, und hoffe, das mir mein Gott, vor Unglück mag bewahren, und Gesundheit schenken, soo zweifele ick nicht, ich werde einen schönen Gewinst darauf haben, das ich mir dan in mein Vater-landt niedersetzen, und mein Brot dann, zu landen haben kann, als mich mein Gott das Leben schencken tut.* Alas, Johan Andreas Muller died in the East in February 1752, leaving his mother with a plethora of difficulties to recover his legacy on products worth at least 2200 'Hollandische Gulden'.
11 Patterns of labour migration have been developed by economic and demographic historians, one of whom, J. Lucassen, is a specialist on the North Sea Migration System. I

refer to his thesis *Naar de kusten van de Noordzee. Trekarbeid in Europees Perspektief, 1600-1900* (Utrecht, 1984).

12 Van Gelder, R., *Het Oost-Indisch avontuur. Duitsers in dienst van de VOC (1600-1800)* (Nijmegen, 1997), 62.

13 Leuftink, A.E., *Harde Heelmeesters. Zeelieden en hun dokters in de 18e eeuw* (Zutphen 1991), 37.

14 It also appears that each type of shipping, be it coastal, merchant, Admiralty or East India Company, had its own specific recruitment pattern, influenced by specific demographic, geographic, economic, social and political factors. P.C. van Royen, 'The "National" Maritime Labour Market: Looking for Common Characteristics', in Van Royen, P., Bruijn, J.R. and J. Lucassen (eds.), "*Those Emblems of Hell?" European Sailors and the Maritime Labourmarket, 1570-1870*, Research in Maritime History 13 (Newfoundland, 1997), 9. The geographical origin of seafarers has received attention from historians in recent decades. To name a few: Bruijn, J.R., and J. Lucassen 'Op de schepen der Oost Indische Compagnie'; Van der Woude, A.M., *Het Noorderkwartier. Een regionaal historisch onderzoek in de demografische en economische geschiedenis van westelijk Nederland van de late middeleeuwen tot het begin van de negentiende eeuw* (Wageningen, 1972); Van Royen, P.C. van, *Zeevarenden op de koopvaardijvloot omstreeks 1700* (Amsterdam, 1987); Knotter, J. and J.L. van Zanden, 'Immigratie en arbeidsmarkt in Amsterdam in de zeventiende eeuw', *Tijdschrift voor Sociale Geschiedenis*, 13 (1987) 4, 403-431; Hart, S., *Schrift en Getal. Een keuze uit de demografische-, economische- en sociaal-historische studieën op grond van Amsterdamse en Zaanse archivalia, 1600-1800* (Dordrecht, 1976); Boon, P., *Bouwers van de Zee: zeevarenden van het Westfriese platteland, c. 1680-1720* (Leiden, 1996); Beers, J.K., and C. Bakker, *Westfriezen naar de Oost. De kamers der VOC te Hoorn en Enkhuizen en hun recruteringsgebied 1700-1800* (Schagen, 1990); Bruijn, J.R., and F.S. Gaastra (eds.), *Ships, Sailors and Spices, East India Companies on their Shipping in the Sixteenth, Seventeenth and Eighteenth Centuries* (Amsterdam, 1993); Massée, Cl., *Les chirurgiens navigants originaires des dioceses de Bordeaux et Bazas dans les ecoles Saint-Côme entre 1752 et 1791* (s.l., n.d.).

15 De Vries, J., and A. van der Woude, *The First Modern Economy: Success, Failure, and Perseverance of the Dutch Economy, 1500-1815* (Cambridge, 1997), 47.

16 De Vries, J., *De economische achteruitgang der republiek in de achttiende eeuw* (Leiden, 1968), 29.

17 Ibid., 167.

18 Israel, J., *The Dutch Republic. Its Rise, Greatness, and Fall 1477-1806* (New York, 1995), 999.

19 Van der Woude, *Het Noorderkwartier* II, 613.

20 Israel, *The Dutch Republic*, 1009.

21 Schutte, G.J., *Een Hollandse dorpssamenleving in de late achttiende eeuw: de banne Graft 1770-1810* (Franeker, 1989).

22 De Vries, *De economische achteruitgang*, 72.

23 Slicher van Bath, B.H., *Een samenleving onder spanning. Geschiedenis van het platteland in Overijssel* (Utrecht, 1977), 741-746.

24 Israel, *The Dutch Republic*, 1000.

25 Ibid., 1017.

26 De Vries and Van der Woude, *The First Modern Econnomy*, 46-47.

27 Van der Woude, *Het Noorderkwartier*, II, 612.

28 Slicher van Bath, B.H., 'The economic situation in the Dutch Republic during the seventeenth century', in: M. Aymard (ed), *Dutch Capitalism and World Capitalism* (Cambridge, 1982), 26,27.

29 Boon, P., *Bouwers van de Zee*, 23. Van der Woude, *Het Noorderkwartier*, I, 99: Population decreased from 190,000 to 128,000.

30 Van Royen, P. , *Zeevarenden*, 149.

31 Schutte, *Een Hollandse dorpssamenleving*, 13.

32 Van der Woude, *Het Noorderkwartier*, II, 613.

33 Schutte, *Een Hollandse dorpssamenleving*, 25. It is not exactly clear why this demographic contraction occurred. Again, there are several contradictory facts for the village Graft:

although the Protestant church recorded more burials than baptisms, the Roman Catholic church showed the reverse. Although in all probability youngsters left the village, the records show a positive balance of migration (Schutte, *Een Hollandse dorpssamenleving*, 28).

34 Van der Woude, *Noorderkwartier*, I, 190-191.

35 Slicher van Bath, B.H., *Een samenleving onder spanning;Geschiedenis van het platteland in Overijssel* (Utrecht, 1977), 53.

36 Page Moch, L., *Moving Europeans. Migration in Western Europe since 1650* (Indiana University Press, 1992), 22.

37 Ibid., 14.

38 Ibid., 25.

39 Ibid., 16.

40 Lucassen, *Migrant Labour in Europe, 1600-1900* (London, 1987), 53, 148-153.

41 Page Moch, *Moving Europeans*, 17.

42 Hart, *Schrift en Getal*, 120.

43 Van Gelder, *Het Oost-Indisch avontuur*, 131.

44 Lucassen, *Naar de kusten van de Noordzee*, 145-149.

45 Page Moch, *Moving Europeans*, 47.

46 Ibid., 32.

47 Lucassen, *Naar de kusten van de Noordzee*, 18.

48 Ibid., 18. Alongside the North Sea System, Lucassen distinguishes six other systems in action around 1811. There was one between London and the Humber; one in the Paris Basin; one between Provence, Languedoc, and adjacent Catalonia; one in Spain around Castile; and two in Italy, in Piedmonte in northern Italy and in southern Tuscany and Lozio in central Italy.

49 Lucassen, J., 'The International Maritime Labour Market', in Van Royen, P.D., Bruijn, J.R., and J. Lucassen (eds.), "*Those Emblems of Hell"? European Sailors and the Maritime Labour Market, 1570-1870* (New Foundland, 1977), 17.

50 Broeze, F.J.A, Bruijn, J.R., and F.S. Gaastra (eds), *Maritieme Geschiedenis der Nederlanden* III (Bussum, 1977), 147.

51 Lucassen, 'The International Maritime Labour Market', in "*Those Emblems of Hell*"?, 17, note by Lucassen.

52 Keevil, J.J., Lloyd, Chr., and J.L.S. Coulter, *Medicine and the Navy 1200-1900*, 4 vols. (Edinburgh, 1957-1963), I: 141.

53 thus it is incorrect to conclude that of the circa 1,000,000 who left the Dutch ports during the seventeenth and eighteenth centuries, circa 700,000 men died in the service of the Company.

54 Broeze, F.J.A, Bruijn, J.R., and F.S. Gaastra (eds.), *Maritieme Geschiedenis der Nederlanden* III (Bussum, 1977), 150

55 This graph is based on the numbers provided in Bruijn, J.R., et al. (eds.), *Dutch Asiatic Shipping in the seventeenth and eighteenth centuries* (The Hague, 1987) I, 144.

56 Broeze, Bruijn, and Gaastra (eds), *Maritieme Geschiedenis der Nederlanden* III (Bussum, 1977), 147-148.

57 Boxer, C.R.*The Dutch Seaborne Empire, 1600-1800* (London, 1973).

58 Broeze, Bruijn, and Gaastra (eds.), *Maritieme Geschiedenis der Nederlanden* III (Bussum, 1977), 151.

59 Lucassen, 'The International Maritime Labour Market', in "*Those Emblems of Hell*"?, 18.

60 Van Royen, Bruijn, and Lucassen (eds.), "*Those Emblems of Hell*"?, 30.

61 Schutte, *Een Hollandse dorpssamenleving*, 25.

62 Boon, *Bouwers van de Zee*, 128, 129.

63 Ibid., 144

64 Page Moch, *Moving Europeans*, 16.

65 *Nederlands Tijdschrift voor Geneeskunde* 123, 46 (1979).

66 Van Gelder, *Het Oost-Indisch avontuur*, 135.

67 My gratitude to H. de Vos of Schoorl in the Netherlands, who supplied me with his data on the vacancies and applicants at the Chamber in Hoorn.

68 Bruijn, and Gaastra (eds.), *Ships, Sailors and Spices*, 200.
69 Gaastra, F., *De Geschiedenis van de VOC* (Zutphen, 1991), 81.
70 Lucassen, 'The International Maritime Labour Market' in: *"Those Emblems of Hell"?*, 19.
71 Ibid., 17.
72 Bruijn, J.R., 'Commandanten van Oost-Indiëvaarders in de achttiende eeuw', in: *Tijdschrift voor Zeegeschiedenis*, 20 (2001), 1, 4-14.
73 Beers, and Bakkers, *Westfriezen naar de Oost.*, 77-78.
74 NA, VOC 13.987.
75 Van Gelder, *Het Oost-Indisch avontuur*, 289-292.
76 Ibid., 56.
77 Von Roemer, L.S.A.M., *Historical Sketches. An introduction to the Fourth Congress of the Far Eastern Association of Tropical Medicine* (Batavia, 1921), 61.
78 Van Gelder, *Het Oost-Indisch avontuur*, 290.
79 Van Gelder, *Het Oost-Indisch avontuur*, 292.
80 Westfrisan Archives in Hoorn: *Werkdocumenten van bewindhebbers van de Oost-Indische Compagnie ter Kamer Enkhuizen* of which the dates concerning the applicant ship's surgeons have been provided by H. de Vos.
81 I refer to the appendix. The central question of this chapter is whether we can discern any patterns of surgical recruitment on the vessels of the Company in the eighteenth century, with the understanding that for the non-Dutch ship's surgeons no baptismal registers have been checked and that their statements of place of origin have been taken here at face value. The emphasis of non-Dutch ship's surgeons will be on Germany. However, no specific research has been done on the economic and demographic history of the German states. What is presented in this chapter in connection with the non-Dutch ship's surgeons are 'merely' the results of the queries for Sample S, and any conclusions about these surgeons' geographical origins should be interpreted with caution.
82 This table excludes the surgeons of unknown origin. The numbers on which this table is based are presented in Appendix 1.
83 The method of the sample is explained in appendix 1.
84 Hart, *Schrift en Getal.*, 122.
85 Ibid., 124.
86 Heringa, J., et al, *Geschiedenis van Drenthe* (Meppel, 1985), 496.
87 Ibid., 485, 495.
88 De Vries and Van der Woude, *The First Modern Economy*, 54-55.
89 De Vries, *De economische achteruitgang*, 43.
90 De Vries and Van der Woude, *The First Modern Economy*, 55.
91 Ibid., 56.
92 Ibid., 64.
93 Beers, and Bakkers, *Westfriezen naar de Oost.*, 13.
94 De Vries and Van der Woude, *The First Modern Economy,* 64.
95 Ibid., 494.
96 Dillo, I.G., *De nadagen van de Verenigde Oostindische Compagnie, 1783-1795* (Amsterdam, 1992), 89.
97 Palmer, R. and J. Colton, *A History of the Modern World* (New York, 1978), 134.
98 Boockmann, H. et al, *Mitten in Europa. Deutsche Geschichte* (Berlin, 1984), 166.
99 Ibid., 182.
100 Ibid., *185*
101 Lindemann, M., *Health & Healing in Eighteenth Century Germany* (Baltimore, 1996), 192. Frederick William I was the second Prussian king who transformed his country from a second-rate power into the efficient and prosperous state that his son and successor (Frederick II the Great) made a major military power on the Continent.
102 Temkin, O., 'The role of surgery in the rise of modern medical thought', *Bulletin of the History of Medicine* 25 (1951), 248-259.
103 Van Gelder, R., *Het Oost-Indisch avontuur. Duitsers in dienst van de VOC (1600-1800)* (Nijmegen, 1997), 220.

104 Bruford, W.H., *Germany in the eighteenth century. The social background of the literary revival* (Cambridge, 1959), 167.
105 Lindemann, M., *Patriots and Paupers. Hamburg, 1712-1830* (Oxford, 1990), 5, 35.
106 Ibid., 35,36.
107 Ibid., 51-53.
108 Bruford, W.H., *Germany in the eighteenth century*, 181.
109 Bruijn, J.R. and F.S. Gaastra (eds.), *Ships, Sailors and Spices*, 135.
110 Bruford, *Germany in the eighteenth century*, 181.

Notes to Chapter 5

1 Madura foot is a chronic, progressive, local infection caused by fungi or bacteria, involving the feet, upper extremities, or back, and is characterised by tumefactions and the formation of multiple sinus tracts.
2 Broeze, F.J.A., Bruijn, J.R., and F.S. Gaastra (eds.), *Maritieme Geschiedenis der Nederlanden* (Bussum, 1977), III, 177; Voegen van Engelen, J., *De Surinaamsche Artz 1786-1788* (Facsimili, Utrecht, 1982), 84.
3 The most significant books and articles have been named in note 13 to the introduction.
4 McNeil, *Plaques and Peoples*, 239.
5 Dorren, G., *Eenheid en verscheidenheid. De burgers van Haarlem in de Gouden Eeuw* (Amsterdam, 2001), 36.
6 Van Deursen, A.Th., *Een dorp in de polder: Graft in de zeventiende eeuw* (Amsterdam, 1994), 113.
7 Ketting, H., *De Amsterdamse chirurgijns: van ambacht naar professie.1750-1798* (Amsterdam, 1988), unpublished masters' thesis, 62-63.
8 Kool-Blokland, J.L., *De zorg gewogen. Zeven eeuwen godshuizen in Middelburg* (Middelburg, 1990), 120.
9 Some 95 professions are known.
10 Kooijmans, L., *Onder regenten: de elite in een Hollandse stad. Hoorn 1700-1780* (Amsterdam, 1985), 289-372.
11 Lindemann, , M., *Health & Society*, 122.
12 Bruijn, J.R., 'Commandanten van Oost-Indiëvaarders in de achttiende eeuw', *Tijdschrift voor Zeegeschiedenis* 20 (2001) 1, 6.
13 Rodger, N.A.M., *The Wooden World*, 20.
14 Nash, G., 'Naval Uniform', *Mariner's Mirror* 41 (1956), 99.
15 NA, VOC 6242, 6320, 6364, 6389, 6422, 6451, 6484, 6515, and Ringoir, D.J., *Plattelandschirurgijns in de zeventiende en achttiende eeuw. De rekeningboeken van de 18e eeuwse Durgerdamse chirurgijn Anthonij Egburts* (Bunnik, 1977), 236.
16 NA, VOC 5995.
17 Ringoir, *Plattelandschirurgijns in de zeventiende en achttiende eeuw*, 279-280.
18 NA, VOC 6090 and 6145.
19 Ringoir, *Plattelandschirurgijns in de zeventiende en achttiende eeuw*, 21-22.
20 Ketting, *De Amsterdamse chirurgijns*, unpublished masters' thesis, 39, 41, 44. After 1760, the pupils take about eleven to twelve years to graduate their master's examination.
21 NA, VOC 14.204, 14.209, 14.217. Date of birth was retrieved by J. Leenders in the municipal archive of Rotterdam. Municipal archive of Schiedam: chirurgijnsgilde OAA 3077, 1-6-1742.
22 NA, VOC 6515, 6476, 6580. Municipal archive of Amsterdam, GAA, inventory 255: 14/10/1754. Inventory 247: 22-2-1770, 1-3-1770, and 4-3-1770.
23 Research of Group F.
24 Again, my gratitude to H. de Vos of Schoorl in the Netherlands.
25 The data that De Vos was retrieved from documents called *Werkdocumenten van bewindhebbers van de Oost-Indische Compagnie ter Kamer Enkhuizen*, which are kept in the archives of Hoorn, and consist of two sets. One set of papers lists the candidates for vacancies of the outward-bound vessels, the other set consists of those candidates who were employed.

26 NA, VOC 6524. GAA, inventory 255: 9/4/1753. Inventory 247: 22/6/1762, 29/6/1762.
27 OAH: 1815(a).
28 My gratitude to P. Poortvliet of Den Helder, who kindly provided me with his data on the seafarers of the province of Zeeland.
29 Poortvliet, Den Helder.
30 Koninkx, C., *The First and Second Chapters of the Swedish East India Company (1731-1766)* (Kortrijk, 1980), 329.
31 Alsop, J.D., 'Sea Surgeons, health and England's maritime expansion: The West-African Trade 1553-1660', *Mariner's Mirror* 76 (1990) 3, 218.
32 Van Royen, P., Bruijn, J.R. and J. Lucassen (eds.), "*Those Emblems of Hell*"?, 28.
33 Bruijn, 'Commandanten van Oost-Indiëvaarders in de achttiende eeuw', 5.
34 NA, VOC 1372, folio 815-817: *vrij groote imaginatie van in India te konnen substitueren opgenomen hebbende als de waarheijdt daarvan in effecte melissig wanckel in zijn opinie ...misleijt en waarlijk komt te bespeuren dat hij met de winsten die de Compagnie aan een ieder na zijn qualiteijt is toe te leggen ... geenszins van kan bestaan.*
35 NA, VOC 130, *Resolutien Heeren XVII*, 29.03.2760 and 2.10.1760.
36 NA, VOC 6145.
37 See chapter 3.
38 Bruijn, J.R., Gaastra, F.S., and I. Schöffer (eds.), *Dutch-Asiatic shipping in the seventeenth and eighteenth centuries*, (The Hague, 1987), I, 150.
39 Taylor, Jean Gelman, *The Social World of Batavia: European and Eurasian in Dutch Asia* (London, 1983), 16.
40 Van Royen, Bruijn,and Lucassen, "*Those Emblems of Hell*"?, 37.
41 Municipal archives of Delft, baptismal registers New Church, inventory 60, folio 176v.
42 NA, VOC 13.997; 14.001; 14.007; 14.020; 14.024; 14.030.
43 Municipal archives of Schiedam; date of baptismal obtained from J. Leenderts.
44 NA, VOC 13.878; 13.882.
45 These figures are based on research done by H. Ketting on Amsterdam's surgeons' estates. Ketting, *De Amsterdamse chirurgijns*, 58-59.
46 Oberschelp, R., *Niedersachsen 1760-1820. Wirtschaft, Gesellschaft, Kultur in Land Hanover und Nachbargebieten* (Hildesheim, 1982), 2 vols., Veröffentlichungen der historischen Kommission für Niedersachsen und Bremen. XXXV Quellen und Untersuchungen zur allgemeiner Geschichte Niedersachsens in der Neuzeit, Band 4, I, 282.
47 Frijhoff, W., and M. Spies, *1650: Bevochten Eendracht* (The Hague, 1999), 18, 23.
48 Bruijn, Gaastra, and Schöffer (eds.), *Dutch-Asiatic shipping*, I, 151.
49 Van Eijck van Heslinga, E.S., *Van Compagnie naar koopvaardij. De scheepvaartverbinding van de Bataafsche Republiek met de koloniën in Azië 1795-1806* (Amsterdam, 1988), 20.
50 NA, VOC 124: 29.3.1745.
51 NA, VOC 14.840.
52 NA, VOC 14.825.
53 NA, VOC 14.826.
54 NA, VOC 14.823.
55 NA, VOC 14.822.
56 Bruijn, Gaastra, and Schöffer (eds.), *Dutch-Asiatic shipping*, I, 151.
57 Taylor, *The Social World of Batavia*, 71.
58 NA, VOC 14.766.
59 NA, VOC 14.866.
60 NA, VOC 14.205.
61 Arsip Nasional, Fam. H958, Notary Gousset, 15.09.1763.
62 Ibid., 27.7.1763.
63 Arsip National, Fam. H959, Notary Gousset.
64 Ibid., nos 07.09.1763; 24.07.1763; 02.05.1764; 14.07.1764.
65 Alsop, 'Sea Surgeons, health and England's maritime expansion', 220.
66 Taylor, *The Social World of Batavia*, 5.

67 NA, VOC 12.741; 12.749; 12.761; 12.788; 12.807.
68 NA, VOC 12.819; 12.843; 12.862; 12.876.
69 NA, VOC 12.875; 12.893; 12.909.
70 NA,VOC 13.191; 13.212; 13.232; 13.252; 13.265. The data on the non-surgical career received from P. Poortvliet.
71 See the appendix.
72 According to modern statistics ('Chi-Square Tests'), this is a significant trend. I would like to thank Dr Nico Nagelkerke of the Statistical Medical Department of Leiden University for his assistance in the interpretation of the data and the creation of the graphs.
73 NA, VOC 14.708.
74 See note 72 to chapter 5.
75 Moreover, the trend in the first three periods is significant. See note 671.
76 The numbers and percentages presented in the tables of T5.14 and T5.15 do not offer any significant trend according to Chi-Square Tests. See note 671.
77 Price, C.H., 'Medicine and pharmacy at the Cape of Good Hope, 1652-1807', *Medical History* 6 (1962), 169-176, 170.
78 Burrows, E.H., *A History of Medicine in South Africa up to the End of the Nineteenth Century* (Cape Town/Amsterdam, 1958), 34.
79 Van Gelder, R., *Het Oost-Indisch avontuur. Duitsers in dienst van de VOC (1600-1800)* (Nijmegen, 1997).
80 Wagenaar, L., Galle, *VOC-vestiging in Ceylon. Beschrijving van een koloniale samenleving aan de vooravond van de Singalese opstand tegen het Nederlandse gezag, 1760* (Amsterdam, 1994), 102-103.
81 For instance, in Semarang, see the table below, which is based on Van der Boom, J.H., 'Genealogisch onderzoek in de archieven van de Verenigde Oostindische Compagnie in het Algemeen Rijksarchief te 's-Gravenhage', *De Indische navorscher*. Orgaan van de Indische Genealogische Vereniging, 10 (1997) 1, 38. This table lists the names of Eurasians and/or Asians who entered the surgical profession, alongside the other medical employees in Semarang in 1798. They rarely if ever succeeded in climbing the hierarchical ladder of the Company, because of the criteria the Company authorities imposed concerning nationality, race, and religion, namely being European and a practicing Protestant. These surgeons certainly cannot be accused of having a lack of experience. It should be noted that all of these cases are from the end of the eighteenth century, when, after 1795, the shipping connections between the Republic and the trading settlements in East India were temporarily suspended. This might have also been the reason for the significantly high number of former soldiers who became surgeons as well as the influx of many Eurasians into the surgical profession.

Medical employees in Semarang in 1798

Name	*Arrival Asia*	*Function*	*Function Semarang*
Chr. Fr. Evers	1787	First surgeon	First surgeon and hospitalier
J.C.W. Hornoff	1773	Soldier	City-physician
J.F.D. Herwich	1786	Surgeon's mate	Surgeon
F.M. Geerling	1778	Surgeon's mate	Surgeon
R. van Leeuwen	1794	Surgeon	Surgeon
G.L. Kaijzel (born in Asia)	1786	'Pupil at the surgery'	Surgeon
Fr. Ruijsendaal	1787	Soldier	Surgeon
G. Elk	1787	Soldier	Surgeon

C.F. Cramer	1791	Surgeon's mate	Surgeon's mate
F.L. Wolff	1792	Sailor	Surgeon's mate
J. de Loo	1788	Sailor	Third surgeon
J.F. Geerling (born in Asia)	1793	'Pupil at the surgery'	Third surgeon

82 NA, VOC 14.766.
83 Bruijn, Gaastra, and Schöffer (eds.), *Dutch-Asiatic shipping*, I, 152.
84 Ibid., I, 157.
85 Bruijn, J.R., 'De personeelsbehoefte van de VOC overzee en aan boord, bezien in Aziatisch en Nederlands perspectief', *Bijdragen en mededelingen van de geschiedenis der Nederlanden*, XCI (1976), 218-248.
86 Bruijn, Gaastra, and Schöffer (eds.), *Dutch-Asiatic shipping*, I, 162.
87 Ibid., I, 152.
88 In this table, the numbers of ship's surgeons whose geographical origins are not clear are excluded.
89 Oberschelp, R., *Niedersachsen*, Band 4, II, 71-72.
90 Again, I am indebted to Dr. N. Nagelkerke for his invaluable grasp of statistics.
91 Keevil, J.J., Lloyd, Chr., and J.L.S. Coulter, *Medicine and the Navy 1200-1900*, 4 vols. (Edinburgh, 1957-1963), III, 49.
92 Dekkers, O. (ed.), *Een Bunschoter VOC chirurgijn. 'Dagelijkse aantekeningen; van de reis naar Oost-Indië in 1654 door Gijsbert Heeck (1619-1669)* (Bunschoten, 2001).
93 NA, VOC 14.722. The data concerning his Texel life I owe to Ms. M. Claassen.
94 NA, VOC 5898, 5973, 5939. The data concerning his Texel life, I owe to Ms. M. Claassen.
95 NA, VOC 14.842; the data concerning his post-VOC life, I owe to Ms. M. Teunissen.
96 NA, VOC 6675, 6735, and 6764.
97 NA, VOC 5930, 5970. Rijksarchief Overijssel, RAO Dalfsen, inv. 67. I would like to extend my gratitude to D. van Zuidam and P. Leising who have supplied me with these data.
98 NA, VOC 13.104, 13.118, 13.136, and 13.163; 's Lands Schip *Zuid Beveland* Amiraliteit Zeeland, rek. C 7924; ISIS: Archief Bevolking Zeeland 1796-1799, Inventaris Gew. Besturen 256.
99 NA, VOC 13.053, 13.070, 13.103, 13.137, 13.151; MCC Nieuwe Hoop MCC0821, and Breedveld, P.H., and J.L.M. Hendrikx, *Het journaal van de scheepschirurgijn J.W. Daman (1735-1783). Gezondheid en ziekten aan boord van een oostindiëvaarder*, Scripta Tironum 12 (Nijmegen, 1987).
100 NA, VOC 6014, and SISIS Velsen.
101 NA, VOC 14.186, and De Jong, J.J., *Met goed fatsoen: de elite in een Hollandse stad (Gouda 1700-1780)* (Amsterdam, 1986), 305-307.

Notes to Chapter 6

1 The senior surgeon on board did not sleep in a hammock as the crew, but was allotted a cabin. He did have to bring his own mattress and cushions, though some surgeons brought along their own hammocks, others their own bed.
2 NA, VOC 6524.
3 NA, VOC 6524.
4 NA, VOC124: 29-3-1745.
5 Van Gelder, R., *Naporra's Omweg: Het leven van een VOC-matroos (1731-1793)* (Amsterdam, 2003), 335.

6 Van Leur, J.C. *Indonesian Trade and Society: Essays in Asian Social and Economic History*, Selected Studies on Indonesia by Dutch Scholars I (The Hague, 1955), 261.

7 Gaastra, F.S., *De Geschiedenis van de VOC* (Zutphen, 1991), 144-145.

8 National Archives Indonesia (ANRI), Buitenland 99: 1,931.50 Dutch guilders were 1,287 Arcat rupiahs.

9 Nicolaas de Graaff describes this custom in his journal. In *Oostindische Spiegel* page 65, see: Warnsinck, J.C.M. (ed.), *De Reisen van Nicolaus de Graaff gedaan naar alle gewesten des werelds. Beginnende 1639 tot 1687 incluis*, Werken uitgegeven door de Linschoten-Vereeniging, XXXIII (The Hague, 1930).

10 NA, VOC 14.813.

11 Van Gelder, R., *Naporra's Omweg*, 243.

12 Dekkers, O. (ed.), *Een Bunschoter VOC chirurgijn. 'Dagelijkse aantekeningen; van de reis naar Oost-Indië in 1654 door Gijsbert Heeck (1619-1669)'* (Bunschoten, 2001).

13 NA, VOC 14.866.

14 NA, VOC 14.466.

15 NA, VOC 6524.

16 NA, VOC 14.475.

17 Scheepvaartmuseum Amsterdam (Maritime Museum Amsterdam), A.0451(39)[nr.0014]. The vessel's carpenter on board, busy with the preparing of cots and other things, had promised to make a case for the salmon the moment he was at leisure.

18 De Haan, F., *Uit de nadagen van de 'Loffelijke Compagnie'. Een keuze uit de geschriften samengesteld door Rob Nieuwenhuijs* (Amsterdam, 1984), 154-155.

19 Taylor, J. Gelman, *The Social World of Batavia: European and Eurasian in Dutch Asia* (Madison, WI, 1983), 86.

20 I hereby would like to express my gratitude to the members of the staff of the Arsip Nasional of Jakarta. They have supplied me with all the testaments relating to the surgeons in Batavia during the seventeenth and eighteenth centuries.

21 Annema, J.T., 'Het erfrecht in Friesland', *Jaarboek van het CBG* 55 (2001), 57. De Blécourt, A.S., and H.F.W.D. Fischer, *Kort begrip van het oud-vaderlands burgerlijk recht* (Groningen, 1950), 20. The influence of Roman law has been very profound on legislation and jurisprudence in the Netherlands, especially in the fields of contract law and succession law. Roman-Dutch law is the legal system that was applied to varying degrees in the provinces of the Republic and its overseas territories in the early modern period, until it was replaced by the Napoleonic Code. This influence was quite strong in Friesland, Holland, Zeeland and Utrecht, but less so in Gelderland, Overijssel and Drenthe. Moreover, the areas and provinces of the Republic were governed by local customs.

22 Many thanks to the erudite Amsterdam notary R. van Helden (LLM) who kindly enlightened me on numerous aspects of notarial problems.

23 The true difference between the two was only apparent if an estate had to be divided without a will and without one parent. Under *Aasdom* Law 'the nearest blood inherits the goods'. Succession, under *Aasdom* Law, first moved directly down the family tree, then directly up, only finally moving across to collaterals. So, for example, if a woman died without having any children or any surviving parents, her property would devolve completely to her surviving parent, or, next in line, any surviving grandparent(s); lastly her brothers and sisters would be benefactors. In the case of inter-state succession under the *Aasdom* Law (absent children and one parent), property followed the lineal kin of the deceased first, then the collateral kin.

Schependom Law operated under the maxim that *het goed moet gaan van daer het gekomen is*, or 'the goods must go from whence they came'. The guiding assumption made by *Schependom* Law is that upon the death of a parent, half of the family estate would pass to the surviving offspring. Upon the death of the son or daughter of the deceased parent, that son or daughter's estate would go to the other remaining offspring of the deceased parent and not to the surviving parent. Since, in theory, the legacy did not come from the surviving parent, they 'must go from whence they came', first to the children of the deceased, then to deceased's side of the family. It has also been observed of *Schependom* Law that 'the goods do not like to climb', pointing to the fact that collaterals or brothers and sisters inherited before grandparents.

24 Jones, E., *Wives, Whores, and Concubines: Early Modern Dutch Marriage Law and the Transmission of Family Wealth in Asia* (Berkeley, 2000). This book is published at: http://aghistory.ucdavis.edu/Jonespaper.html.
25 Gehlen, A.F., *Notariële akten uit de 17e en 18e eeuw: handleiding voor gebruikers* (Zutphen, 1986), 12.
26 Ibid., 36.
27 Ibid., 36.
28 ANRI, FAM J 87.
29 Gehlen, *Notariële akten*, 44.
30 Ibid., 54.
31 Ibid., 45.
32 ANRI, Notarieel, Testamenten: 1772/73.
33 ANRI, Notarieel, Testamenten: 8-11-1725.
34 ANRI, Notarieel, Testamenten: 23-2-1767.
35 ANRI, Notarieel, Testamenten: 30-6-1654.
36 ANRI, Notarieel, Testamenten 1769/70: 12-4-1760.
37 ANRI, Notarieel, Testamenten TB 25: 23-5-1681.
38 ANRI, Notarieel, Testamenten TB 1664/66: 5-6-1666.
39 ANRI, Notarieel, Testamenten: 8-8-1653.
40 ANRI, Notarieel, Testamenten 1664-66: 16-4-1664.
41 In the end, it was essentially a quite preposterous idea, certainly in light of population figures: Among a population of 350 million people in Asia during the second half of the seventeenth century, the European population at that time of circa 12,000 (on all Asian settlements) was less than a drop in a bucket: F.S. Gaastra, *De geschiedenis van de VOC*, 85.
42 Taylor, *The Social World of Batavia*, 11.
43 Ibid., 12.
44 NA, VOC 155: 13-3-1690.
45 NA, VOC 155: 12-12-1689.
46 NA, VOC 155: 13-3-1690.
47 NA, VOC 114: 5-3-1705.
48 Taylor, *The Social World of Batavia*, 29-30.
49 Ibid., 71-72.
50 An example of which has been admirably described in Leonard Blussé's *Bitters bruid. Een koloniaal huwelijksdrama in de Gouden Eeuw* (Amsterdam, 1997).
51 Van der Chijs, J.A., *Nederlandsch-Indisch Plakaatboek, 1602-1811*, Uitgegeven door het Bataviaasch Genootschap van Kunsten en Wetenschappen, I (The Hague, 1885), 173.
52 The 340 documents represent the bulk of the surgeon's deeds in, mostly, Batavia.
53 ANRI, Notarieel, Testamenten 1725/26: 14-5-1725.
54 ANRI, Notarieel, Testamenten, 1751/53: 15-7-1752.
55 ANRI, Notarieel, Testamenten TB 31, 1699/1700: 2-2-1700.
56 ANRI, Notarieel, Testamenten: 15-8-1788.
57 ANRI, Notarieel, Testamenten 1726/27: 9-8-1726.
58 ANRI, Notarieel, Testamenten 1727/29: 27-9-1727.
59 ANRI, Notarieel, Testamenten1727-29: 20-2-1728.
60 ANRI, Notarieel, Testamenten TB 33: 2-12-1702.
61 ANRI, Notarieel, Testamenten 1733: 18-11-1730.
62 ANRI, Notarieel, Testamenten TB 63: 25-2-1746.
63 ANRI, Notarieel, Testamenten, TB 78: 30-8-1769.
64 ANRI, Notarieel, Testamenten 27-4-1786.
65 ANRI, Notarieel, Testamenten: 28-8-1726.

66 This graph is based on the following table: Numbers of surgeons whose legal deeds were deposited at the Batavian *Weeskamer*.

Period	*Number of surgeons drawing up a legal document*	*Period*	*Number of surgeons drawing up a legal document*
1643-1650	6	1721-1730	34
1651-1660	7	1731-1740	21
1661-1670	10	1741-1750	19
1671-1680	10	1751-1760	39
1681-1690	24	1761-1770	47
1691-1700	26	1771-1780	29
1701-1710	20	1781-1790	26
1711-1720	16	1791-1793	6

67 ANRI, Notarieel, TB 1, 7-9-1643.
68 This percentage is calculated as follows: those who did not return to the Republic within three years on their first voyage (and did not die in the mean time) and of those who did not return to the Republic within three years on their second voyage (and did not die in the mean time). As a result, the number is a minimum, as there were also some, though not many, who first made some short voyages, and later on remained behind in Asia for longer periods.
69 After their first departure from the Republic.
70 De Haan, F., *Uit de nadagen van de 'Loffelijke Compagnie'*, 19-20.
71 ANRI, Notarieel TB 22, 1686-1688.
72 ANRI, Notarieel, Testamenten ,14-6-1774.
73 ANRI Notarieel, Testamenten, 27-1-1750.
74 ANRI, Notarieel, Testamenten 26-11-1699.
75 Taylor, *The Social World of Batavia*, 16.
76 Ibid., 17.
77 ANRI, Notarieel, Testamenten 6-10-1687.
78 ANRI, Notarieel, Testamenten 13-5-1727.
79 ANRI, Notarieel, Testamenten 13-2-1749.
80 ANRI, Notarieel, Testamenten 23-7-1780.
81 ANRI, Notarieel, Testamenten 9-10-1783.
82 ANRI, Notarieel, Testamenten 23-12-1745.
83 ANRI, Notarieel, Testamenten 8-6-1752.
84 ANRI, Notarieel ,Testamenten 31-10-1757 and 18-6-1766.
85 ANRI, Notarieel, Testamenten 29-5-1686 and 26-11-1687.
86 ANRI, Notarieel, Testamenten 21-6-1670 and 31-10-1678.
87 Surgeons J. Haas, L. Kreps, G. Croese, and J. de Alsetaer.
88 ANRI, Notarieel, Testamenten, 10-4-1693.
89 ANRI, Notarieel, Testamenten, 17-9-1751.
90 Ketting, H., *De Amsterdamse chirurgijns: van ambacht naar professie.1750-1798* (unpublished thesis Amsterdam, 1988), 58.
91 ANRI Notarieel, TB 63.
92 De Haan, F., *Uit de nadagen van de 'Loffelijke Compagnie'*, 154.
93 ANRI, Notarieel, Testamenten: 18-2-1728.
94 ANRI, Notarieel, Testamenten: 9-3-1728.

95 Though some surgeons also made some provisions with respect to their corpses. The surgeon's mate, Cornelis Peekstok, bequeathed twenty *rijksdaalders* to a *ziekentrooster*, provided he laid out Peekstok's body and Hendrik Hollesloot donated to each of the bearers and grave-diggers a golden ducaton.

96 Peters, M., and F. André de la Porte, *In Steen Geschreven. Leven en sterven van VOC-dienaren op de kust van Coromandel in India* (Amsterdam, 2002), 90.

97 ANRI Notarieel, Testamenten 1745/46: 3-9-1744.

98 ANRI, Notarieel, Testamenten TB85: 22-3-1775.

99 ANRI, Notarieel, Testamenten 1729/30: 25-10-1729.

100 ANRI, Notarieel, Testamenten TB 83: 19-3-1774.

101 ANRI, Notarieel, Testamenten TB 1740: 7-6-1741. A ducat was 78 *stuivers.*

102 NA, VOC 14.813.

103 De Haan, F., *Uit de nadagen van de 'Loffelijke Compagnie'*, 54-56.

104 Blussé, J.L et al (eds), *De Dagregisters van het kasteel Zeelandia, Taiwan 1629-1662*, IV: 1655-1662 (The Hague, 2000), 351. The kidnapping of Joost, Leendert Bollekeus's (or Bollekens) son, is, however, not mentioned in this daily journal of the Company headquarters of Taiwan.

105 ANRI, Notarieel, Testamenten 5-12-1663. Nothing about this kidnapping is to be found in the Dagregister Taiwan.

106 ANRI, Notarieel, Testamenten 1704/5, 3-11-1703.

107 ANRI Notarieel, TB 45, 22-11-1722.

108 ANRI, Notarieel, Testamenten, 9-11-1754, 27-12-1778 and 19-7-1752.

109 Watt, J., 'Surgeons of the Mary Rose. The practice of surgery in Tudor England', *Mariners Mirror* 69 (1983), 10.

110 Jacobs, J., *Een zegenrijk gewest. Nieuw-Nederland in de zeventiende eeuw* (Amsterdam, 1999), 352.

111 Ringoir, D.J., *Plattelandschirurgijns in de zeventiende en achttiende eeuw. De rekeningboeken van de 18e eeuwse Durgerdamse chirurgijn Anthonij Egberts* (Bunnik 1977), 44.

112 Van Loon, L., 'Het Rotterdamsche chirurgijnsgilde "S. Cosmas et Damianus" van 1467 – 1798', I, *Nederlands Tijdschrift voor Geneeskunde* 83 (1939) II, 3912. The surgical books mentioned were: *Der chirurgien Instructie; Antidotarium; Chirurgie Felix; d'Examen der chirurgijns; Corte bereijdinge der medicijnen; Dispensatorium novum; chirurgie van Guido de Cauliaco; Enscheiridium authonicum; Joh. Beverwijck Heelkonst; Joh. Beverwijck Schadt der Ongesondtheijt; Joh. Beverwijck Schadt der gesontheijt; Het licht der apothekers; Handtboeck der chirurgie; De cleine chirurgie; Het tweede handtboeck chirurgijns; De vier consten der medicijnen; De melancolie verdriver; Het constigh suijver boeck; Het constigh disteleerboeck; Nieuvelt Scheerdersconst; Bloeme, daarmede d'chirurgie enz;* and *Anatomie ofte ontledinge van 't verderf.*

113 NA, VOC 1342, folio 760-772.

114 Louis Vlasbloem or Ludovicus Vlasblom lived and worked in the seventeenth century. Wrote *Claare beschrijvinghe van de zee-custen, sanden, gronden ende diepten van het geheele Christenrijck, verdeelt in vijff boecken*, published in 1650. The title mentioned here has not been found.

115 Johannes Calvijn (1509-1564), or *Calvinus*, French church reformer.

116 The Moravian, Johann Amos Comenius (1592–1671) played a prominent role in familiarising Europe with the idea of national education systems, covering the entire field from the teaching of infants to the instruction given in universities. His projects epitomise contemporary reform; the introduction of modern studies, especially that of the mother tongue, the belief in the extraordinary power of method and the search for psychologically grounded principles of teaching are characteristic features of his *Didactica Magna,* whose contents seem to have been well known before its inclusion in his *Opera Didactica Omnia* (1657). Travelling to London in 1641, and meeting René Descartes in 1642, he lived mostly in Lissa, Poland, though he fled to Amsterdam in 1655, where he died in 1670. The title mentioned here is Comenius's *Didactica magna universalis omnes omnia doc.. artificium exhibens*, 1638.

117 Johannes Strauch, lawyer. Title unidentified.
118 This must be Johannes Christian Frommann, and the title of the book mentioned here is *Tractatus de fascinatione, in quo fascinatio bulgaris profligatur, naturalis confirmatur et magica examinatur*, published in 1675 in Neurenberg.
119 Hieronymus Fracastorius Veronensis (1484-1553) and Athanasius Kircher (1601-1680) were the first in history to state that "micro-organisms" caused infectious diseases. R.H. Major, *Classic Descriptions of Disease* (Springfield, IL, 1939), 7-50.
120 The physician and author of German-language pharmacopaeias Johann Hiskia Cardilucius (1630-1697), a representative of the iatrochemical school. The title of the work mentioned here is his *Officina sanitatis sive praxis chymiatrica*, published in Neurenberg, 1677.
121 Unidentified.
122 Thomas Bartholinus (Copenhagen 1616-1680), anatomist.
123 Schneegass, Elias (?-1697), lawyer.
124 The author Franciscus Silvius De le Boe (1614-1672) or Francois de le Boë Sylvius was the most prominent representative of the so-called iatrochemical or chemiatric school which attempted to explain physiological and pathological phenomena on the analogy of the processes that take place in chemical retorts. He was a Leiden professor of medicine. The title mentioned in the text is *Totius medicinae idea nova, seu Francisci Silvii De le Boe … Opera omnia : novas potissimum super morborum causis symptomatis & curandi ratione meditationes & disputationes continentia; accessere Chymia …* (1671).
125 This is probably the *Miscellanea Curiosa Sive Ephemeridum Medico-Physicarum Germanicarum Academiae Ceasareo-Leopoldinae Naturae Curisorum, Decuriae III. Annus primus, anni 1670*. Misceallaneous documents from the Leopoldinian-Carolinian Academy of Scientists.
126 Unidentified.
127 This can be Giulio Cesare Benedetti, whose *Julii Ceasaris Benedicti epistolae medicinales: libri X* was published in Rome, 1649.
128 Unidentified.
129 Goosen van Vreeswijck (1626-circa 1689), a seventeenth-century alchemist.
130 Antoine Le Grand (1629-1699) was a philosopher and theologian (Roman Catholic) who played a significant role in propagating Cartesian philosophy in England during the latter half of the seventeenth century. Born in Douai, and early in life associated with an English community of Franciscans who had a college in Douai, Le Grand became a Franciscan Recollect friar prior to his leaving for England as a missionary in 1656. In England, he taught philosophy and theology, advocating Roman Catholicism and eventually Cartesianism, the latter being as unpopular as the former was perilous. It is not clear how Le Grand came to Cartesianism, but the first evidence of his adoption of the new philosophy was in his *Institututio Philosophiae*, published in London in 1672. It is this book that is mentioned in Cleijer's library.
131 Unidentified.
132 Franciscus Bayle. The title is *Dissertationes physicae: in quibus principia proprietatum in mistia, oeconomia corporum in plantis et animalibus … demonstratur* and was published in 1678.
133 The author is Dirk Graswinckel (1601-1666) and the title is *Theod.I.F. Graswinkelii J.C. Delphinensis stricturae ad censuram Ioannis à Felden … ad libros Hugonis Grotii de jure belli ab pacis*, published in Amsterdam in 1654.
134 Though a book by Io. Georg. Otto. Fried. Conradi does exist (*Dissertatio inauguralis medico-chirurgica de oesteomalacia*), it was published in 1796, so it cannot be the one mentioned here. In all probability, this is a work by Isr. Conradt, *Dissertatio medico-physica de frigoris natura et effectibus*, which was published in 1677.
135 Unidentified.
136 The eminent Dutch lawyer Hugo Grotius or Hugo de Groot (Delft 1583-Rostock 1645).
137 Unidentified.
138 Cook, H.J., *Trials of an Ordinary Doctor: Joannes Groenevelt in Seventeenth-Century London* (London, 1994), 215.

139 Cornelis Herls (?-1625) wrote a very popular textbook especially composed for apprentices in the form of questions and answers, though edited by others after Herls' death: *Examen der chirurgie* (in 1725?) and *Chirurgijns scheepskist* (Surgeon's Sea Chest, in 1672).
140 Both the Helvetius, father and son, taught anatomy and surgery in Middelburg for a period of more than 40 years in the eighteenth century.
141 Cornelis van de Voorde (c. 1630-1678), M.D., was the author of *Lichtende fakkel der chirurgie* (Shining Torch of Surgery, 1664) which, after Herls' textbook, was very popular among apprentices. The last reprint was in 1742. The book confirms that the scientific progress of medicine in the seventeenth century mainly took place in the field of anatomy and the physiology of individual organs.
142 Abraham Titsing (1684-1776), surgeon. Prior to establishing himself in his native Amsterdam, he was for many years a ships' surgeon. He became the City-Surgeon of Amsterdam, and was attached to various orphanages as surgeon.
143 Kool-Blokland, J.L., *De Zorg Gewogen. Zeven Eeuwen Godshuizen in Middelburg* (Middelburg, 1990), 434.
144 Johannes Hoogvliet, born around 1730, published this book in Rotterdam in 1749.
145 ANRI, Buitenland 99.
146 Ringoir, D.J., *Plattelandschirurgijns in de zeventiende en achttiende eeuw. De rekeningboeken van de 18e eeuwse Durgerdamse chirurgijn Anthonij Egberts* (Bunnik 1977), 43-44.
147 NA, VOC 6524.
148 NA, VOC 6536.
149 NA, VOC 6536.
150 NA, VOC 6424.
151 NA, VOC 14.764.
152 NA, VOC 14.139.
153 NA, VOC 14.787.
154 NA, VOC 14.496.
155 NA, VOC 14.489.
156 NA, VOC 14.435.
157 NA, VOC 14.475.
158 NA, VOC 6296.
159 NA, VOC 14.766.
160 NA, VOC 14.486.
161 NA, VOC 14.514.
162 NA, VOC 6464.
163 NA, VOC 6447.
164 NA, VOC 5794.
165 NA, VOC 5767.
166 NA, VOC 13.053 and VOC 13.071.
167 Lorenz Heister (1683-1758), physician, whose name is also latinised as Laurentius Heisterus. He wrote one of the first systematic illustrated textbooks on surgery (1718), which was translated into many languages.
168 Paulus Barbette (1619-1665), physician.
169 Cornelis van Solingen (1641-1687).
170 Hendrick van Roonhuijse (1622-1672), surgeon. His *Genees en heel-konstige aanmerkingen* were translated into German (1674) and into English (1676). Before establishing himself in Amsterdam as surgeon, he went on a study tour to Paris and London, specifically to receive training in obstetrics. He was a professional friend of Job van Meekeren. See the next note.
171 Petrus Nijlandt (c. 1635-c1675), physician (M.D.).
172 Job van Meekeren (1611-1666), City-Surgeon of Amsterdam, as well as surgeon attached to the Amsterdam Admiralty, he was also a warden of the surgeon's guild and a surgeon in the Amsterdam hospital. His main interest was in anatomy. Together with Barbette, he dissected at the St. Pieters Gasthuis. His carefully recorded observations were brought together in his published (1) *Heel- en geneeskonstige aenmerkingen* (Rotterdam, 1728) and

(2) *Observationes medico-chirurgicae*; ex Belgico in Latinum translatae ab Abr. Blasio (Amsterdam, 1682). One of the two is meant here.

173 Johannes de Gorter (1689-1762), master-surgeon and physician.

174 Jan Kouwenburgh: *Zeechirurgie, of matroozen troost in zeer veel gebreken, den zeevarende overkomende ...* ; *Begrepen in drij deelen* (Middelburg, 1726; Amsterdam, 1726)

175 Two vols. on the art of distillation.

176 Arent Blankert (eighteenth century) wrote *Scheeps-geneesoeffening, of Naaukeurige aantekeningen en aanmerkingen, wegens de voornaamste ziektens en quaalen, die op de Oost Indische vaart, en in Indie voorkomen. Hier komt bij een beschrijving van de krachten der geneesmiddelen, die ten meerendeele in de medicijnskisten der Oost Indische Maatschappij gevonden worden* (Amsterdam, 1722).

177 *Pharmacopaeia Amstelredamensis*, or *d'Amsterdammer apotheek* (1686).

178 NA, VOC 14.813.

179 Johannes Jacob Woijt (1671-1709), physician.

180 Sir Richard Steele (1672-1729) studied in Oxford, became a soldier and later "Whig" in the Parliament in London. He criticised the excesses on the royal court of Charles II. He was the founder of two periodicals: *The Tatler* (1709-1711), and *The Spectator* (1711-?), which were written for an upper-middle-class readership.

181 Dr A.G. Richter, MD (1742-1812) was an eminent German physician and surgeon and founder of the periodical *Chirurgisch Journal* (1771-1796).

182 Albrecht von Haller (1708-1777) was from Bern and studied under Boerhaave, to eventually become a physiologist, physician, philosopher, and poet.

183 Samuel Schaarschmidt (1709-1747) temporarily taught at the Berlin *Collegium medico-chirurgicum* in 1735, worked in the field of surgical training, and was also a *Garnisonsmedikus*. Together with his brother August Schaarschmid (1720-1791), he edited a popular periodical *Medicinisch-Chirurgische Berlinische Nachrichten* as well as a series of much used teaching tables, which both reveal the enduring merits of the brothers Schaarschmid.

184 David Samuel Madai (1709-1780), a physician – though better known as a numismatist – who composed the three-vol. *Vollständige Thaler-Cabinett* (Königsberg) between 1765-1774, the most expansive overview on thaler-sized silver coins of Germany and adjacent lands. He also wrote the *Kurtze Nachricht von dem Nutzen und Gebrauch eniger bewährten Medicamenten*, which Jager read in a translated Dutch version.

185 Who else but William Harvey (1578-1657), whose brilliant proof of the constant circulation of the blood within a contained system was the seventeenth century's most significant achievement in physiology and medicine. He published his findings in *De Motu Cordis* (1628).

186 Percival Pott (1714-1788) was a famous surgeon and chief surgeon at the St. Bartholomew's Hospital in London for more than forty years. With William Cheselden (1688-1752), he dominated the field of surgery in England during much of the eighteenth century. Pott is known for several medical conditions, including "Pott's fracture" and "Pott's paralysis". The title which is mentioned in Jager's bookcase is the study on the anal fistula of 1765 translated into German.

187 NA, VOC 6170.

188 NA, VOC 5742.

189 NA, VOC 5891.

190 NA, VOC 5738.

191 NA, VOC 5767.

192 NA, VOC 5596.

193 NA, VOC 6592.

194 NA, VOC 14.466.

195 NA, VOC 14.764.

196 NA, VOC 6552.

197 Eloy, J., 'Rélations de Voyages de Charles-Ghislain Wilmet. Chirurgien major à la Cie Maritime des Indes Neêrlandaises', *Annuaire d'Hisoire Régionales et Locales « Le Vieux Châtelet »* (1984), 131.

198 Eloy, 'Rélations de Voyages de Charles-Ghislain Wilmet', 127.
199 ANRI, Notarieel, Testamenten, 30-12-1765.
200 GAA (Municipal Archives of Amsterdam).
201 ANRI, Buitenland 99.
202 ANRI, Buitenland 99.
203 This brewery 'De Hooijbergh' was already in existence in 1599 (GAA, notarial archive 10-07. Notary S. Henrix, 15.4.1599). Though it changed ownership in the course of some 300 years, its ultimate owner appears to have been Heineken, who was charged with the safekeeping of the archive of the *Brouwerscollege* (council of breweries in Amsterdam) when this *college* dissolved itself in 1871. Heineken, who has lent his name to one of today's most famous Dutch beers, was then the owner of the brewery 'De Hooijberg'.
204 ANRI, Fam. K.290.
205 GAU (Municipal Archives of Utrecht), Notariële akten, nr. U122a4-137, d.d. 30-11-1718.
206 GAU, Notariële akten, nr. U120a3, d.d. 17-12-1725.
207 NA, VOC 14.473.
208 Public Records office HCA 32 351/13. Thanks to Dr. I.G. Dillo.
209 NA, VOC 6447.
210 Rijksarchief Friesland, Trouwregister Hervormde Gemeente Dokkum, 15 June, 1738: the marriage documents of Marten Berger to Sike Gerardus state that Marten Berger was a *chirurchus* or surgeon.

Notes to Appendices

1 Page Moch, L., *Moving Europeans. Migration in Western Europe since 1650* (Indiana University Press, 1992), 49.
2 Boon, P., *Bouwers van de Zee*, 85.
3 http://geneaknowhow.net/digi/bronnen.html
4 The twenty-two proven and corrected POBvís:
Aldert Strantvliet, van Alkmaar (POBr: Haarlem)
Engel van Tongeren, van Amsterdam (wife lives in *De Rijp*)
Leendert Wuijster, van Charlois (POBr: Rotterdam)
Pieter Bruegels, van Delfshaven (POBr: Rotterdam)
Pieter Albertus Tulp, van Delfzijl (POBr: Appinga)
Jan Willem van Eerten, van den Ham (POBr: Zwolle)
Josua Spelle, van Wolfaarsdijk (POBr: Goes)
Johannes Bothael, van Goude (POBr: Rotterdam, after marriage migrates to Rotterdam)
Johannes Dobbelaar, van Koudekerke (POBr: Middelburg)
Daniel Gravius, van Tessel (POBr: Leiden)
Arnoldus op de Ool, van Alphen ad Rijn (POBr: Leiden)
Willem Patijn, van Maasland (POBr: Maassluis)
Cornelis Mouthaan, van Medemblik (POBr: Haarlem)
Huijbregt Huijbregtsen, van Westkapelle (POBr: Middelburg)
Jan Leendertse, van Amerstol (POBr: van Middelburg)
Arnoldus Plomp, van Alblasserdam (POBr: van Middelburg)
Hendrik Ooijkaas, van Naaldwijk (POBr: van Rijswijk)
Hubertus de Gester, van Nijmegen (POBr: van De Graaf)
Lourens Elderbeek, van Noordwijkerhout (POBr: van Haarlem)
Hendrik van der Casteele, van Swaanshals (POBr: van Rotterdam)
Pieter Servaas, van Axel (POBr: Tholen)
Jacob van Solingen, van Naaldwijk (POBr: Waalwijk)
5 Hart, S., *Geschrift en Getal* (Dordrecht, 1976).
6 ANRI, Notarieel, Testamenten.

Indices

Geographical index

A
Achterhoek 145
Africa 52, 58, 87, 255
Alkmaar 128, 146-47, 264
Alphen aan den Rijn 126
Alsace 156
Amboina 82, 85-86
Amersfoort 125, 146
Amsterdam 34-39, 42-45, 48, 57-63, 67, 76, 86-95, 103-05, 128, 132-33, 138, 141, 143-149, 151-153, 155, 165, 169, 171-176, 179, 185, 187-88, 200, 206, 209-10, 221-222, 224-226, 228, 236-238, 241-42, 245, 247, 253-254, 263
Angké 108
Aquitaine 49
Aragon 50
Archangel 139
Arnhem 39, 43, 145
Ascension 79
Austria 140, 157
Austrian Netherlands 43, 64, 138, 146, 161, 163-64, 254

B
Baltic Sea 139, 261
Banda Islands 85
Bangkok 69
Bantam 111, 230
Basel 32
Batavia 20-21, 52, 64, 67, 71, 75, 79-81, 85-87, 89, 95-110, 112-15, 117-23, 163, 170, 184-85, 187-90, 192, 196-98, 203-05, 207, 209-213, 215-30, 232, 236, 240, 243, 248, 250-51, 256
Batticaloa 111
Bavaria 156, 159
Beemster 130
Bengal 81, 86, 102, 111, 232, 236, 238
Bentheim 159
Bergen op Zoom 145, 178
Berlin 35, 159
Biscay, Bay of 49
Black Forest 159
Bohemia 140
Bologna 27
Bordeaux 49
Brabant 128-29, 133, 145-46, 155, 164, 252
Brandenburg 156, 159
Breda 45, 145, 226
Bredevoort 145
Bremen 133-34, 139
Brunswick 159-60, 166
Brussels 32

C
Cadiz 31, 54
Calais 133-34
Calicut 51
Canton 79, 81
Cape of Good Hope, Cape Town 17, 51, 64, 67, 71, 73, 75, 77-78, 85-87, 89-90, 111-12, 120, 137, 169, 183, 185, 196, 198, 209, 211, 213, 216, 238, 241, 246, 249
Cape Verdian Islands 82
Castres 163
Ceylon 52, 85-86, 89, 102, 111-113, 185, 197, 236-37, 241
Cheribon 86
Chinsurah 111
Cleves 36
Cochin 190, 192
Colombo 86, 96, 111, 113, 192
Copenhagen 31, 162
Coromandel 86, 229

D
Dalfsen 145, 206
Damman 216
Danzig 157
Delden 205
Delfshaven 61, 263

Delft 59, 61, 68, 87-88, 93, 99, 141, 147-48, 152, 154-55, 166, 184-85, 253, 260, 263
Den Bosch 145
Den Briel 148
Den Haag (The Hague) 148, 152
Den Helder 91, 94, 251
Denmark 31, 84, 134
Deshima 87, 111-12, 169, 249, 255
Deventer 34, 37, 144-45
Doesburg 145
Doetinchem 145
Dokkum 58, 143, 236, 243
Dordrecht 41, 129, 148
Drammen 139
Drenthe 127, 129, 132, 134, 143, 152, 164, 166, 252, 259
Dunkirk 259
Durgerdam 173
Dutch Republic 15, 19, 33-35, 42, 47, 55-56, 58, 62-63, 71, 77, 81, 84, 87, 98, 110, 122, 128-30, 134-36, 144, 148, 159-60, 170, 210, 245, 251-52

E
East Frisia 132
Edam 173
Eifel 133
Elburg 45, 145
England 15, 19, 25, 29, 40-41, 46, 49-50, 54-55, 58-59, 81, 128, 134, 183, 205, 232, 235
Enkhuizen 35, 48, 58-59, 61-63, 87-88, 94, 129-30, 139, 144, 146-47, 149, 151, 153-55, 163, 165, 173, 175, 187-89, 206, 212, 234, 251, 253
Enschede 159

F
Flushing 37, 63-64, 94, 138, 177, 216
Formosa 85
France 15, 25, 30-31, 49-50, 74, 78, 128-30, 134, 163-64, 254
Franconia 156
Franeker 34
Frankfurt 159, 175
Friesland 33, 71, 91, 127-30, 133, 143, 152, 164-65, 214, 243, 252, 260

G
Galle 111, 185, 97
Gedeh 116
Gelderland 33, 128-29, 142, 144-45, 152, 154, 164, 166, 252-54
Gembloux 64, 138, 236
Generaliteitslanden 128
Germany 57, 72, 80, 127, 130, 132-34, 139-40, 155-60, 163-64, 166, 171, 178, 209, 226, 254, 259-60
Goa 52-54, 79, 82, 216
Gorinchem 37
Gouda 37, 43, 88, 206
Graft 35, 129, 131, 137, 171
Great Britain 134
Groenlo 145
Groningen 34, 37, 127, 132-33, 143-44, 152, 164-64, 172, 252
Guinea 138

H
Haarlem 39-40, 128-29, 132, 147, 170, 236, 252, 259, 263
Hainaut 133
Halle 113
Hamburg 133, 159-60, 166, 254
Hanau 82, 159
Hannover 159, 209
Harderwijk 34-35, 42, 138, 173
Harlingen 58, 129, 143
Harz Mountains 159
Hasselt 133, 145
Heeren XVII, Gentlemen XVII \f 59
Helmstedt 206
Hesse 156, 159
Hirado 112
Hirschberg 225
Hoorn 44-45, 58-59, 61, 67, 87-88, 93-94, 128-30, 138-39, 144, 146-47, 149, 151, 153-55, 165, 171, 173, 175, 177, 179, 253, 260
Houghly 86, 111, 210, 236-37
Hunsrück 133

I
Ile d'Aix 74
India 51, 53-54, 82, 96, 236
Island of Edam 115-16
Island of Oléron 49
Island of Onrust 237
Island of Onrust, Batavia 99, 115
Island of Purmerend 108-09, 113
Island of St. Jago 83
Ile de France 78
Italy 25, 27-28, 162

J
Japan 17, 85, 87, 104, 111-12, 169, 192, 249, 255

K
Kalpitya 111
Kampen 43, 46, 144
Kirchheim 159
Königsberg 157

L
Languedoc 163
Leeuwarden 133, 143-44, 260
Leiden 33-34, 38, 46, 97, 108, 113, 126, 128, 148, 152, 156, 169, 252
Liège 133, 146, 162
Lima 54
Limburg, Neth. 128, 145-46, 155, 164, 252
Lingen 159, 241, 259
Lisbon 55
London 29-30, 36, 55-56, 134-35, 200, 238
Lower Saxony 132-33, 156-60, 164, 206
Lübeck 157
Lüneburg 134

M
Maastricht 146
Macassar 86, 192, 211, 229, 234
Madras 55
Magdeburg 156
Magdenburg 139, 175, 196
Malabar 86
Malacca 51, 85-86
Mannar 111
Marseilles 50
Mattara 111
Mecklenburg 134, 156, 158
Meppel 144, 259
Meppen 159, 259
Meuse 93
Mexico City 54, 96
Middelburg 15, 35, 37, 39, 42, 44, 58-59, 61-63, 68, 73, 78, 87, 93, 149-50, 171, 178, 191, 206, 217, 232, 245, 247, 252-53
Minden 134
Montpellier 27
Mozambique 52
Münster 127, 134

N
Nagasaki 112, 232
Naumburg 205
Netherlands 30, 33, 37, 41, 43, 58, 129, 132, 135, 206
Nieuwe Diep 94
Nijmegen 133, 145
Noorderkwartier 91, 128-31, 146-47, 165, 171
Noord-Holland. See North Holland
Nörenberg 227
North Holland 46, 128, 130, 146-49, 152, 165
North Sea 127, 132-33, 139, 144, 159
Norway 162

O
Oldenzaal 145
Ommelanden, near Batavia 143
Osnabrück 134, 159
Ostheim 260
Oude Pekela 205
Overijssel 33, 128-29, 131, 134, 142, 144, 154, 164, 166, 205-06, 252-54

P
Padua 32, 41-42
Palatinate 156
Palembang 86

Paris 27-28, 30-31, 35, 138, 156, 162, 169
Pattna 232, 237
Persia 26, 86, 111, 216
Pommerania 156, 158
Portugal 51, 54, 57, 59, 82, 134, 139
Potsdam 159
Preanger 116, 119
Prussia 50, 156-57, 159-60, 227
Purmer 130

Q
Quakenbrück 160

R
Rammekens 94-95
Republic. *See* the Dutch Republic
Rhine 57, 133, 159
Rochefort 74
Rotterdam 41-43, 58-59, 61, 63-64, 84, 87-88, 128, 131, 138, 141, 145, 147-49, 152, 154-55, 162, 164, 166, 171, 206, 212, 231, 237, 253-54, 260, 263
Ruhr 159

S

Salak 113, 116
Salerno 27
Saxony 112, 140, 156-57, 159, 254
Saxony-Anhalt 139, 157, 159, 164, 205, 254
Scandinavia 133-34, 162-64, 254
Schermer 130
Schiedam 148, 174, 185
Schlauwen 234
Schleswig 159
Schleswig Holstein 139, 156, 159
Schoonhoven 148
Scotland 58
Semarang 116, 192, 216
Serooskerke 178
Siam 69, 79, 111
Silesia 140, 225
South Holland 128, 131, 142, 147-48, 150-52, 154, 164
Spain 25, 28, 31, 44, 46, 50-51, 53-54, 57-59, 84, 96, 134
St. Helena 79
Stavenisse 234
Stettin 157
Stockholm 139, 175
Surat 54, 190, 192, 216, 238
Swabia 156
Sweden 162
Switzerland 140, 162-64

T

Taiwan 230
Ternate 85-86
Texel 91, 93-95, 205, 237, 251
Thuringia 156, 159, 254
Tjiandjur 116
Tjiliwong River 113, 118
Tjipannas 116-18
Trier 156
Trincomalee 52, 111

U

Utrecht 33-34, 128, 145-46, 252, 263

V

Veere 37, 78
Velsen 206
Veluwe 134
Venice 50, 134
Vlissingen. *See* Flushing
Vollenhoven 129
Vorpommern 158-59

W

Wandersleben 178
Wesel 226
West Africa 58, 139
West Friesland 130, 146-47, 165
West Indies 58, 80-81, 138, 149, 178
Westphalia 130, 132-33, 156-59, 164, 254
Windsheim 140
Winterswijk 145
Wolfenbüttel 159-60
Wormer 130
Württemberg 125, 156, 159, 171

Z

Zaan 129, 132
Zeeland 15, 33, 35, 46, 57, 60, 63, 68, 70-71, 73, 87, 91, 93-95, 128-29, 137, 141-42, 145, 149-51, 155, 162-64, 166, 171, 177-78, 191, 206, 214, 217, 222, 232, 234, 247, 252-53, 261-62
Zierikzee 129
Zuid-Holland. See South Holland
Zürich 162
Zutphen 145
Zuider Zee 130, 132-33
Zwolle 43, 46, 144

Index of Names

A

Aarholt, Johan Policarpus 205
Abbing, Jan 233, 307, 309
Albinus, Bernhard Siegfried 34
Albuquerque, Alfonso 52
Allorath, Johan 175
Alma, Petrus 229
Andeles, Simon 216
Andersen, Jurgen 139
Andreas, Petrus 79, 205
Andriesz, Marcus 227
Ang, Simon 237
Angelocnator, Andreas Hendrik 175
Annica of Ambon 225
Annica of Batavia 225
Anson, George 77
Anspach, J.C. 308, 313
Aquapendante, Fabricius ab 42
Aristotle 24, 245
Auerbach, Andreas 226
Aurous, Francois 163
Avicenna 23, 25-26, 32

B

Badenhausen, Joan George 106
Baillet, Isaak 220, 229
Bakers, Richard 231
Barbette, Paulus 42
Bartholinus, Thomas 41-42
Baten, Carel 41-42
Bekken, Wilhelm Hendrik 187
Belde, Hendrik 64
Belkol, W. 66, 308-07
Bello, family 144, 307
Benraath, Justus Jenning 90
Berg, O. 209
Berger, Jacob 210, 232, 236-38, 242-43
Berger, Marten 372
Berggo, Joseph 237
Blanket, Petronella 189
Blenke, Willem 83
Blok, Jan Hendrik 61, 177
Bloys, Jan of 37
Boerhaave, H. 33-34, 83, 93, 138
Boerrigter, Dirk 187
Bogaard, Cornelis 64
Bolle, Hermanus 144
Bolle, Josephus 144
Bollekeus, Dieuwertje 230
Bollekeus, Joost 230
Bollekeus, Leendert 230
Bolten, Peter 236
Bontekoe, Willem IJsbrantsz 15, 126
Bontius, J. 79, 82, 84, 97-97, 104, 108, 122, 248
Boom, Claas 233, 308, 312
Boon, P. 147, 261
Boorde, Andrew 41
Borstius, Jacobus 231
Bouwens, Adriaan 99
Bovet, Jan 235, 308, 312
Braudel, F. 96
Brauns, Christiaan 66, 209-11, 213, 233, 307, 311
Brauns, Mattheus 218
Bremer, Michael 93
Bruel, Jan 61, 177
Bruijn, J.R. 72
Brunschwig, Hieronymous 40
Brusekom, Jan 259
Brusteijn, Frans 93
Burrows, E.H. 196
Butner, Jan Daniel 113

C

Callenfels, Petrus Wilhelmes 70, 178
Cappellen, Johanna 93
Captain Bencon 109
Cartier, Jacobus 83
Cats, Jan 83
Chaucer, Geoffrey 23-25
Cleijer, Andreas (Andries) 104, 231-32
Clowes, William 55
Coen, Jan Pietersz. 85, 97, 109, 217-18
Coenderdingh, Jan 90
Cogh, J.J. 229
Colbert, Jean-Baptiste 78
Columbus, Christophorus 51
Commelin, Caspar 231
Cortes, H. 96
Costa, Christophorus à 82
Coster, Alida 229
Craan, Jacobus Johannes 190
Crabbenburg, Jan 145
Crabbenburg, Pieter 145
Cruijs, H. 104
Curtis, Charles 52
Curvemaker, Jacob 233, 235, 307

D
Da Gama, Vasco 51, 53
Dake, Jan 235, 308, 213
Dalrymple, William 54
Daman, Johannus Wilhelmus 206
D'Arnaud, David 237-38
Dat, Jan 119
Daum, Jan Meteren 175
De Barnij, Hendrik Hugo 188
De Bils, Louis 42
De Bruas, Hendrik 64
De Bruas, J.H. 138
De Chauliac, Guy 30, 32, 39, 41-42, 47, 245
De Famars, C.J. 94, 249
De Feijter, Susanna 229
De Fuijter, Lodewijk 182, 185
De Gorter, Johannes 35, 42-43
De Graaf, Gerrit 61
De Graaff, Nicolaas 65, 69, 100, 125, 127, 137, 212
De Jager, Adriaen 112
De Klerk, Reijnier 118-19
De la Marre, Christoffel 229
De le Boë Sylvius, Franciscus 33-34
De Leegh, Evert 240
De Monchy, S. 63, 83-84
De Nijs, Jacobus 218
De Put, Hendrik 188
De Put, Jan 116-19
De Reus, Arnoldus 259, 271
De Sille, L. 126
De Sousa, Dionisia 225
De Vigo, Johannes 231
De Vos, H. 175
De Vries, Jan 130, 145
De Vries, Johan 129
De Wind, Paulus 15, 78
De Winter, J. 178, 309
De Wolf, Christiaan 61, 177
Decker, Andries Johan 119
Dekker, Andries 213
Dekker, Pieter 61, 177
Den Engelsman, Johannes 69, 73-73
Derrix, Willem 64
Descartes, René 33
Di Vigo, Giovanni 40-42
Diamantslijper, Pieter Symonsz 217
Diaz, Bartholomeu 51
Dioscorides 23
Dirks, Christoffel 222
Dissel, Steven 237-38
Donk, Jan 144
Donk, Lambertus 144
D'Orta, Garcia 82
Drélincourt, Charles 34

E
Eckhart, Augistinus 176
Edward IV 29, 41
Eekel, Claas 221
Eleanor, Duchess of Aquitaine 49
Elikman, Lambert 235, 307, 310
Elizabeth I 30, 41
Elleputte, Jan 83
Ellerie, Jacobus 172
Enema, B. 309
Engelbert, Bernardus Johannes 241-42
Engelbregt, Johannes 197
Ernesto, Anna Adriana 225
Ernste, Pieter 93
Evertsen, Pieter 178

F
Fallopio, Gabrielle 42
Feber, Jan Jurge 118
Fokking, R. 309
Frederick William I 157, 254
Fresel, Abigail 217
Frik, Christoph 140

G
Gabelhoven, Oswalt 42
Galen 23-27, 29, 32-34, 47, 69, 84, 245
Gallandat, David Henry 137, 162
Gastman, Simon 62
Gelman Taylor, J. 219, 243
Glasenhap, Johannes 64
Goch, Hendrik 98-99
Gousset, J.L. 189
Gouwenaar, Jan Pietersz. 188-89, 197, 233, 307, 312
Grevenraet, Johannis 217
Grimm, Hermanus Nicolaas 113
Groenendijk 220
Groenevelt, Joannes 34-36, 82
Grubee, Albertus 173
Grubee, Anna Catharina 183
Grubee, Arnoldus 183
Gualterius 50

H

Haafner, Jacob 16
Haagelbos, Hendrik 145
Haagelbos, Jan 145
Hanevelt, Johannes 220
Hansen, Paulus 188
Harmens, Jan 105
Harmensz, Reiner 105
Hartman, H. 90
Harvey, William 15, 18, 33
Hasendonk, Christiaan 105
Hay, Gnot 109
Heeck, Gijsbert 69, 79, 84, 125, 212
Heijligers, Hermanus 145
Heijligers, Pieter 145
Heijn, David 230
Heinse, Johan Christoffel 196-97
Heking, Bartholomaeus 140
Helburgh, Joost Pietersz. 231
Helvetius 232
Hendriks, Aeltjen 223
Henke, H.H. 312
Henry II 49
Henry VIII 30, 41
Herls, Andries 58
Herls, Cornelis 42, 232
Hermanus, Paulus 206
Hildanus, Wilhelmus Fabritius 42
Hille, Jan 100
Hink, Pieter Everhard 233, 308, 312
Hinneville, J. 226
Hippocrates 23-26, 34, 42, 245
Hofman, Johannes Paulus 119
Hogewoning, Pieter 226
Holtman, Anna Maria 226
Hoogvliet, Jan 232
Hooijkaas, Pieter 70
Huijberts, Mijndert 197
Huttenus, Albertus Arnoldus 231

I

Israel, Jonathan 128-29, 143-45, 166

J

Jager, Christoph Godfried 66, 211, 229, 234-35, 307, 311
Jagera, Care 109
James I of Aragon 50
Jansen, Caspar 105
Jansz, Isaac 96
Jansz, Pieter 228
Jaspers, Johannes 145
Jaspers, Lucas Johannes 145
Johnstone, George 241
Jongedijk, Pieter 238
Josse, P. 66, 312
Julius II 40

K

Kaempfer, Engelbert 117
Kakelaar, Jan 68
Kamelaar, Valentijn 93
Karreman, Hendrik 213
Keijser, Jan 308
Keil, Johannes 226
Kemper, Gabriel Hendrik 197
Ketting, H. 66, 174, 176
Kloot, Pieter 221, 224
Koedijk, Johannes, Lambertus 230
Kreps, L.D. 239-40
Kriel, Samuel Christiaan 107, 119-20
Kruijs, Frederick 238, 240, 243
Kuilenburg, Gerrit 145
Kuilenburg, Hendrik 145

L

Lambert, E. 311
Lameij, N. 66, 312
Lammers, Cornelis 178
Landuis, Johannes 99
Langsable, Jan 221
Lanre, Jessebert 105
Laurentsy, Andreas 217
Lembroek, Claas 83
Leo X 51
Liesthout, Anna 229
Liesthout, Jan 228
Lind, James 78
Lindemann, Mary 19, 125
Littre, Alexis 31
Livingstone, Frank 80
Livy 231
Louis VII 49
Louis XIV 34, 130
Louwers, Pieter 99
Lubbertsz, Hermen 45
Ludeker, Caspar 119

M
Maas, F. 308
Maas, Gerardus 119
Maas, V. 312
Magellan, Ferdinand 51
Maria of Bengalen 225
Martijn, Hendrik 99
Mary, Queen 41
Massener, Johan Philip 221
Maurenbrechen, J.St.L. 188
Maurice of Nassau 46
Mazade, Jan 205
Mazee, Willem 237
Meijer, J.F. 307, 311
Meijer, Petrus 107
Meijer, Wessel 66, 235, 312
Merklein, Johan Jacob 140
Mester, Werner August 235, 307, 309
Methwold, William 54
Middeldijk, A. 230
Ming-Kong, Su 109
Miseroy, Benjamin 62
Molanus, Margaretha 226
Molhuijsen, Willem 218
Molière 24
Morell, Abraham 228
Mossel, Jacob 116, 188-89, 213
Mouthaan, Cornelis 259
Muller, J.F. 309
Muller, Johan Andreas 126, 139, 212, 357
Munninkhuijsen, Johannes 216
Munt, Jan 226
Musculus, Philip Pieter 140

N
Nack, Albert 237
Nasbij, Christiaan 236, 312
Nebbens, Bartholomeus 178
Neddermans, Anthonij 221
Neiman, Jacob 233, 307, 311
Neuman, Daniel 225
Newton, Isaac 18
Nicht, Hendrick 178
Nies, Jacobus Adolph 187
Nietsch, James Fredrik Christiaan Hendrik 187
Noordervliet, Willem 220

O
Oldenzeel, Hendrik 230
Olthof, Isaac 39-40
Oostwalt, Jan August 230
Op den Ool, Arnoldus 189-90, 212, 226, 236, 238
Otteleben, Coenraadt, Hendrick 206

P
Page Moch, L. 131-32
Pannekoek, Catharina 206
Paracelsus 32-33, 41, 47, 84
Paré, Ambroise 30-32, 41, 231
Pasqualsen, David 226
Patijn 84
Perrera, Nicolaas 225
Philip II 38, 58
Pieterse, Piet 90
Pietersz, Pellegrom 97, 103
Pigre, Pieter 42
Pijl, Albert 192
Pijl, Lucas 217
Pinket, Jan Baptista 220
Piscator, H. 307
Planket, Petronella 190
Poortvliet, P. 178
Porter, Roy 96
Pott, Percival 234
Poupart, Francois 31
Pourier, Abraham 206
Provo, Cornelis 226
Pruijs, Johannes Matthijs 217
Puthuijs, Frans 237

Q
Quickelenburg 225

R
Raben, R. 96
Radermacher, Hendrik 226
Radermacher, J. 120
Rau, Johannes 34
Reijn, Michiel 236
Richard the Lionheart 49
Ringoir, D.J. 231
Robbé, Frans 221
Robertson, Thomas 56
Rodrip, Maria 226
Roelofs, Jan 213, 307, 309
Roemers, Johannes 99
Roger, Isaak 308
Rombouts, Abraham 230

Ros, Siwert 173
Rosendaal, Abraham 188
Rottink, Gerrit 205
Rumphius, G.E. 82
Runstorff, Bared Frederik 197

S
Saltsman, Johan David 260
Sarij of Bougis 224
Sarcharson, Johan 231
Sas, Anthonij 83
Schambergen, Caspar 169
Scharl, Bernardus 232-33, 235, 308, 312
Scheffens, Francois 218
Scheffer 221
Schepen, J.F. 188
Schilham, I. 46
Schopper, Johan 227, 242
Schoute, C. 220
Schouten, Sybrand 226
Schouten, Wouter 82, 169
Schreuder, Hendrik Ernst 119
Schrijver, Leopoldus 221
Schuijl, Florentius 34
Schuts, Johan 224
Sculteus, Johannes 42
Severinus, Marcus Aurelius 42
Shakespeare, William 24
Sion, J.G. 308, 313
Slicher van Bath, B.H. 129, 145
Sluijs, Gerrit Jansz 62
Smits, Cornelia 226
Snoek, Aegidius 76
Speelman, C. 182
Spenolt, J.A. 119, 213, 226
Spies, Johan 235, 313
Stadius van Halm, A. 209
Stellingwerf, Petronella 226
Stevens, Hendrik 221
Stilzer, J.W. 66, 233, 307, 311
Strantvliet, Aldert 264
Swart, Hille 235, 308, 313
Swerus, Cecilia 205

T
Taas, Aletta 229
Taffin, Jean 231
Takens, Jan 220-21
Tavernier, Jean Baptiste 54, 126
Teijling, Simon 172
Teisseire, Guillaume, C. 163
Ten Berge, George 205
Ten Berge, Harm Dirks 206
Ten Cate, Bernardus 233, 311
Ten Holder, Stephanus 191
Ten Rhijne, Willem 82, 106
Theering, Jonas 197
Thuinzaad, Andries 232, 237
Thunberg, Carl Peter 169, 177
Timmers, Willem 185
Titsing, Abraham 63, 232
Tooreman, Arnoldus 173
Troef, Martinus 227, 242
Tulp, N. 38, 79, 231
Twent, S.H. 235, 308, 312

U
Ulman, M. 233, 242, 307, 310
V
Van Berthem, Pieter 104
Van Beverwijck, Jan 41-42
Van Brakel, Adriaan 184-85
Van Breemen, M.L. 80
Van Broekhuijs, Gerrit 229
Van Brugge, Matthijs 174
Van Buren, Jacobus 240
Van Coopstad, Leendert 216
Van Dam, Pieter 101
Van de Coppello, Servaas 74
Van de Sande, P. 233, 308
Van de Voorde, Cornelis 42, 99, 232
Van Deijl, B. 188
Van den Abeele, Dingenis 70, 206
Van den Berge, Angila 229
Van den Berge, Joseph 189
Van den Spiegel, Adriaan 41
Van den Sprenkel, Pieter 189
Van den Vijver, Petronella 228
Van der Baan, Jan Dirksen 83
Van der Brug, P.H. 80-81, 114, 203, 205
Van der Burg, Johanna 229
Van der Duijm, Frans 220
Van der Heuvel, Adriaan 217
Van der Hulst, H. 307
Van der Kemp, Hendrik 66, 197, 233, 307, 312
Van der Leen, Lidia 226
Van der Leer, Elisabeth 216
Van der Niepoort, Florentius 216
Van der Parra, P.A. 117
Van der Riet, Johannes 178

Van der Sande, Pieter 233, 308
Van der Stael, Agita 217
Van der Steege, Jacobus 213
Van der Woude, Ad 130-31, 145
Van Diemen, Anthonij 217
Van Dijk, Christoffel 217
Van Driel, Elisabeth Anna 228
Van Esten, Anna 227
Van Ette, Hendrik 174
Van Geel, Gerrit 237
Van Gelder, R. 196
Van Goens, François Rijkloff 189, 216
Van Groenenberg, Gerrit 221
Van Hedin, R. 190, 283
Van Hoeke, Johanna 93
Van Horne, Joannes 34
Van Imbrock, Gijsbert 230
Van Imhoff, G. 116, 122
Van Laarbeek, Gillis 181
Van Leur, J.C. 210
Van Linschoten, Jan Huijghen 52
Van Luepken, Claudicis Anthonij 118
Van Melligem, J. 66, 312
Van Mellingen, Jan 223, 235, 308
Van Meteren 231
Van Nier 240
Van Ossenbergh, W.H. 189
Van Outhoorn, Cornelia 240
Van Putten 64
Van Riebeeck, Jan 77, 85, 112
Van Rostok, Jan 100
Van Royen, P. 130
Van Rustingh, Salomon 42
Van Santen, H. 105
Van Snellenberg, Maria 240
Van Soest, Geertruijda 217
Van Soest, Hermanus 206
Van Solingen, Cornelis 42
Van Sorgen, Cornelis 234, 307, 309
Van Tongeren, Douwe 206
Van Tongeren, Engel 220-21
Van Waveren, Robert 217
Van Willemsvaart, Johannes 233, 308
Van Zeilighem, Elias 178
Vegnerus, Johannes 226
Velthuis, Henricus 35-36
Veltjes, Georg 233, 307
Vernerius, Johannes 308
Verwoert, Johannes 67, 187
Verzeijl, Jan 307
Vesalius, Andreas 32-33, 41
Vicary, Thomas 41
Vink, Adriaan 83
Virgili, Pedrol 31
Vlaming, Simon 220
Voegen van Engelen, Jacob 16
Vogelzang, Adrianus 118
Vollé, Gerrit 119
Von der Behr, Johan 139
Von Gersdorff, Hans 41
Voskuil, Mathijs 226
Vuijstingh family 126

W

Walmeester, Simon 188-89, 197, 213, 308
Webrigh, Abraham 99
Weemeijer, H.D. 233, 307, 310
Weesing, Joseph 187
Weidner 230
Weijers, Mathijs 233, 308, 313
Werick, Anthonij 240
Wervel, Fredrik 113
Wijthof, Gerardus 209
Wildermans, Hendrik 216
Willebrinck, Cornelis 190
Willemsvaart, J. 233, 308
William III 46
Wilmet, Charles-Ghislain 64, 138, 162, 236
Winkelaar, Johannes 70, 190-91
Wirtsung, Christoph 231
Witsen, Cornelis 99
Woijt, Johannes Jacob 234
Woodall, John 56-57, 65, 77
Worms, Wijnand 233, 308, 313
Würtz, Felix 41-42

Z

Zas, Nicolaas 41-42
Zeeukes, Aaltje 217

Index on Ships

A
Aurich 67

B
Baanman 175
Barbestein 83
Bleijswijk 73-74
Buis 83, 175

D
d'Jonge Wilhelm 83

G
Geertruid 175
Groenendaal 91

H
Held Woltemade 241
Herstelde Leeuw 64
Honkoop 91
Huis ter Meije 91

K
Kasteel van Tilburg 237

L
Land van Beloften 175
Langewijk 175
Leijden 90
Lycochton 209

M
Mary Rose 55

N
Noordwijkerhout 83

O
Oost Capelle 213
Opperdoes 83, 216
Orangezaal 197, 233

P
Petronella Alida 70

R
Rebecca Jacoba 238
Rotterdam 64

S
Salisbury 78
St. Jehan 58
Steenhoven 83
Suzanna Helena 94-95

V
Velzen 70
Vrouwe Petronella 175

W
Walvis 69, 79
Westcappel 83
Westhoven 126
Willem de Vijfde 70
Woestduijn 93

Z
Zorgewijk 83

Index on Subjects

A
Aasdomsrecht 214
Académie Royale de Chirurgie 31, 138
Admiralty 45-46, 58-59, 63, 70, 90, 137, 146, 149, 171, 174, 178, 206
Anglo-Dutch wars 59, 129, 150-51, 241
Apprentice 15, 25, 29-30, 37, 41-42, 46-47, 56, 60-61, 127, 151, 174, 178, 246, 251, 254, 260
Artikelbrief, General Instruction 65, 98

B
Barber-surgeons 24, 27, 29, 37-41, 45-46, 55-56, 61, 156, 160, 245
Batavia Castle 64, 97-107, 117, 119, 163
Batavia Hospital, *Binnenhospitaal* 17, 64, 81, 86, 98-103, 105-107, 114-117, 121, 185, 196, 207, 220-21, 226, 240
Batavian Deeds 214, 219-220, 223-225, 228, 230, 242
Beriberi. *See* Diseases
Binnengasthuis 38, 44-45, 67, 90-91
Binnenhospitaal. *See* Batavia Hospital
Black Death. *See* Diseases
Books 20, 30-32, 35, 41-42, 45, 56, 64, 68, 174, 209, 211, 230-235, 241
Bottomry transactions, *Bodemerij* 238
Brede Burgerij, Upper Bourgeoisie 171
Brewery, *Hooijbergse Princesse Royal*, Heineken 236, 238
Burger- en Aalmoezeniershuis 44
Burgher (*burger*) 40, 43, 45-46, 102, 105, 107-108, 205, 220-21, 225, 241

C
Chatham Chest 55
Cholera. *See* Diseases
City Apothecary (*Stadsapotheek*) 104-05, 120
City Physician, *Stadsdoctor* 35, 41, 43-44, 63-64, 83, 106-07, 119-21, 138
City Surgeon, *Stadschirurgijn* 43-44, 63-64, 90-91, 101, 106-10, 120-121, 138, 140, 217
Collegium Medicum 35-36, 38, 160
Compagnons 127, 133
Council of the Indies, *Raad van Indie* 87, 95, 98-100, 104-06, 108-10, 113, 115, 117-23, 182, 207, 218-19, 248
Country Surgeon 45-46, 56, 172-73
Crimps 72, 91, 116, 131

D
Diseases
- Beriberi 18, 20, 53, 79, 82, 84, 100, 205
- Black Death 25, 28, 43, 50
- Cholera 52
- Dysentery 52-53, 67, 73, 76-77, 116, 198
- Insanity 44
- Leprosy 19, 25, 44, 52, 82, 108-09, 227, 255
- Madura Foot 82, 169
- Malaria 18, 20, 52, 80-81, 114, 122, 198, 203-04, 255
- Measles 52
- Rickettsia virus 75
- Scurvy 18, 40, 51-53, 76-79, 81, 83, 92, 115-16
- Skin Diseases 29, 40, 47
- Smallpox 52, 213
- Syphilis 32-33, 44, 52
- Typhoid Fever 20, 52
- Typhus 53, 72, 75, 79-80, 92, 122, 198-99
- Ulcers 18, 20, 29, 39-40, 61, 97
- Yellow Fever 52, 81

Dispensary, Medicinale Winkel 98, 103-07, 112, 121
Dolhuis 45
Dresser, *Verbandmeester* 100-01, 115-16, 121
Dysentery. *See* Diseases

E
East India Company (English), EIC 96, 180, 246
Edict of Nantes 130
Empirics 27, 30, 36, 47
Enkhuizen Ordinance 62
Examiner of the roadstead, *visitateur ter rheede* 101, 103, 227

F
Feldscher, Wundarzte 156

G
Guild 17, 28-30, 34-43, 45-47, 56, 61-63, 96, 98, 151, 156-57, 172, 174-77, 179, 193, 206-07, 238, 245, 252-55

H
Head of Surgery, *Hoofd der Chirurgie* 97-98, 100, 103-05, 107, 116, 118-19, 121-23, 198, 205, 207, 213, 226, 248

Heeren XVII, Gentlemen XVII 59, 64-65, 68-70, 87, 91-95, 97, 106, 110, 118-22, 182-83, 207, 217, 223, 249
Hoge Regering, High Government 95
Hortus Medicus 38, 174
Hospital for the Elderly, *Oude Mannen- en Vrouwengasthuis* 44
Hospital Ship, *Hulk* 58, 91, 94-95, 99, 121, 251
Hospital, *Gasthuis* 43-44
Hospitalier, First Surgeon 211, 229, 234-35
Humoral Pathology 26, 33, 255
Humours 23, 26-28, 32, 39, 69

I
Immigration 44, 130, 218-19, 265
Imperial Trade Edict 156-57
Insanity. *See* Diseases
Instruments 27, 37, 45, 59, 66-67, 69-71, 89, 92, 98, 103-04, 174, 184-85, 209, 211, 230, 235, 247

J
Journeyman 29, 37-38, 45, 61, 137, 174, 251

K
Krankenhaus 97

L
Labour 21, 37, 63, 127-28, 130-36, 142-44, 186-87, 199, 229, 253-55
Labour Migration 131, 133, 135, 140, 143-44, 146, 254, 265
Lapdoos 58, 65, 68
Leerbrief 37, 174, 176, 251
Lepers Hospital, *Leproserie* 43, 52, 108-10
Leprosy. *See* Diseases

M
Madura Foot. *See* Diseases
Malaria. *See* Diseases. *See* Diseases
Maritime Medicine 49-50, 53, 62
Master's Examination, *Huisproef* 29, 37-39, 45-46, 48, 61-62, 172, 174-76, 245-46, 251-52
MCC 58, 178
Measles. *See* Diseases
Medical Chest 53, 56-59, 64-65, 67-70, 74, 78, 84, 88-89, 91-92, 96, 103, 105, 184, 247
Merchant Fleet 45, 48, 63, 72, 137-39, 146-47, 174, 206
Migration System 132
Moorish Hospital, *Moorse Ziekenhuis* 117, 120
Morshandel, Spillage Trade 186, 212

O
Operater, *Operateur* 100
Operating Theatre 69, 101
Ordinance for Surgeons 105
Ordre en Instructie 92
Orlop 69, 73
Outer Hospital, *Buitenhospitaal* 115-16, 118-20

P
Palatinate War 156
Parish Relief Board 107-10, 116
Peace of Utrecht 173
Peace of Westphalia 130, 156
Pesthuis 45
Pharmacist 60, 67, 87-92, 95, 100, 104-05, 144, 247
Pharmacopeia 32, 36, 89, 93, 95, 105
Political Council 90, 112
Poorhouse 68, 102, 189, 216, 225, 227
Practitioner, *praktizijn*103, 105, 107, 115-17, 120-21, 135, 159-60, 172, 251

Q
Quarantine 50

R
Recruitment 71, 130, 134-35, 137-38, 141-52, 154-56, 158-59, 161-66, 179, 199, 249, 251-54
Rolls of Oléron 50

S
Schependomsrecht 214
Scurvy. *See* Diseases
Seven Years' War 156, 160, 166, 246
Sick bay 69
Skin Diseases. *See* Diseases
Slave Trade 52
Smalle Burgerij, Petty Bourgeoisie 171, 207, 218
Smallpox. *See* Diseases
St. Caecilia Gasthuis 34
Statutes of Batavia 217
Superintendent 99, 103, 107, 115-18, 120-21, 185
Surgeon-Examiner 60, 63, 87, 89-92
Surgeon-General 52, 58-59, 65, 77, 79, 104
Surgeon's Journal, *Chirurgijns Journaal* 65
Syphilis. *See* Diseases

T

Thirty Years' War 156, 158
Tjipannas Spa 117
Travelling Brothers 127
Treatment 20, 24-25, 27, 29, 31, 33, 37, 39-40, 46-47, 49-50, 53, 59-61, 67, 69, 71, 76, 82-83, 90, 98, 100, 103, 107-08, 116, 120, 122, 213, 245
Treaty of Tordesillas 51
Typhoid Fever. *See* Diseases
Typhus. *See* Diseases

U

Ulcers. *See* Diseases
University 24, 27-28, 30, 32-35, 47, 54, 83-84, 88, 93, 95, 113, 133, 138, 157, 169, 231, 245, 247

V

Veldscheer, Field Barber 46, 48, 174
Vitamins 73, 77, 79

W

Wanderburschen 133, 254
Wanderschaft 45, 159, 174
War of the Austrian Succession 156
Weeskamer 213, 215-16, 219-20, 222, 227
WIC 58, 178

Y

Yellow Fever. *See* Diseases

Z

Zeeproef 48, 61-63, 88, 174-75, 193